THE CANCER PREVENTION DIET_____

THE CANCER PREVENTION DIET

Michio Kushi's Nutritional Blueprint for the Prevention and Relief of Disease

By MICHIO KUSHI
with ALEX JACK

St. Martin's Griffin
New York

To the Spirit of George Ohsawa

Note to the reader:

It is advisable for the reader to seek the guidance of a
physician and appropriate nutritionist before implementing the approach to health suggested by this book.
It is essential that any reader who has any reason to
suspect cancer or illness, contact a physician promptly.
Neither this nor any other book should be used as a
substitute for professional medical care or treatment.

Library of Congress Cataloging-in-Publication Data

Kushi, Michio.
    The cancer prevention diet / Michio Kushi with Alex Jack.
        p.   cm.
    ISBN 0-312-11245-9 (pbk.)
    1. Cancer—Diet therapy. 2. Cancer—Prevention. 3. Macro-
biotic diet. I. Jack, Alex. II. Title.
RC271.D52K86   1994
616.99′4052—dc20   94-28110
                                                           CIP

10 9 8 7 6 5 4 3

Contents

Preface

Each year since *The Cancer Prevention Diet* first appeared in 1983, the relation between diet and cancer has become more widely recognized. Following publication of the historic report, *Diet, Nutrition, and Cancer*, commissioned by the National Cancer Institute (NCI), the American Cancer Society issued dietary guidelines for the first time in 1984, calling for increased consumption of whole grains, vegetables, and other fresh foods and for corresponding reductions in intake of fat, sugar, and highly processed foods. The American Cancer Society subsequently launched an impressive public campaign to "Cook Up a Defense against Cancer" and in the years since has promoted nutritional research and "chemoprevention"—including the use of food and traditional healing substances to prevent cancer. Over the last ten years, the American Medical Association, the American Dietetic Association, and other scientific bodies have issued similar recommendations. In 1989 the National Research Council (NRC) published *Diet and Health*, a comprehensive 749-page review of the relation between diet and degenerative disease, marshaling even more evidence that the modern way of eating is associated with cardiovascular disease, major forms of cancer, and other illnesses. In 1992 the American Cancer Society announced plans to conduct the first large dietary intervention study in which people at high risk for colorectal cancer would be given a high-fiber diet. As a result of macrobiotic influence, leading scientific and medical organizations are becoming increasingly interested in the role of soybeans and soybean products, including tofu, miso, and tempeh (a fermented soyfood), in reducing the risk of cancer. The American Cancer Society and *Oncology Times* have highlighted this research, and the NCI recently sponsored a special workshop on the role of soy products in cancer prevention.

The NRC, the nation's highest scientific body, endorsed organic farming in its 1989 report, *Alternative Agriculture*, linking modern agriculture with rising cancer rates and with environmental pollution. The NRC found that insecticides accounting for 30 percent, herbicides accounting for 50 percent, and fungicides accounting for 90 percent of all agricultural use have been found to cause tumors in laboratory animals. As an example of a healthy, environmentally clean, and productive alternative, the report included a case history of the Lundberg Family Farm in Richvale, California, the largest source of organically grown brown rice eaten in macrobiotic households in this country today. Dozens of international organizations have issued similar findings on personal and planetary health. For example, in a study on diet, nutrition, and the prevention of chronic diseases released in 1991, the World Health Organization warned developing countries about adopting the rich diet of the industrialized world:

> Compared with the diet that fueled human evolution, today's affluent diet has twice the amount of fat, a much higher ratio of saturated to unsaturated fatty acids, a third of the daily fibre intake, much more sugar and sodium, fewer complex carbohydrates, and a reduced intake of micronutrients. Throughout the world, the adoption of such a diet, foreign to human biology, has been accompanied by a major increase in the incidence of chronic diseases. . . . An epidemic of cancers, heart disease and other chronic ills need not be the inevitable price paid for the privilege of socioeconomic progress.

In Europe, researchers announced plans in 1991 to launch "the world's largest-ever in-depth investigation into diet and cancer." For five years, more than 250,000 people in seven European countries would keep detailed food diaries and provide blood samples to scientists. In the former Soviet Union, medical researchers for the first time have begun to investigate the environmental and dietary causes of cancer. In a 1991 study, scientists speculated that "a Western type of diet and sedentary jobs" may contribute to elevated cancer rates in the European part of Russia and in the Baltic republics compared with the Asian republics, where more traditional food is eaten and cancer rates are low. Dietary and cancer research has also come to China. In the early 1990s, the directors of the China Health Study, a large epidemiological study of diet and degenerative disease sponsored by the U.S. NCI and the Chinese Institute of Nutrition and Food Hygiene, found that in rural Chinese counties where the diet included a high proportion of cereals and vegetables and a low amount of animal food, fewer than 1 percent of deaths were caused by coronary heart disease, and breast cancer, colon cancer, lung cancer, and other malignancies common in the West (and increasingly in urban China) were rare.

Each year modern science and medicine move closer to the macrobiotic approach. In 1992 the U.S. Department of Agriculture adopted the Food Guide Pyramid (see illustration), calling for Americans to consume a majority of their daily food as whole grains and vegetables and substantially cut down on meat, dairy products, fats, oils, and sweets. The graphic replaced the Basic Four Food Groups (centered around meat and dairy food), which had served as the standard since the 1950s, and the U.S. government will distribute the Food Guide Pyramid to millions of schools, hospitals, Native-American communities, nursing homes, and other segments of society in the years ahead. The recommended servings of whole grains (equalling about 40 percent) and vegetables and other fresh foods (about 30 percent) in the Food Guide Pyramid are very similar to that in the standard macrobiotic diet. The principal difference is the recommended amount of fat in the diet (about 30 percent versus 15 percent) and the quality of protein (largely animal versus plant quality). In 1990 the Physicians Committee for Responsible Medicine (PCRM), a newly formed

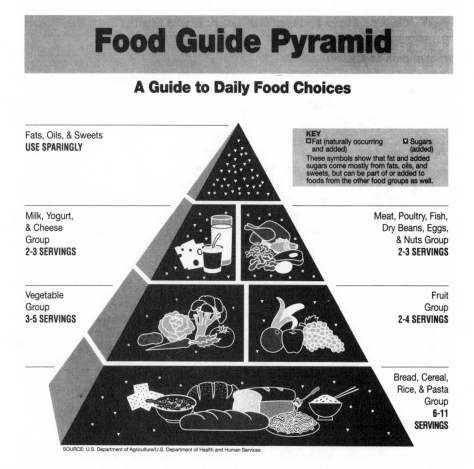

Food Guide Pyramid

A Guide to Daily Food Choices

Fats, Oils, & Sweets
USE SPARINGLY

KEY
□ Fat (naturally occurring   ▣ Sugars
and added)   (added)
These symbols show that fat and added
sugars come mostly from fats, oils, and
sweets, but can be part of or added to
foods from the other food groups as well.

Milk, Yogurt,
& Cheese
Group
2-3 SERVINGS

Meat, Poultry, Fish,
Dry Beans, Eggs,
& Nuts Group
2-3 SERVINGS

Vegetable
Group
3-5 SERVINGS

Fruit
Group
2-4 SERVINGS

Bread, Cereal,
Rice, & Pasta
Group
**6-11
SERVINGS**

SOURCE: U.S. Department of Agriculture/U.S. Department of Health and Human Services

national group of three thousand medical doctors, called for the adoption of a grain-and-vegetable–based diet with an optimal intake of 15 to 20 percent fat. Drawing upon macrobiotic medical studies, the PCRM cited recent cancer studies showing that there was no difference in breast cancer incidence between women following the standard modern diet (40 percent or more fat) and those following the prudent diet advocated by the major medical associations (30 percent fat). The World Health Organization and other groups have also called for further cutbacks in fat consumption, ideally to under 20 percent, to protect against cancer. Such recommendations have begun to take effect. In 1992 the American Cancer Society announced the first low-fat dietary intervention study for breast cancer in which participants would be limited to only 15 percent of calories from fat.

Researchers at Tulane University, the University of Michigan, Boston University, the University of Minnesota, and other institutions have begun to study the macrobiotic approach to cancer since the first edition of this book appeared. Some of the results published over the last ten years have been very impressive. For example, in the Tulane study, twenty-four pancreatic patients who adopted a macrobiotic diet survived an average of 17.3 months compared with 6.0 months for matched controls from a national tumor registry. The one-year survival rate was 54.2 percent in the macrobiotic patients versus 10.0 percent in the controls. Other cancer specialists at Harvard University, the University of Alabama, the University of Wisconsin, and elsewhere have begun to study the protective effects of miso, shoyu (soy sauce), seaweed, and other foods in the standard macrobiotic diet. (See a summary of these studies in Part I, Chapter 5.) In Washington, D.C., a Congressional House Subcommittee on Health and Long-term Care reviewed the macrobiotic approach and concluded: "The macrobiotic diet appears to be nutritionally adequate. . . . The diet would also be consistent with the recently released dietary guidelines of the National Academy of Sciences and the American Cancer Society in regard to possible reduction of cancer risks." In 1990 a report by Congress's Office of Technology Assessment recommended further research on the macrobiotic approach to cancer: "If cases such as Newbold's [a medical doctor who documented the recovery of six patients with advanced malignancies who adopted a macrobiotic diet] were presented in the medical literature, it might help stimulate interest among clinical investigators in conducting controlled, prospective trials of macrobiotic regimens, which could provide valid data on effectiveness." In New York, a macrobiotic program to prevent and relieve AIDS was started in the mid-1980s. Members of the gay community with Kaposi's sarcoma, a form of skin cancer associated with this disorder, sought dietary counseling. Generally, their condition stabilized or improved on the new diet, and immunologists from some of the medical schools collected their blood samples and monitored their progress for documentation. Overall, the macrobiotic group outlived all other AIDS control groups being monitored, with some men experiencing complete recoveries. (See Part II, Chapter 28, for further details.) In a review of special diets, the American Medical Association noted: "In general, the macrobiotic diet is a healthful way of eating." In Germany, a cancer treatment center has incorporated macrobiotics into its approach and macrobiotic teachers and cooks work side by side with oncologists.

Nearer to home, thousands of individuals and families have come to the Kushi Foundation's new home in the beautiful Berkshire Mountains to attend seminars and classes during the last ten years. The seven-day Way to Health Seminar, the most popular program, offers daily "hands on" cooking classes and lectures in theory and practice, with an emphasis on preventing cancer and other degenerative diseases. There have been many wonderful recoveries as a result of these and other classes (some of which are summarized in the personal accounts in Part II). Around the world, *The Cancer Prevention Diet* has appeared in many foreign editions over the last ten years, including British, French, German, Italian, Spanish, Norwegian, Danish, Swedish, Hungarian, Czechoslovakian, Yugoslavian, and Russian, and is helping to stimulate awareness of a more natural approach to health in these societies. Macrobiotics spread quickly throughout Eastern Europe and the Soviet Union in the 1980s.

In 1990 Alex Jack and several other macrobiotic teachers organized an airlift of macrobiotic foods to Moscow and Leningrad (now Saint Petersburg) and lectured to doctors at the Cardiology Center, the Cytology Center (the chief cancer research institute), and other Soviet scientific and medical associations. Medical doctors, who head up the macrobiotic movement across Russia and other former Soviet republics, continue to use miso, seaweed, and other foods that have been shown to be effective against radiation-related cancers to treat adults and children exposed to contamination from Chernobyl and other nuclear accidents. (See the new chapter on radiation- and environmentally related cancers [Chapter 27] for further information.) At a governmental level, during the last decade I have been asked to advise health and food and agricultural ministries in several European countries, including Hungary (which has the world's highest cancer death rate); Central America; Africa; and the Middle East.

All the statistics, research, and other supporting material in this new edition have been updated to reflect current societal trends and medical findings. In addition, my own approach to cancer has gradually changed over the last decade. Each year I continue to see several thousand individuals and families with cancer who come to me for personal guidance and direction. In follow-up visits, through letters and faxes, and on the telephone and at seminars and conferences, I observe their progress, in some cases, over the course of years and decades. I have made many fine adjustments in dietary recommendations, special dishes and drinks, compresses and other home cares, and way-of-life suggestions that are incorporated in this new edition of the book.

Lastly, new chapters have also been added on exercise and lifestyle factors that may reduce cancer risk, including meditation and visualization exercises to complement the healing process; on the environment and the relation of personal and planetary health; on children and cancer; and on AIDS-related cancers. The glossary, bibliography, resource section, and other material in the back of the book have been completely revised, and an appendix summarizing the dietary guidelines of the major scientific and medical associations has been added.

Life moves in a spiral, and each generation faces in slightly different form the obstacles and challenges of the past. In his 1849 book, *Cancerous and Cancroid Growths*, British physician John Hughes Bennett proposed a nutritional approach to preventing malignancy. "It seems to be a prudent step to diminish all those dietetic substances easily converted into fat, including not only oily matters themselves but starch and sugar. . . . These are points which, although at present unknown, will, I trust, erelong be investigated and understood," the onetime president of the Royal Medical Society continued, "and then we shall begin to have glimpses of what ought to constitute a sure and certain guide to the constitutional treatment of numerous diseases of nutrition, and, among the rest, of cancer."

Only in the last couple decades has modern medicine begun to investigate systematically a daily diet high in fat, refined flour, and sugar and its relationship to cancer, heart disease, and other degenerative illnesses. The exact mechanism of tumor formation at the cellular level is still imperfectly understood. However, in the last ten years, most of the major American, Canadian, and

European medical associations have recommended that, pending further research, the general public adopt a prudent diet low in saturated and unsaturated fat, cholesterol, and refined carbohydrates and high in whole grains, vegetables, and fresh fruit.

Virology, genetics, and immunology have commanded most of the attention and grants in cancer research until now. However, after a century of neglect, nutrition, the perennial stepchild of modern medicine, is finally gaining recognition as a potential Cinderella science in this effort. There is reason to believe that the slipper of dietary common sense, in combination with other lifestyle and environmental factors, will eventually be found to fit the relevant epidemiological, laboratory, and clinical data. If this holistic approach wins widespread acceptance, the chapter on cancer, one of the most sorrowful in human history, will have a happy ending.

Even though most of the prudent diets advanced during the last decade are moving in the right direction, some are more prudent than others. A few are based on the nutritional requirements of experimental animals, which may not always be appropriate for humans. Others are derived from computer analyses programmed by people themselves suffering the same diseases that they hope to eliminate. However, perhaps the weakest link between dietary guidelines and their implementation is in the lack of adequate recipes and menus. How does an ordinary person, family, school cafeteria, or hospital kitchen translate general proposals to lower fat and increase fiber into daily meals? The nation's food writers and cooking columnists have moved to fill this vacuum by publishing various menu plans to help protect against cancer. Basically they call for consuming a little less of everything that people already are eating and suspect is not particularly good for them. The menus do not reflect the fundamental change in the quality of food selection, preparation, or cooking that is needed if cancer, heart disease, and other degenerative illnesses are truly to be eliminated.

The approach to health presented in this book has evolved naturally in both East and West. We call it the Cancer Prevention Diet because it has protected most of the human family from cancer and related diseases for more than a hundred generations. During the last generation, hundreds of thousands of people around the world have successfully adopted this way of eating, under the name macrobiotics, and found that it not only protects them from serious disease, but also is delicious and satisfying. This includes hundreds of people from all walks of life who have relieved already existing cancers with the recipes and menus developed by Aveline Kushi and introduced in this volume.

Over the centuries, many individuals, communities, and cultures have contributed to the approach presented in this book. The authors would especially like to express their deep appreciation and gratitude to the late Yukikazi Sakurazawa (George Ohsawa) and his wife, Lima, who have inspired modern macrobiotics, and to the few remaining traditional societies that have kept alive the intuitive culinary wisdom of the past. This year marks the one hundredth anniversary of George Ohsawa's birth, and we are happy to dedicate this book to him.

Also, we are thankful to the many practitioners down through the ages, both Eastern and Western, traditional healers and medical doctors, therapists and researchers, who have devoted their lives to studying diet and disease. We appreciate all current medical, educational, and governmental efforts, as well as individual initiatives, to improve personal, family, and public health. We wish to work together with all organizations and people concerned with the problem of cancer and modern society. We hope that this book serves as a contribution to this common goal and we welcome any comments or suggestions on cooperation in the future.

Natural foods and holistic healing practices are gradually entering the mainstream of American society. This book also represents the unfolding experience and insight of thousands of contemporary macrobiotic health and dietary counselors, teachers, cooks, organic farmers and gardeners, natural foods store personnel, authors, and artists who are actively involved in transforming world health through a return to whole foods and a more natural way of life.

New directions in medicine are also emerging as we prepare for the century ahead. We are grateful to the many doctors, nurses, nutritionists, public health educators, medical journalists, and cancer patients and their families who have participated since 1977 in the East West Foundation's annual conference on a nutritional approach to cancer and other degenerative diseases, and related activities. These include the late Robert S. Mendelsohn, M.D., author, syndicated columnist, and former chairman of the Medical Licensure Committee for the State of Illinois; Nicholas Mottern, a congressional staff member, who contributed to the U.S. Senate Select Committee on Nutrition and Human Needs' report *Dietary Goals for the United States;* the late Dr. Edward Kass and Dr. Frank Sacks of Harvard Medical School; Marilyn Light, president of the American Hypoglycemia Foundation; Marian Tompson, founder of the La Leche League; and William Castelli, M.D., director of the Framingham Heart Study.

Participants also included Stephen Appelbaum, Ph.D., of the Menninger Foundation; Jonathan Lieff, M.D., of the Shattuck Hospital, Boston; Frederic Ettner, M.D., of the American International Hospital, Zion, Illinois; Norman Ralston, D.V.M., from Dallas; Marc Van Cauwenberghe, M.D., a teacher at the Kushi Institute; Keith Block, M.D., from Evanston, Illinois; Christiane Northrup, M.D., from Portland, Maine; Peter Klein, M.D., from Rockville, Maryland; Kristen Schmidt, R.N., from Cincinnati; Chandrasekhar Thakkur, M.D., from Bombay; Hideo Ohmori of the Japan C.I. Foundation; Shizuko Yamamoto, a shiatsu teacher in New York; William Dufty, author of *Sugar Blues;* the late Gloria Swanson, film star, author, and inspirational example of a healthy way of life; the late Jean Kohler, professor of music at Ball State University, and his wife, Mary Alice, authors of *Healing Miracles from Macrobiotics;* and Peter Barry Chowka, medical journalist.

Useful assistance in preparing this book has been provided by our families and friends. We would especially like to thank my wife, Aveline, for developing the recipes and menus in this book and my son, Lawrence, an epidemiologist at the University of Minnesota, who has been involved in many scientific and medical research studies of the relation between diet and degenerative disease. Alex's parents, Homer and Esther Jack; his wife, Gale; his sister, Lucy; and her late husband, Jonathan Williams, also contributed their support and encouragement to this book.

Research was conducted at the Boston Public Library, the Brookline Public

Library, and the Harvard University Medical School Library. We are fortunate to have these resources in the Boston area. At the back of this book, we include our own reference section. Please turn to the glossary to look up any medical terms and food items that may be unfamiliar.

Various other colleagues deserve mention for their ongoing work in this field. These include Edward Esko, a senior teacher at the Kushi Institute, who made helpful suggestions and provided some material for the section on launching a health revolution and the material on meditation and visualization. Carolyn Heidenry, Charles Millman, Bill Tara, Olivia Oredson, Sherman Goldman, Tom Monte, Karin Stephan, David Brisson, Eric Zutrau, and Frank Salvati, and other past and present associates at the Kushi Institute and *East West Journal* also contributed to various parts of this work. We are grateful to the many medical associates who are currently active in promoting research into the macrobiotic approach to degenerative disease, including Martha Cottrell, M.D., director of the macrobiotic AIDS project in New York and co-author with me of *AIDS, Macrobiotics, and Natural Immunity;* Dr. Robert Lerman, director of clinical nutrition at University Hospital in Boston; Elinor Levy, Ph.D., and John Beldakas, Ph.D., of the Department of Immunology and Microbiology at Boston University's School of Medicine; Vivien Newbold, M.D., a physician in Philadelphia who has pioneered in the study of the macrobiotic approach to cancer; Dr. Hugh Faulkner, a British physician who recovered from pancreatic cancer using the approach in this book and is the author of *Physician, Heal Thyself;* Neal Barnard, M.D., founder of the PCRM, who actively participates in our conferences; and Dr. Benjamin Spock, the pediatrician and author, who changed his way of eating in his late eighties and is now actively spreading the macrobiotic way.

In seeing this book into final form, we wish to thank Flo Nakamura and Anna Picchioni for secretarial help. We are especially grateful to Julia Coopersmith, our literary agent, and our editors at St. Martin's: Ashton Applewhite and Barbara Anderson. Their prudent editorial guidelines, enthusiasm, and gracious help all along the way are deeply appreciated.

Society as a whole is on the threshold of a breakthrough in its application of diet to disease. Despite a trend toward artificialization—including genetically altered food, irradiated food, and microwaved food—the health revolution is essentially over. It may take another generation for even the current modest dietary guidelines of the major scientific and medical associations to be fully implemented. But modern society and macrobiotics are clearly moving in the same direction. Making fundamental changes in our way of eating will eventually lead not only to an end to cancer and tragedy for millions of families, but also to the return of a safe, clean environment and the realization of a healthy, peaceful world.

Michio Kushi
Becket, Mass.
Summer 1992

PART I

Preventing Cancer Naturally

1

Cancer, Diet, and Macrobiotics

When I first came to the United States nearly forty-five years ago, the expected rate of people who would get cancer in their lifetime was about one out of eight. Today this rate has risen to nearly one out of every three people (see Table 1). This year more than 520,000 Americans will die of cancer and another 1,130,000 new cases will be detected. Between 1973 and 1988, the incidence of cancer at all sites in the body combined climbed nearly 17 percent (20 percent among men and 13 percent among women). Altogether, according to the American Cancer Society, 83 million Americans now living will eventually get the disease. If this increase continues at the present rate, by the beginning of the twenty-first century 40 to 50 percent of the population will develop cancer during their lifetime, and thirty to thirty-five years from now virtually everyone will have the disease at some time before his or her death.

TABLE 1. CANCER INCIDENCE IN THE UNITED STATES

	1900	1962	1971*	1992
New Cases	25,000	520,000	635,000	1,100,000
Selected sites				
Breast	no data	63,000	69,600	175,900
Lung	no data	45,000	80,000	178,000
Colorectal	no data	72,000	75,000	157,500
Prostate	no data	31,000	35,000	122,000
Uterus	no data	no data	no data	46,000
Persons affected	1 in 25	1 in 6	1 in 5	1 in 3

* The year President Nixon declared War on Cancer.
Source: U.S. Vital Statistics and American Cancer Society

While the mortality rate from some cancers—for example stomach, cervix, and rectum—has declined in the United States, it has steeply risen for others—notably lung, melanoma, prostate, multiple myeloma, and brain tumors (see Table 2). Despire ever more sophisticated methods of diagnosis and treatment, the consensus is that the War on Cancer declared in 1971 is being lost. The United States is not unique in this regard. In fact, among the nations of the world, it ranks in the middle (see Table 3). Twenty-three of the fifty countries surveyed had higher mortality rates than the United States for cancer among men and sixteen had higher rates among women. Hungary, Czechoslovakia, and Luxembourg had the highest death rates for men, while Denmark, Scotland, and Hungary had the highest for women.

Clearly, cancer is one of the great levelers of the modern age. It strikes the high and the low, rich and poor, male and female, young and old, black and white, Westerner and Easterner, capitalist and communist, Democrat and Republican, environmentalist and developer, believer and unbeliever, saint and sinner. There is hardly a family today untouched.

Other chronic and degenerative illnesses are also on the rise. In the last ten years, AIDS has spread logarithmically around the world, with the number of

TABLE 2. NEW CASES OF CANCER EACH YEAR*

	Men	Women
1.	Prostate 132,000	Breast 180,000
2.	Lung 102,000	Colon & Rectum 77,000
3.	Colon & Rectum 79,000	Lung 66,000
4.	Bladder 38,500	Uterus 45,500
5.	Lymphoma 27,200	Lymphoma 21,200
6.	Oral 20,600	Ovary 21,000
7.	Melanoma 17,000	Melanoma 15,000
8.	Kidney 16,200	Pancreas 14,400
9.	Leukemia 16,000	Bladder 13,100
10.	Stomach 15,000	Leukemia 12,200
11.	Pancreas 13,900	Kidney 10,300
12.	Larynx 10,000	Oral 9,700
	All Sites 565,000	All Sites 565,000

* Excluding skin cancer and carcinoma *in situ*.
Source: American Cancer Society, 1992

TABLE 3. DEATH RATES FROM CANCER AROUND THE WORLD

Rank	Male	Female
1.	Hungary (235)	Denmark (139)
2.	Czechoslovakia (228)	Scotland (136)
3.	Luxembourg (218)	Hungary (129)
4.	Belgium (205)	England/Wales (127)
5.	France (205)	Ireland (126)
6.	Uruguay (203)	New Zealand (124)
7.	Scotland (201)	Northern Ireland (123)
8.	Netherlands (201)	Czechoslovakia (120)
9.	Poland (200)	Uruguay (118)
10.	Italy (194)	Iceland (116)
11.	USSR (193)	Costa Rica (116)
12.	Denmark (182)	Chile (114)
13.	England/Wales (182)	West Germany (112)
14.	Hong Kong (182)	Canada (111)
15.	Singapore (181)	Belgium (111)
16.	West Germany (181)	Netherlands (110)
17.	Ireland (175)	United States (110)
18.	Northern Ireland (174)	Singapore (110)
19.	Austria (174)	Austria (110)
20.	Switzerland (174)	Luxembourg (109)
21.	New Zealand (172)	Poland (108)
22.	Canada (171)	East Germany (103)
23.	East Germany (166)	Norway (102)
24.	United States (163)	Australia (102)
25.	Australia (163)	Israel (100)
26.	Costa Rica (162)	Italy (100)

TABLE 3.   (*Con't.*)

Rank	Male	Female
27.	Finland (159)	Switzerland (100)
28.	Spain (158)	Sweden (99)
29.	Yugoslavia (154)	Hong Kong (98)
30.	Argentina (152)	Argentina (98)
31.	Korea (150)	Cuba (96)
32.	Japan (150)	USSR (93)
33.	Norway (149)	Finland (91)
34.	China (148)	Malta (91)
35.	Malta (145)	France (90)
36.	Greece (144)	China (89)
37.	Chile (141)	Yugoslavia (89)
38.	Portugal (139)	Ecuador (86)
39.	Bulgaria (138)	Venzuela (85)
40.	Iceland (137)	Bulgaria (84)
41.	Cuba (129)	Portugal (84)
42.	Sweden (128)	Spain (79)
43.	Puerto Rico (122)	Greece (79)
44.	Israel (118)	Mexico (78)
45.	Venzuela (92)	Japan (78)
46.	Kuwait (89)	Kuwait (77)
47.	Panama (87)	Puerto Rico (75)
48.	Ecuador (84)	Panama (72)
49.	Mexico (77)	Korea (65)
50.	Thailand (54)	Thailand (36)

Age-adjusted rates per 100,000 population
Source: *World Health Statistics Annuals,* 1987–90
Note: This data was compiled prior to the reunification of Germany and the breakup of the USSR.

deaths doubling nearly every two years. Over 100,000 Americans have died of this disease, and several million others carry the HIV virus and may become sick. In Africa, Latin America, Asia, and other regions, especially in tropical latitudes, AIDS has reached epidemic proportions. Though primarily an immune-deficiency disorder, AIDS is related to cancer, and many AIDS patients come down with Kaposi's sarcoma (a form of skin cancer), lymphoma, and other malignancies. By the year 2000, according to the most recent estimates, 120 million persons will be infected with the virus. During the 1990s, an estimated 10 million children will suffer the loss of one or more parents from AIDS.

Thirty years ago the incidence of mental illness in the United States was one out of twenty. It has now more than doubled to over one out of ten. Forty-two million people in this country have cardiovascular disorders, 37 million have high blood pressure, 35 million have allergies, 14 to 28 million suffer from alcoholism, tens of millions abuse drugs, 13 million have birth defects, 11 million are diabetic, 5 million are mentally retarded, 2 million have epilepsy, about 1 million have Parkinson's disease, and one-half million have multiple sclerosis.

One of the most dramatic increases in recent decades has been in the area of sexual disorders. In 1982 the British Medical Association, for example, reported that the number of new cases of venereal disease recorded in Great Britain had risen 1,700 percent since 1957. In the United States, the incidence of syphilis in 1990 was the highest since 1949 and represented a 75 percent increase from 1985. In both Europe and North America, herpes and other sexually transmitted diseases (STDs) have assumed epidemic proportions. In addition, infertility is on the increase. Since the 1920s, the average sperm count in American males has dropped by 39 percent according to medical tests, and one recent study of otherwise healthy college males showed that 23 percent were functionally sterile. Cesarean sections rose from 5.5 percent of deliveries in 1970 to 22.7 percent in 1990. Moreover, about 800,000 American women, many of childbearing age, currently have their ovaries or uteri surgically removed each year because of cancer or the fear of cancer. By age sixty-five, a majority of American women have lost their wombs.

A host of new diseases has developed to challenge medical science and national health. Toxic shock syndrome, Legionnaires' disease, chronic fatigue syndrome, and the Epstein-Barr virus, to mention a few, have affected thousands of people, and millions of others are afraid of developing these disorders. Meanwhile, old illnesses are coming back in more virulent form. New varieties of pneumonia and other infectious diseases have been reported for which there is no medical relief on the horizon. Malaria, once believed to have been eradicated by modern medicine, has proven invulnerable to drugs and is spreading across the world, with 270 million new infections each year and an estimated 2 million deaths annually. Tuberculosis, also once believed to have been eliminated after the introduction of antibiotics after World War II, has returned in new, virulent forms and has caused an estimated 3 million deaths annually around the world. For the first time in a century, cholera appeared in epidemic proportions in the Americas in 1991. A recent Tufts University Medical School study found that 75 percent of the population sampled now carries a significant level of antibiotic-resistant bacteria in their digestive system. Even the simple common cold, despite a much publicized medical campaign begun over thirty years ago under President Kennedy, remains largely immune to effective treatment. In fact, few major sicknesses, if any, can really be cured by modern methods. In some cases pain and other discomfort can be relieved and the symptoms temporarily diminished or controlled, but, fundamentally, illness cannot be cured and sooner or later reappears.

Altogether, disease accounts for 80 percent of all deaths worldwide. The rest are caused primarily by accident—often resulting from physical or mental decline—and social violence, including war, crime, and abuse and neglect of children, spouses, and the elderly. In the United States, over the last four decades, from two to four times more Americans have killed each other than have died on the battlefronts of foreign wars. Violence is also on the rise in other parts of the world.

Like the human family, the planet as a whole is in urgent need of healing. The natural environment is being destroyed by the unchecked spread of modern civilization. Tropical rain forests and thousands of species of plants and animals are vanishing. Desertification is spreading as topsoils become depleted and crops will no longer grow in soil saturated with harmful chemicals. The world's nonrenewable resources are being depleted, radioactive wastes are accumulating, the air is contaminated by industrial pollutants and the buildup of greenhouse gases, and the ozone shield that protects the planet from harmful ultraviolet radiation is thinning. The ubiquity of artificial electromagnetic radiation—from nuclear energy to microwave cooking, from hospital X rays to computer terminals, from satellites orbiting in space to VCRs—is creating a global field of ionizing and nonionizing particles whose effects on health and human evolution may not show up for generations.

Given these and many other trends, we can see that modern civilization as a whole is on the verge of self-destruction as a result of deep-seated chronic biological degeneration. This includes the United States, Canada, the former Soviet republics, Eastern and Western Europe, Japan, Australia, China, and many other parts of Asia, Africa, and Latin America. With the end of the Cold War, the threat of possible extinction from degenerative disease and the inability of humanity in the future to pass life on to future generations have now surpassed the danger posed by the spread of nuclear weapons. The time left to reverse direction and recover personal and planetary health is very short. By the time the current generation grows to adulthood, we may be witnessing the complete decline of our recently developed modern way of life. The final collapse may come within the next twenty-five or, at most, thirty-five years.

The cancer problem, however, offers us the chance to rethink our present understanding of health and sickness. It provides the opportunity to reexamine the basic premises of our way of life and to work together as members of a common planetary family to build one healthy, peaceful world.

CANCER IN THE ANCIENT WORLD

The history of cancer goes back 2,500 years to ancient Greece, where Hippocrates first identified and described the illness. In Greek the word *karkinos*, from which our word *cancer* comes, originally meant "crab." The Father of Western Medicine evidently chose the image because of the disease's crablike spread through the body. Though known and classified since ancient times, cancer was an extremely rare illness. Through most of recorded history it has affected only a tiny fraction of the world's population. For instance, cancer is not mentioned in the Bible, nor is it included in the *Yellow Emperor's Classic of Internal Medicine*, the ancient medical book of China. In most traditional societies, cancer was completely unknown. However, about the time of the Industrial Revolution, beginning in the seventeenth century, cancer gradually began to emerge in the West. In the 1830s Stanislas Tanchou, a French scientist who pioneered in the field of vital statistics, tabulated the mortality rates around Paris and reported that cancer deaths comprised about 2 percent of the total. At the beginning of the twentieth century, the annual mortality rate from cancer in the United States had reached about 4 percent. As recently as a generation ago, many forms of cancer common today were rare.

"In 1919, during my junior year at Washington University, a patient with cancer of the lung was admitted to the Barnes Hospital," Alton Oschner, M.D., recalls of his medical training in an article in *American Scientist*. "As was usual, the patient died. Dr. George Dock, our Professor of Medicine, who was not only an eminent clinician and scientist but also an excellent pathologist, insisted upon the two senior classes witnessing the autopsy, and he stressed that the condition was so rare he thought we might never see another case as long as we lived." Dr. Oschner adds that he saw his next case of lung cancer in 1936, seventeen years later.

As modern civilization spread across the world, a legion of explorers, medical doctors, missionaries, and other travelers marveled at the almost complete absence of degenerative disease in native societies. In 1908 W. Roger Williams, a Fellow of the Royal College of Surgeons, chronicled the absence of cancer in overseas territories of the British Empire in his book, *The Natural History of Cancer*. In the 1920s Sir Robert McCarrison, director of nutritional research in India, wrote about his discovery of the remote Hunza culture where disease was virtually unknown and people lived to an exceedingly old age. In the 1930s Japanese educator George Ohsawa began his study of indigenous cultures culminating in his book, *Cancer and the Philosophy of the Far East*. Dental surgeon Weston Price performed fieldwork among the Indians of North America, the Eskimo, the Polynesians, and the Australian Aborigines and reported no trace of cancer in his 1945 publication, *Nutrition and Physical Degeneration*.

These four medical detectives and others tried to explain why traditional peoples living in the tropics, polar regions, islands, and other cultures removed from modern civilization remained immune to cancer, heart disease, and even tooth decay. After careful observation and research, including laboratory testing in some cases, they each independently concluded that cancer was a disease of overnutrition caused by intake of sugar, white flour, and other refined foods, as well as excess protein and fat. When these items were introduced into primitive societies, cancer and other degenerative diseases followed close behind.

A few professional cancer researchers drew the obvious conclusions from reports such as these, as well as from epidemiological studies comparing diets and incidence of disease among different populations. In the July 1927 medical journal *Cancer*, William Howard Hay, M.D., conjectured:

> Think back over the years of cancer research, of the millions spent, the time consumed, the pains expended . . . and where are we today? Is it not time to take stock of our basic conception of cancer to see if there is not something radically wrong with this, to account for the years of utter and complete failure to date? . . . Cancer has been consistently on the increase. . . . Is it possible that the cause of cancer lies in our departure from natural foods? It would surely look so to any man from Mars, but we have lived so long on processed foods deficient in vitamins and tissue salts that we are in a state of unbalanced nutrition almost from birth. . . . We have come to regard our [refined] foods as the hallmark of civilization, when it is a fact that these very foods set the stage for every sort of ill, including cancer.

THE STAFF OF LIFE

All civilizations prior to ours recognized the primacy of food and agriculture and enshrined dietary concerns in their household economies, religions, and literature and art. Cooked whole grains, in particular, have constituted humanity's staple food for thousands of years, and, until fairly recently, were eaten as the staple food throughout the world. For example, rice and millet were principal foods in the Orient; wheat, oats, and rye in Europe; buckwheat in Russia and Central Asia; sorghum in Africa; barley in the Middle East; and corn in the Americas. In fact, the English word for "food" is *meal*, or ground grain, while in Japanese, the term used for meal is *gohan*, which means "cooked rice."*

In the ancient world, nutritional therapy formed the core of medical understanding and practice. Hippocrates' writings, for example, are permeated with dietary considerations, and he frequently emphasizes the importance of wheat and barley, the two principal grains of the Hellenistic world. "I know too that the body is affected differently by bread according to the manner in which it is prepared," he explains in *Tradition in Medicine*. "It differs according as it is made from pure flour or meal with bran, whether it is prepared from winnowed or unwinnowed wheat, whether it is mixed with much water or little, whether well mixed or poorly mixed, overbaked or underbaked, and countless other points besides. The same is true of the preparation of barley meal. The influence of each process is considerable and each has a totally different effect from another. How can anyone who has not considered such matters and come to understand them, possibly know anything of the diseases that afflict man-

---

* The Old English word *meat* also originally meant daily food, staple fare: oats, barley, rye, wheat, and the edible part of nuts and fruits. Later the word took on four connotations: 1) green meat or grains and vegetables, 2) baked meat or bread (cf. *Hamlet*: "The Funerall Bakt-meats/ Did coldly furnish forth the Marriage Tables"), 3) sweetmeats or pastries, and 4) butcher's meat (also known as red-, dark-, horse-, and hard-meat). Later, when the generic words for stable food in the Bible were translated into the vernacular, confusion about the original meaning of the concept *meat* arose. In the King James Version, it refers to staple food, as this passage from Genesis makes clear: "Behold, I have given you every herb bearing seed, which is upon the face of all the earth, and every tree, in the which is the fruit of a tree yielding seed; to you it shall be for meat."

kind? Each one of the substances of a man's diet acts upon his body and changes it in some way and upon these changes his whole life depends. . . ."

The matter of food became so important to the founder of Western medicine that he coined another new word, *diaita,* to refer to a way of life. From this Greek word our modern word *diet* comes. Today its meaning has narrowed to signify weight loss or a restricted eating regimen, but the proper meaning is a mode of living of which food selection and preparation is the main factor.

In treating serious illnesses in the fifth century B.C., Hippocrates stressed the importance of using dietary methods. In *The Book on Nutriment* he declares: "Let food be thy medicine and medicine thy food." The Hippocratic Oath, still taken by modern medical doctors, states, in part: "I will apply dietetic measures for the benefit of the sick according to my ability and judgment; I will keep them from harm and injustice. I will neither give a deadly drug to anybody if asked for it, nor will I make a suggestion to this effect. . . . I will not use the knife. . . ." His favorite remedy was cooked whole-grain barley cereal. He hailed this broth as "smooth, consistent, soothing; slippery and fairly soft; thirst-quenching and easily got rid of; doesn't produce constipation or rumbling or swell up the stomach." He described various ways the barley meal could be modified for different illnesses and supplemented dietary adjustments with simple, safe compresses made of grains, vegetables, and herbs, which could be prepared in the home. In the case of cancer, he warned against surgery: "If treated the patients die quickly; but if not treated, they hold out for a long time."

CANCER IN MEDIEVAL TIMES

Hippocrates' careful attention to diet and environment won widespread renown. His conviction that disease had a natural rather than a supernatural origin represented a break with the past and set the direction for the medicine of the future. Until the seventeenth century, his natural healing methods and those of Galen, the second-century Roman physician, were widely practiced in the European and Arab worlds. In the Middle Ages, Maimonides, the famous Jewish physician, formulated a similar dietary philosophy and cautioned against eating "any kind of meal so completely sifted that not a trace of bran remains in it."

The *Divine Comedy* alludes to the origin of cancer. The key passage comes in a discussion between Dante and Virgil, his guide through the Inferno and Purgatory, on the necessity of heeding Nature's teaching and following "her laws, her fruits, her seasons." Dante characterizes the approach to life that ignores or scorns Nature as "a canker to every conscience" and throughout the early fourteenth-century epic extols the harmonious souls who followed a simple diet during their lifetime. For example, from the Bible he singles out Daniel for refusing the meat of the Babylonian king's table, and he locates the followers of Hippocrates atop the summit of the Earthly Paradise. As late as Shakespeare's day, the sixteenth century, Sir Thomas Elyot's *The Castle of Health,* a popular guide to home remedies, cataloged the effects of different foods upon the human body and recommended the consumption of cereal grains, principally rye and barley, to relieve serious illnesses.

Food selection and proper cooking also served as the cornerstone for preventing and relieving illness in the Far East. In the *Yellow Emperor's Classic of Internal Medicine*, Ch'i Po (the Hippocrates of the Orient) recommended that a broth of brown rice be eaten for ten days to cure cases of chronic disease. The *Caraka Samhita*, India's chief medical text, dating to the first century A.D., equated the rise of illness in Hindu society with deterioration in diet. Other works warned against a departure from simple, whole foods, which then as now tended to be neglected by the rich and upper classes of society. For example, during the Song Dynasty, nearly a thousand years ago, a Chinese philosopher named Yang Fang complained that the children and grandchildren of officials "will be unwilling to eat vegetables and will look on greens and broth as coarse fare, finding beans, wheat, and millet meager and tasteless, and insisting on the best polished rice, and the finest roasts to satisfy their greedy appetites, with the products of the water and the land and the confections of human artifice set out before them neatly in ornamentally carved dishes and trays."

Farther east, in 1714 Ekiken Kaibara, a Japanese physician and Confucian scholar, completed *Yojokun*, a book on health and longevity describing the wisdom of adopting a brown rice diet and disapproving of all symptomatic treatments for disease, including surgery.

THE RISE OF MODERN SCIENCE AND MEDICINE

Despite the calls for dietary common sense by Yang Fang, Maimonides, Sir Thomas Elyot, Ekiken Kaibara, and others, the spice trade generated by the Crusades and the discovery of the New World transformed traditional patterns of eating in East and West and ushered in the scientific age. With the overthrow of Hippocrates, Galen, Aristotle, and Ptolemy in the seventeenth and eighteenth centuries, the philosophy of natural healing, which had prevailed for two thousand years, declined, and Descartes' view of the world as a machine laid the conceptual groundwork for modern science and medicine. The doctrine of humors, which animated medicine in ancient Greece, the Middle Ages, and the Renaissance, quickly faded. Under this system, human constitutions and conditions, body organs, and different foods were classified according to varying combinations of Earth, Air, Water, and Fire, and an imbalance in these energies and their respective humors was believed to give rise to disease, including cancer. With the invention of the microscope and lifting of Church sanctions against dissection of the human body, a new view developed that saw illness as a manifestation of a chemical change in the body's tissues, usually localized in a particular organ. Treatment, according to this perspective, could also be chemical, directed to the diseased organ.

In the first laboratory experiment with cancerous tissue, Jean Astruc, a physician to eighteenth-century French and Polish monarchs, incinerated a piece of a human breast tumor and a piece of beefsteak in a retort and found they tasted the same. He concluded that cancerous growth had no more salty or bitter taste than ordinary cow's meat, the staple diet of royalty, and that the traditional humoral theories, which connected cancer with foods containing excess bile salts or acid, were wrong. On the basis of this test, future cancer researchers tended to dismiss the dietary hypothesis, which, in actuality, it had confirmed.

In other developments, Lavoisier laid the foundation for empirical study of respiration, oxidation, and caloric measurement. In France and England, the first hospitals devoted exclusively to cancer opened. In America, Dr. Benjamin Rush's treatment of yellow fever with calomel in 1793 ushered in the modern era of medical intervention and massive purging, bloodletting, blistering, and use of caustic dyes to root out disease. The eminent signer of the Declaration of Independence blamed Hippocrates for relying too much on the patient's own recuperative powers and held that "the work [of healing] must be taken out of nature's hand."

With the spread of the Industrial Revolution, traditional agriculture and food technology changed. By the early nineteenth century, steam-driven mills replaced water- and windmills, and nearly all aspects of breadmaking were mechanized and out of human hands. Tuberculosis, stomach ailments, and cancer increased as refined flour became widely available. A few eloquent health reformers warned against the declining use of whole grains. They include Rev. Sylvester Graham, popularizer of the whole wheat Graham bread and Graham cracker; Mary Gove Nichols, leader of the Boston Ladies Physiological Society; and Ellen Harmon White, a founder of the Seventh-Day Adventists, who championed unbolted flour and helped introduce soyfoods to this continent. However, these prophetic voices were ultimately lost in the analytical din of the nineteenth century as the engine of industrial society forged full steam ahead.

European society witnessed continued quantification and specialization in medical science and the rise of metabolic theory. The German scientist Liebig classified nourishment into protein, carbohydrate, and fat. The Austrian biologist Virchow developed cellular pathology and, as a scientific model, likened the cells of the body to citizens of a republic. In his view, disease represented a civil conflict among cells brought about by the intervention of outside forces. In the field of cancer, the Russian researcher Novinsky performed the first transplants of tumors in laboratory animals. In Vienna, Billroth introduced surgical removal of cancerous inner organs. In the Far East, Japanese medical studies avidly turned to Western medicine following contact with Portuguese, Spanish, and Dutch surgeons. By 1868, under the Meiji rulers, Japan officially adopted the German medical system and prepared to assume its role in the technological forefront of the modern world. In China, government edicts outlawed the teaching and practice of traditional medicine as it had existed for thousands of years.

CANCER TREATMENT IN THE TWENTIETH CENTURY

With the rise of the petrochemical industry in the United States and Western Europe in the early part of the twentieth century, surgery and pharmacology consolidated their triumph over other approaches to medicine. The spread of chemical agriculture and factory farming revolutionized patterns of food consumption in the industrialized world. Nutrition became relegated to the back Bunsen burner as genetics, biochemistry, and radiation techniques dominated medical research.

Despite the general neglect of dietary concerns, a host of international population studies emerged during the middle part of the century linking cancer with high fat intake, refined carbohydrates, chemical additives, and other nutritional variables. Building on the earlier reports of the colonial medical doctors and anthropologists, epidemiologists concluded that cultures and subcultures eating a traditional diet of whole grains, cooked vegetables, and fresh seasonal fruit remained largely cancer-free.

One of the clearest warnings was sounded by Frederick L. Hoffman, LL.D., cancer specialist and consulting statistician for the Prudential Life Insurance Company. In his 1937 volume, *Cancer and Diet,* he stated:

> I have come to the essential conclusion that there has been a decided increase in the cancer death rate and progressively so during the last century ending with 1930. From this I reflect that the profound changes in dietary habits and nutritional condition of the population taking place during the intervening years have been world wide and due to the rapid and almost universal introduction of modified food products, conserved or preserved, refrigerated or sterilized, colored or modified, aside from positive adulteration by the addition of injurious mineral substances close to being of a poisonous nature. To a diminishing extent food is being consumed in its natural state, at least by urban populations everywhere, and to a lesser degree also among persons in rural communities.

In the 1940s and 1950s, laboratory studies on mice and other animals began to confirm these findings. Also, several European countries experienced a significant drop in cancer mortality rates during World Wars I and II when meat, dairy food, and eggs became scarce and local populations were forced to survive on brown bread, oats and barley meal, and home-grown produce.

Following World War II, frozen and enriched foods became more widely available, many tropical and subtropical foods such as oranges, grapefruits, and pineapples found their way to the daily breakfast table, and soft drinks, ice cream, candy bars, pizza, hamburgers, french fries, potato chips, and other fast foods became a way of life. As cancer rates climbed, the medical profession stepped up its technological arsenal. In 1971 President Nixon formally declared war on the disease and commissioned the National Cancer Institute (NCI) to eradicate it. However, this mobilization largely excluded dietary means.

In 2,500 years, since cancer was first described in ancient Greece, medicine had come full circle. In *Epidemics,* Book I, Hippocrates cited factors for the physician to consider in making diagnoses and recommending treatment. At the head of the list comes "what food is given to him [the patient] and who gives it," followed by conditions of the climate and local environment, the patient's customs, mode of life, pursuits, age, speech, mannerisms, silences, thoughts, sleeping patterns, and dreams. Last on the list is physical symptoms. The priorities of modern medicine were just reversed. In 1973, according to a Harvard School of Public Health study, only 4 percent of the nation's medical schools had an independent course in nutrition.

A RETURN TO WHOLE FOODS

In nature, just as day follows night and valleys turn into mountains, societies regenerate after a long period of decay. In the modern world, the turning point came in the 1960s and 1970s when awareness of the deficiencies of the contemporary way of life and eating generated the natural foods and holistic health movements. Vegetarian and health foods had long been available, but their quality was often low and they appealed only to a tiny market. Suddenly, the postwar generation, which had become active in integrating southern lunch counters and preserving the rice fields of Vietnam from destruction by bombs and chemical reagents, became conscious of the food they ate, and organized Food Days to consider the impact of modern agriculture on world hunger, energy conservation, and the quality of the environment.

By 1976 the concern for healthy food echoed through the halls of Congress. In its historic report, *Dietary Goals for the United States*, the Senate Select Committee on Nutrition and Human Needs listed cancer as one of the six major degenerative diseases associated with improper nutrition. The report sent shock waves through the American food industry and medical profession. The cattle- and hog-growers' associations, the poultry and egg producers, and the refined salt institute condemned the report.

However, at the highest national level, the door had been opened for a return to healthy food. Within the next five years, dozens of medical and scientific associations corroborated the link between diet and degenerative disease. In his 1979 report, *Healthy People: Health Promotion and Disease Prevention*, the U.S. Surgeon-General stated: "People should consume . . . less saturated fat and cholesterol . . . less red meat . . . more complex carbohydrates such as whole grains, cereals, fruits and vegetables." The American Heart Association, the American Diabetes Association, the American Society for Clinical Nutrition, and the U.S. Department of Agriculture issued similar statements. In 1981 a panel of the American Association for the Advancement of Science reported on the social impact of a change to a whole-grain diet. The scientists declared that changes in our eating habits could have significant beneficial effects on everything from land, water, fuel, and mineral use to the cost of living, unemployment, and the balance of international trade as well as reduce coronary heart disease by 88 percent and cancer by 50 percent.

In 1982 the National Academy of Sciences issued a 472-page report, *Diet, Nutrition, and Cancer*, calling upon the general public to reduce substantially consumption of foods high in saturated and unsaturated fat and increase daily intake of whole grains, vegetables, and fruit. The panel reviewed hundreds of current medical studies associating long-term eating patterns with the development of most common cancers, including those of the colon, stomach, breast, lung, esophagus, ovary, and prostate. The thirteen-member scientific committee suggested that diet could be responsible for 30 to 40 percent of cancers in men and 60 percent in women. The flood of interest and activity in the relation between diet and cancer in the last ten years has been recounted in the preface to this newly revised edition.

LAUNCHING A HEALTH REVOLUTION

While along with George Ohsawa and early macrobiotic pioneers we had been promoting natural foods and a dietary approach to cancer, heart disease, and other ills since the 1950s, the role of the macrobiotic community in helping to launch the health revolution of the 1970s and 1980s is not widely known. In 1972 my wife, Aveline, invited Sadayo Kita, one of the leading No actors in Japan, to come to the United States to perform under the auspices of the East West Foundation (EWF), a cultural and educational foundation that we founded to promote international friendship and world peace. Mr. Kita's public performances in Boston and New York were so successful that he returned on a regular basis. In connection with the EWF's No program, I had the opportunity to meet Edwin Reischauer, one of the world's leading scholars of Far Eastern culture. Professor Reischauer, who passed away a few years ago, was born and grew up in Japan. He spoke fluent Japanese and served as ambassador to Japan under Presidents Kennedy and Johnson in the 1960s and after returning to Harvard headed up the East Asian studies program. In 1973 my wife and I met with Professor Reischauer at the Seventh Inn, a macrobiotic restaurant in Boston. While our meeting, and others between Reischauer and my associates, focused largely on the meeting of East and West, the dialogue often turned to a discussion of macrobiotics in the United States and the relation of diet and health.

In *The Japanese*, published several years later by Harvard University Press, Professor Reischauer addressed the role that diet played in modern Japanese culture and history: "The traditional Japanese diet of rice, vegetables, and fish, which contrasts with the heavy consumption of meat and fat in the West, would be almost a perfect health diet if the Japanese did not insist on polishing their rice. This diet may account in part for the low incidence of heart disease as compared with Americans."

Noting the increase in size and weight of Japanese children following World War II, he went on: "Since World War II, Japanese children have increased several inches in height and many pounds in weight. Part of the increased height may be attributed to the straightening of legs, as Japanese sit on the floor and more on chairs, but, like the weight, it may be chiefly due to a richer diet, which now includes dairy products and more meat and bread. Young Japanese today are quite visibly a bigger breed than their ancestors, and fat children, which were formerly never encountered, have become a commonplace sight."

Another of our friends at Harvard, Edward Kass, M.D., was one of the nation's leading researchers on cardiovascular disease. As director of Channing Laboratories, Dr. Kass oversaw research, beginning in 1973 and extending on and off for more than a decade, on macrobiotic people living in Boston. With Frank Sacks, M.D., of Harvard Medical School; William Castelli, M.D., director of the Framingham Heart Study; and other colleagues, Dr. Kass reported on the protective health benefits of the macrobiotic dietary approach, particularly in lowering cholesterol and high blood pressure. These studies were published in the *American Journal of Epidemiology*, the *New England Journal of Medicine*, the *Journal of the American Medical Association*, *Atherosclerosis*, and other professional journals and were the turning point in the medical profession's recognition of the relation of diet and heart disease. Popular publications such as *Vogue*, the *Boston Globe*, and the *New York Times* also ran articles featuring this research, and the notion that diet was connected to heart disease and thus it could be prevented—and possibly relieved—spread throughout society.

Meanwhile, in 1976 the *East West Journal* (*EWJ*), a monthly magazine that my associates and I started several years earlier, began publishing special issues devoted to cancer and diet. The editors, Sherman Goldman and Alex Jack, introduced case histories of individuals with cancer who had recovered using a macrobiotic diet, as well as theoretical articles by me and a series of investigative reports on the NCI, the American Cancer Society, and the pharmaceutical industry by journalist Peter Barry Chowka. The *EWJ* issues received national attention and helped to focus public attention on what was being done—or not being done—to end the cancer epidemic.

In 1976 the Senate Select Committee on Nutrition and Human Needs in Washington, D.C., responding to this grass roots movement to address causes rather than symptoms of disease, began to hold hearings and take scientific testimony linking diet with heart disease, cancer, and other degenerative diseases. One of the star witnesses was Dr. Gio B. Gori of the NCI. In his testimony (and subsequent candid interview with *EWJ* for which he got in trouble with his superiors), he suggested that diet was possibly the most important factor in the development of cancer and that more research should be focused in this direction. In Boston, meanwhile, the EWF, under the guidance of Edward Esko, published the first book-length report on macrobiotics and cancer, titled *A Dietary Approach to Cancer according to the Principles of Macrobiotics*. Through the EWF, we also began to contact and, in some cases, meet with government policymakers, medical researchers, and scientists throughout the world in order to let them know about our approach, including many researchers who appeared before the dietary goals hearings or later became part of the National Academy of Sciences panel that compiled the landmark report, *Diet, Nutrition, and Cancer*.

We received many encouraging replies to our letters, books, and other educational materials. For example, Sen. Edward Kennedy wrote:

Thank you for your letter and the enclosed reports on food policy and the relationship between our diet and our health.

As you know, I share your deep concern over this important issue and during future consideration of legislation relating to the importance of nutrition to proper health care in the nation, the reports prepared by the Foundation will continue to be most helpful.

On the Republican side, Robert Dole, vice chairman of the Senate Select Committee on Nutrition, responded:

Thank you for sharing with me copies of your organization's publications, *A Nutritional Approach to Cancer* and *Food Policy Recommendations for the United States*. I am sure the documents will serve as significant resources in future congressional discussions in these areas.

Your comments on the work of the Select Committee are appreciated. After December 31, many of the functions and responsibilities of that body will transfer to the new Subcommittee on Nutrition of the Senate Agriculture Committee. As ranking minority member of this Subcommittee, I would like to be kept informed of the nutrition and health related concerns of your foundation.

Among scientists we met with Mark Hegsted, M.D., of the Department of Nutrition at the Harvard School of Public Health, who was one of the key witnesses before the Senate dietary goals hearings, and Dr. Gori of the NCI. At one meeting at Boston City Hospital, I introduced Dr. Kass to Jean Kohler, a professor of music at Ball State University in Muncie, Indiana. Professor Kohler had developed pancreatic cancer in 1973 and completely recovered his health after adopting a macrobiotic diet. Medical documentation, based on tests performed by the Indiana University Medical Center in Indianapolis, was very persuasive, as was the fact that Jean Kohler was still alive. About 90 percent of all pancreatic patients die within the first year, and the disease is considered almost invariably terminal. Now almost five years had passed since his original diagnosis.

Dr. Kass became very interested in Professor Kohler's case and suggested ways that future research could be carried out. He recommended that a group of twenty-five patients with the same type of cancer begin to eat macrobiotically under the supervision of the EWF and that after a period of time their status be compared to that of a control group with the same type of cancer eating the standard modern diet. Afterward, Dr. Kass introduced me to Dr. Emil Frei, the director of the Dana Farber Cancer Center in Boston, one of the leading cancer research institutes in the world. My associates and I introduced several macrobiotic case histories and discussed with Dr. Frei the possibility of conducting future research on the macrobiotic approach. He seemed very open-minded to our suggestions and said he felt the subject warranted further study.

In March 1977 the EWF sponsored its first conference on a nutritional approach to cancer at Pine Manor College, outside of Boston. Many medical doctors and researchers attended the gathering, including Dr. Robert Mendelsohn, one of the nation's best-known pediatricians and author of a popular newspaper column, "The People's Doctor." The Pine Manor Conference brought together for the first time leading scientific and medical researchers, leading teachers of the international macrobiotic community, and ordinary men and women from many walks of life who had recovered from cancer following adoption of a macrobiotic diet. An active public program followed, with annual diet and cancer conferences, public symposiums, and television and radio interviews with EWF staff in New York, Boston, Philadelphia, Baltimore, Miami, Atlanta, Dallas, and other big cities.

In the summer of 1977, influenced by the Senate's report *Dietary Goals for the United States,* which came out earlier in the year, President Carter ordered an official review of governmental food policy. In September, along with Dr. Mendelsohn and several staff of the EWF and *EWJ,* I met with members of the president's domestic policy staff at the White House. We presented the advisers with a series of food policy recommendations and warned that unless the nation changed its national food policy a wave of epidemic diseases would threaten the survival of the nation within the next generation. In subsequent meetings with the president's advisers in the areas of health and consumer affairs, as well as with members of the U.S. Department of Agriculture, my associates presented further information and policy recommendations. (Some of the research on macrobiotic people was cited by the U.S. Surgeon-General in his report, *Healthy People,* in 1979.)

At a personal as well as professional level, macrobiotics began to have an impact on key government policymakers. When President Carter's sister, Jean Stapleton, was diagnosed with pancreatic cancer, she came to me for advice.

In 1985 the NCI reported that radiation therapy and chemotherapy were ineffective and in some cases produced toxic side effects as follow-ups to surgery in the treatment of cancer: "Except possibly in selected patients with cancer of the stomach, there has been no demonstrated improvement in the survival of patients with the ten most common cancers when radiation therapy, chemotherapy, or both have been added to surgical resection." The ten most common cancers are lung, colorectal, breast, prostate, uterus, bladder, pancreas, stomach, skin, and kidney. Shortly after the report was published, the author, Dr. Steven A. Rosenberg, the NCI's chief of surgery, operated on President Ronald Reagan's colon cancer and instead of chemotherapy or radiation treatment put him on a modified whole-grain diet.

Macrobiotic food was prepared at United Nations functions by Laura Masini, who had recovered from breast cancer with the help of macrobiotics and who served as hostess for her brother, Vernon Walters, the U.S. ambassador, who was a bachelor. In Washington, Blande Keith, wife of a former Republican congressman from Massachusetts, was influential in introducing macrobiotics to the family and staff of other government officials. Over the years, many governors, senators, congressmen, and heads of state have come to me for advice, especially when cancer struck themselves or their families.

As a result of the EWF and *EWJ*'s pioneering activities, the awareness of diet and health began to spread throughout the United States. Articles on our approach appeared in the *Saturday Evening Post, Life* magazine, and other publications, as well as on radio and television. The health revolution of the late 1970s and 1980s was the successor to the natural foods movement of the 1960s. Leading scientific and medical associations began to take a serious interest in studying the relation between diet and degenerative disease and for the first time issued dietary guidelines to protect against cancer and other degenerative diseases. As the 1970s ended, the mass media began to focus on diet and nutrition as the most promising avenue for future medical study. In an article at the start of the new decade, *Newsweek* noted:

The rich and abundant U.S. diet had recently been linked to a growing number of serious illnesses, and the worst may be to come. For researchers are now becoming convinced that the foods Americans put on their tables play a major part in the most frightening disease of all—cancer.

THE MACROBIOTIC APPROACH

It is important to understand that macrobiotics is not just a diet in the modern sense of the term, but a way of life encompassing all dimensions of living. From such diverse phenomena as the size and shape of distant galaxies to the movements of subatomic particles, from the periodic rise and fall of civilizations to the patterns of our own individual lives, macrobiotic philosophy offers a unifying principle to understand the order of the universe as a whole.

Translated literally, *macro* is the Greek word for "great" or "long" and *bios* is the word for "life." Macrobiotics means the way of life according to the greatest or longest possible view. The earliest recorded usage of the term is found in the writings of Hippocrates. In the essay, *Airs, Waters, and Places*, the Father of Western Medicine introduces the word to describe a group of young men who are healthy and relatively long-lived. Other classical writers, including Herodotus, Aristotle, Galen, and Lucian, also used the term, and the concept came to signify living in harmony with nature, eating a simple balanced diet, and living to an active old age. In the popular imagination, macrobiotics became particularly associated with the Ethiopians of Africa, who were said to live 120 years or more, the biblical patriarchs, and the Chinese sages. In *Pantagruel and Gargantua*, the sixteenth-century French humanist Rabelais mentions a fabulous Isle of the Macreons where his adventurers meet a sage named Macrobius who guides them along their way. In 1797 the German physician and philosopher Christoph W. Hufeland, M.D., wrote an influential book on diet and health titled *Macrobiotics or the Art of Prolonging Life*.

In the Near and Far East, the macrobiotic spirit also guided and shaped civilization. Dietary common sense and principles of natural healing underlie the Bible, the I Ching, the Tao Te Ching, the Bhagavad Gita, the Kojiki, the Koran, and many other scriptures and epics. Down through the centuries, as we have seen, cultural movements surfaced in Asia to extol the benefits of the traditional way of eating and caution against increasingly artificial ways.

In the late nineteenth and early twentieth centuries, macrobiotics experienced a revival originating in Japan. Two educators, Sagen Ishitsuka, M.D., and Yukikazu Sakurazawa, cured themselves of serious illnesses by changing from the modern refined diet then sweeping Japan to a simple diet of brown rice, miso soup, sea vegetables, and other traditional foods. After restoring their health, they went on to integrate traditional Oriental medicine and philosophy with Vedanta, original Jewish and Christian teachings, and holistic perspectives in modern science and medicine. When Sakurazawa came to Paris in the 1920s, he adopted George Ohsawa as his pen name and called his teachings *macrobiotics*.

Thus macrobiotics today is a unique synthesis of Eastern and Western influences. It is the way of life according to the largest possible view, the infinite order of the universe. The practice of macrobiotics is the understanding and practical application of this order to our lifestyle, including the selection, preparation, and manner of eating of our daily food, as well as the orientation of consciousness. Macrobiotics does not offer a single diet for everyone but a dietary principle that takes into account differing climatic and geographical considerations, varying ages, sexes, and levels of activity, and ever-changing personal needs. Macrobiotics also embraces the variety and richness of all the world's cultures and heritages.

Broadly speaking, dietary practice according to macrobiotics is the way of eating that flourished from before the time of Homer to the Renaissance. It is the diet that Buddha ate under the tree of enlightenment and that Jesus shared with his disciples at the Last Supper. It is the diet that helped Moses free his people from bondage and that sustained the Pilgrims upon their arrival in the New World. Most of all macrobiotics is the way of life followed by ordinary people throughout history: farmers, shepherds, fishermen, merchants, traders, artisans, scribes, monks, bards. From the earliest campfires in the Ice Age to the latest space launches in the Atomic Age, countless mothers, fathers, daughters, sons, babies, and grandparents have shared nourishing food together and saved the seeds to plant the following spring.

To the eye of Heaven, our era is but a day. The spread of cancer and the proliferation of nuclear weapons are only passing shadows in humanity's prolonged adolescence. One day future generations will look back at the cult of modern civilization and regard its unnatural food and artificial way of life as a fad that flared up and extinguished itself in the relatively short span of four hundred years. Under many names and forms, macrobiotics will continue as long as human life continues to exist, as its most fundamental and intuitive wisdom. It offers a key to restoring our health, a vision for regenerating the world, and a compass for charting our endless voyage toward freedom and enduring peace.

2

Cancer and Modern Civilization

Over the last thirty-five years, modern medical science has mounted a tremendous campaign to solve the problems of cancer and other degenerative illnesses. To date, however, this large-scale effort has produced no lasting, comprehensive solutions.

In the field of cancer research, for example, modern medicine has pioneered such techniques as surgery, radiation therapy, laser therapy, chemotherapy, hormone therapy, and others. But these treatments are, at best, successful in achieving only temporary relief of symptoms. In the majority of cases they fail to prevent the disease from recurring, as they do not address the root cause or origin of the problem.

We believe that this biological decline is not irreversible, but that to prevent such a catastrophe from occurring we must begin to approach such problems as cancer with a new orientation. Specifically, we must begin to seek out the most basic causes and to implement the most basic solutions rather than continue the present approach of treating each problem separately in terms of its symptoms alone. The problem of degenerative disease affects us all in one way or another in all domains of modern life. Therefore, the responsibility for finding and implementing solutions should not be left only to those within the medical and scientific communities. We believe that the recovery of global health will emerge only through a cooperative effort involving people at all levels of society.

The epidemic of degenerative disease, the decline of traditional human values, and the decomposition of society itself are all clear indications that something is deeply wrong with the modern orientation of life. At present, we tend to value the development of civilization in terms of our advancing material prosperity. At the same time, we tend to undervalue the development of human consciousness, intuition, and spiritual development. But this viewpoint is out of proportion with the very nature of existence. The world of matter itself is a small, fragmental, and almost infinitesimal manifestation when compared to the vast currents of moving space and energy that envelop it and out of which it has come into physical existence.

Not only is the material world infinitesimally small by comparison, but also, as modern quantum physics has demonstrated, the more we analyze and take it apart, the more we discover that it actually has no concrete substance. The search for an ultimate unit of matter, which began with Democritus's assumption that reality could be divided into atoms and space, has ended in the twentieth century with the discovery that subatomic particles are nothing but charged matrixes of moving energy. Einstein's formulation that $E = MC^2$ signifies that matter is not solid material at all but ultimately waves of energy or vibration.

However, our limited senses easily delude us into believing that things have a fixed or unchanging quality, in spite of the fact that all of the cells, tissues, skin, and organs that comprise the human body are continuously changing. The red blood cells in the bloodstream live about 120 days. In order to maintain a relatively constant number of these cells, an astounding 200 million new cells are created every minute, while an equal number of old cells are continuously destroyed. The entire body regenerates itself about every seven years. As a result, what we think of as today's "self" is very different from yesterday's "self" and tomorrow's "self." This is obvious to parents who have watched their children grow. However, our development does not stop when we reach physical maturity: our consciousness and judgment also change and develop during the entire period of life.

ENLARGING OUR PERSPECTIVE

In reality, there is nothing static, fixed, or permanent. Yet modern people frequently adopt an unchanging and inflexible attitude and, as a result, experience repeated frustration and disappointment when faced with the ephemerality of life. Today's culture, which overemphasizes competition and material acquisition, is based primarily on consumer values, and the successful production of consumer goods depends largely on mass marketing. In order to succeed, a product must stimulate or gratify our physical senses. Of itself, sensory satisfaction is not necessarily destructive; everyone is entitled to satisfy their basic senses. However, trouble arises when sensory gratification becomes a society's driving motive. This causes a society to degenerate, since the realm of the senses is extremely limited in comparison to our comprehensive native capacities, including emotion, intellect, imagination, understanding, compassion, insight, aspiration, and inspiration.

In the past, most people appreciated the simple, natural taste and texture of brown bread, brown rice, and other whole natural foods. Now, in order to stimulate the senses, whole wheat bread has been replaced by soft, often sugary white bread, while brown rice is usually refined and polished into nutritionally deficient white rice.

At the same time, a food industry has developed to enhance sensory appeal by adding artificial colorings, flavorings, and texture agents to our daily foods. Over the last fifty years, this trend has extended to many items necessary for daily living, including clothing, cosmetics, housing materials, furniture, sleeping materials, and kitchenware. As many people have discovered, however, the application of technology to the production of synthetic consumer goods often results in lower quality, poorer service, less material satisfaction, and is ultimately hazardous to our health. All in all, we have created a totally artificial way of life and have moved further and further from our origins in the natural world. By orienting our way of life against nature, we are separating ourselves from our evolutionary environment and threatening to weaken and destroy ourselves as a species that is naturally evolving on this planet.

Cancer is only one result of this total orientation. However, instead of considering the larger environmental, social, and dietary causes of cancer, most research up to now has been oriented in the opposite direction, viewing the disease mainly as an isolated cellular disorder. Most therapies focus only on removing or destroying the cancerous tumor while ignoring the overall bodily conditions that caused it to develop.

Cancer originates long before the formation of a malignant growth, and is rooted in the quality of the external factors that we select and consume in our day-to-day life. When a cancerous symptom is finally discovered, however, this external origin is overlooked, and the disease is considered to be cured as long as the symptom or tumor has been removed or destroyed. But because the cause has not been changed, the cancer will often return, in either the same form or some other form and location. This is usually met by another round of treatment that again ignores the cause. This type of approach represents an often futile attempt to control the disease by suppressing its symptoms.

In order to control cancer, we need to see beyond the immediate symptoms and consider larger factors such as the patient's overall blood quality, the types of food that have contributed to create that blood quality, and the mentality and way of life that have led the patient to consume those particular foods. It is also important to see beyond the individual patient and into the realm of society at large. Factors such as the trends of the food industry, the quality of modern agriculture, and our increasingly unnatural and sedentary way of life also apply.

For the past thirty years, I have been seriously studying this larger problem with many people. The first conclusion my associates and I reached was: If cancer is to be cured, it must first be understood. If it is to be understood, dualism must be outgrown in favor of a unified perspective. From this more holistic perspective, we can see that no enemy or conflict really exists. On the contrary, all factors proceed in a very harmonious manner, coexisting and supporting each other.

THE BENEFICIAL NATURE OF DISEASE

In our experience, cancer is only the final stage in a sequence of events in an illness through which individuals in the modern world tend to pass because we fail to appreciate the beneficial nature of disease symptoms. A healthy system can deal with a limited amount of excess nutrients or toxic materials taken in the form of daily food. This imbalance can be naturally eliminated through daily activity, sweat, urination, or other means. However, if we overconsume or increase the amount of toxins over a long period of time, the body begins to fall back upon more serious measures for elimination: fever, skin disease, and other superficial symptoms. Such sickness is a natural adjustment, the result of the wisdom of the body trying to keep us in natural balance.

Many people, however, are alarmed by those symptoms and think there is something unnatural or undesirable about them. So they try to suppress or control those natural manifestations with pills, cough syrups, or other medications, which separate them from the natural workings of their own bodies. If minor ailments are treated in this symptomatic way with no adjustment in what we consume, the excess held in the body eventually begins to accumulate in the form of fatty-acid deposits and chronically troublesome mucus, and manifests in vaginal discharges, ovarian cysts, kidney stones, or other troublesome conditions. In this state the body is still able at least to localize the excess and toxins that we continue to take in. By gathering the unwanted material in local areas, the rest of the body is maintained in a relatively clean and functioning condition. That process of localization is part of our natural healing power, saving us from total breakdown. But the modern view looks on those localizations as dangerous enemies to be destroyed and removed. Its attitude is comparable to the behavior of the inhabitants of a city troubled by too much waste. Instead of investigating the source of waste, the city dwellers blame the sanitation department for the accumulation of garbage in designated locations and decide to do away with the sanitation department.

As long as we continue to take in excessive nutrients, chemicals, and other factors that serve no purpose in the body, they must continue to accumulate somewhere in order to continue our normal living functions. If we don't allow them to accumulate in limited areas and form tumors, they will spread throughout the body, resulting in a total collapse of our vital functions and death by toxemia. Cancer is only the terminal stage of a long process. Cancer is the body's healthy attempt to isolate toxins ingested and accumulated through years of eating the modern unnatural diet and living in an artificial environment. Cancer is the body's last drastic effort to prolong life, even a few more months or years.

Cancer is not the result of some alien factor over which we have no control. Rather it is simply the product of our own daily behavior, including our thinking, lifestyle, and daily way of eating. We must go beyond looking at cancer at the cellular level and realize that our cells are constantly changing in quality, being nourished and rejuvenated as a result of nourishment and energy coming into them. Whatever is in the nucleus of a cell is nothing but the end result of what originally came in from the outside and formed the cell components. If the cell is abnormal, something coming in is abnormal, such as the blood, lymph, or vibrational energy, including electromagnetic waves from the environment.

The cell is only the terminal of a long organic process and cannot be isolated from its surroundings and other body functions. Instead of focusing on the cell, we need to change the blood, lymph, and environmental conditions that have created malignant cells. Instead of treating isolated organs in the body, we need to treat the source of nourishment and other factors going into those organs and change the character of those organs. The proper place to perform cancer surgery is not in the operating room after the disease has run its course, but in the kitchen and in other areas of daily life before it has developed. By removing certain foods from the pantry and refrigerator, replacing them with the proper quality and variety of foods, and applying proper cooking methods, together with correcting environmental conditions and our daily way of life, we can ensure that cancer and other degenerative illnesses do not arise.

3

Preventing Cancer Naturally

In considering two people living in the same environment, we often find that one develops cancer while the other does not. This difference must be the result of each person's own unique way of behavior, including thinking, lifestyle, and way of eating. When we bring these simple factors into a less extreme, more manageable balance, the symptoms of illness no longer appear. Accordingly, the following practices are beneficial in restoring balance to our lives.

SELF-REFLECTION

Sickness is an indication that our way of life is not in harmony with the environment. Therefore, to establish genuine health, we must rethink our basic outlook on life. In one sense, sickness results largely from thinking that life's main purpose is to give us sensory satisfaction, emotional comfort, or material prosperity. This more limited view places our happiness above that of those around us. Our daily life becomes competitive, aggressive, and demanding on the one hand or withdrawn, suspicious, and defensive on the other. In either case, we continually take in more than we are able to give out.

A more natural, harmonious balance can only be established by overcoming egocentric views and adopting a more universal attitude. As a first step, we can begin to offer our love and care to our parents, family, friends, and to all members of society, even extending our love and sympathy to those who have hurt us in some way or whom we think of as our enemies. By taking responsibility for all aspects of our lives, we begin to see that failure and illness contribute to our overall development as much as success and well-being. In reality, difficulties and obstacles challenge us to develop our intuition, compassion, and understanding. By appreciating the gift of life in all of its manifestations, we increase the universe's faith in us and life becomes an endlessly amusing and joyful adventure. If we have cancer, for example, we accept what it has to teach us about ourselves. We never lament over our fate and blame it on an accident, karma, evil spirits, or an indifferent cosmos. We look for the source of our problems within ourselves, and when we make a mistake we learn from it and gratefully move on.

Self-reflection involves using our higher consciousness to observe, review, examine, and judge our thoughts and behavior as well as contemplate the larger order of nature or what we might call the law of God. The more we reflect upon ourselves and the eternal order of change, the more refined and universal our awareness becomes. We begin to remember our origin, foresee our destiny, and understand what we came to accomplish upon this earth. As our consciousness develops, our life manifests the spirit of endless giving just as the universe itself expands infinitely. Our motto becomes: "One grain, ten thousand grains." For each seed planted in the soil, the earth returns many thousand seeds. By endlessly distributing our knowledge and insight, our understanding deepens and we become one with the eternal order of creation.

Self-reflection may take many forms, including a short period each day in quiet meditation or prayer. Questions we might ask and areas we might seek guidance in include the following:

1. Did I eat today in harmony with my environment?
2. Did I think of my parents, relatives, teachers, and elders with love and respect?
3. Did I happily greet everyone today and express an interest in their life?
4. Did I contemplate the sky, the trees, and the flowers and marvel at the wonders of nature?
5. Did I thank everyone and appreciate everything I experienced today?
6. Did I perform my tasks faithfully and thereby contribute to a more peaceful world?

RESPECT FOR THE NATURAL ENVIRONMENT

The relation between humanity and nature is like that between the embryo and the placenta. The placenta nourishes, supports, and sustains the developing embryo. It would be bizarre if the embryo were to seek to destroy this protecting organism. Likewise, it is simply a matter of common sense that we should strive to preserve the integrity of the natural environment upon which we depend for life itself. Over the last century, however, we have steadily contaminated our soil, water, and air and destroyed many of the plant and animal species on which our fragile ecology rests. Our daily way of life has also become more unnatural, relying heavily on synthetic fabrics and materials, and exposing us continually to great quantities of artificial electromagnetic radiation. These actually weaken our natural ability to resist disease.

A NATURALLY BALANCED DIET

The trillions of cells that make up the human body are created and nourished by the bloodstream. New blood cells are constantly being manufactured from the nutrients provided by our daily foods. If we eat improperly, the quality of our blood and cells, including our brain cells, and quality of thinking begin to deteriorate. Cancer, a disease characterized by the abnormal multiplication of cells, is largely the result of improper eating over a long period.

For restoring a sound, healthy blood and cell quality, the following dietary principles are recommended.

Harmony with the Evolutionary Order

Nature is continually transforming one species into another. A great food chain extends from bacteria and enzymes to sea invertebrates and vertebrates, amphibians, reptiles, birds, mammals, apes, and human beings. Complementary to this line of animal evolution is a line of plant development ranging from bacteria and enzymes to sea moss and sea vegetables, primitive land vegetables, ancient vegetables, modern vegetables, fruits and nuts, and cereal grains. Whole grains evolved parallel with human beings and therefore should form the major portion of our diet. The remainder of our food should be selected from among more remote evolutionary varieties of plants and may include land and sea vegetables, fresh fruit, seeds and nuts, and soup containing fermented enzymes and bacteria representing the most primordial form of life.

In traditional cancer-free societies, this way of eating is reflected in the natural development of infants and children. After conception, the human embryo develops from a single-celled fertilized egg into a multicellular infant and is nourished entirely on its mother's blood, analogous to the ancient ocean in which biological life began. At birth, mother's milk is the principal food, and as children begin to stand, whole grains become their staple fare.

The exact proportion of plant food to animal food, with the latter being eaten primarily as a dietary supplement, also reflects our ancestors' understanding of nature's delicate balance. The ratio approximated seven parts vegetable food to about one part animal food. Modern views of geological and biological evolution have also found approximately the similar proportion in the evolutionary period of water life, roughly 2.8 billion years, compared to the period of land life, approximately 0.4 billion years. The structure of the human teeth offers another biological clue to humanity's natural way of eating. The thirty-two teeth include twenty molars and premolars for grinding grains, legumes, and seeds; eight incisors for cutting vegetables; and four canines for tearing animal and sea food. Expressed as a ratio of teeth designed for plant use and for animal use, the figure once again is seven to one. If animal food is eaten, it is ideally selected from among species most distant from human beings in the evolutionary order, especially fish and primitive sea life such as shrimp and oysters.

The modern notion that primitive hunting societies lived chiefly on mastadons, deer, birds, and other game has recently been shown by scientists to be exaggerated. Paleolithic cultures hunted mostly for undomesticated cereals and wild grasses and foraged for plants, berries, and roots. Animal life was taken only when necessary and consumed in small amounts. The *New York Times* science section reported in a lengthy article on the early human diet:

> Recent investigations into the dietary habits of prehistoric peoples and their primate predecessors suggest that heavy meat-eating by modern affluent societies may be exceeding the biological capacities evolution built into the

human body. The result may be a host of diet-related health problems, such as diabetes, obesity, high blood pressure, coronary heart disease, and some cancers.

The studies challenge the notion that human beings evolved as aggressive hunting animals who depended primarily upon meat for survival. The new view—coming from findings in such fields as archaeology, anthropology, primatology, and comparative anatomy—instead portrays early humans and their forebears more as herbivores than carnivores. According to these studies, the prehistoric table for at least the last million and a half years was probably set with three times more plant than animal foods, the reverse of what the average American currently eats (see Table 4).

Harmony with Universal Dietary Tradition

According to calculations based on U.S. Department of Agriculture surveys (see Table 5), from 1910 to 1976, the per capita consumption of wheat fell 48 percent, corn 85 percent, rye 78 percent, barley 66 percent, buckwheat 98 percent, beans and legumes 46 percent, fresh vegetables 23 percent, and fresh fruit 33 percent. Over this same period, beef intake rose 72 percent, poultry 194 percent, cheese 322 percent, canned vegetables 320 percent, frozen vegetables 1,650 percent, processed fruit 556 percent, ice cream 852 percent, yogurt 300 percent, corn syrup 761 percent, and soft drinks 2,638 percent. Since 1940, when per capita intake of chemical additives and preservatives was first recorded, the amount of artificial food colors added to the diet has climbed 995 percent.

TABLE 4. PALEOLITHIC AND MODERN DIETARY COMPOSITION

	Paleolithic Diet	Standard American Diet	Current Dietary Recommendations
Dietary Energy (%)			
Protein	33	12	12
Carbohydrate	46	46	58
Fat	21	42	30
Poly/Sat Lipid Ratio	1.41	0.44	1
Fiber (g)	100–150	19.7	30–60
Sodium (mg)	690	2300–6900	1000–3300
Calcium (mg)	1500–2000	740	800–1500
Ascorbic Acid (mg)	440	90	60

Source: *New England Journal of Medicine,* 1985

TABLE 5.   FOOD CHANGES 1910–1976
Per capita annual consumption in pounds unless noted otherwise

Category	1910	1976	Change
Grains	**294**	**144**	**−51%**
Wheat	214	112	−48%
Corn	51.1	7.7	−85%
Rice	7.2	7.2	none
Barley	3.5	1.2	−66%
Oats	3.5	3.5	none
Vegetables	**188**	**144.5**	**−23%**
Cabbage	23.2 (1920)	8.3	−64%
Fresh potato	80.4	48.3	−40%
Frozen potato	6.6 (1960)	36.8	+457%
Tomato Products	5.0 (1920)	22.4	+348%
Canned Vegetables	12.6 (1920)	53.0	+320%
Frozen Vegetables	.57 (1940)	9.9	+1,650%
Fresh Fruit	**123**	**82.0**	**−33%**
Processed Fruit	20.5	134.6	+556%
Frozen Citrus	1.0 (1948)	117.0	+11,600%
Frozen Foods	3.1 (1940)	88.8	+2,764%
Meat	**136.2**	**165.2**	**+21%**
Beef	55.5	95.4	+72%
Poultry	18.0	52.9	+194%
Eggs	**305 whole**	**276 whole**	**−10%**
Fish	**11.4**	**13.7**	**+20%**
Dairy	**320.2**	**354.3**	**+11%**
Whole Milk	29.3 gal.	21.5 gal.	−27%

TABLE 5. *(Con't.)*
Per capita annual consumption in pounds unless noted otherwise

Category	1910	1976	Change
Low Fat Milk	6.8 gal.	10.6 gal	+56%
Cheese	4.9	20.7	+322%
Ice Cream	1.9	18.1	+852%
Frozen Dairy	3.4	50.2	+1,376%
Sweeteners	**89.0**	**134.6**	**+51%**
Corn Syrup	3.8	32.7	+761%
Sugar	73.7 (1909)	94.8	+29%
Soft Drinks	1.1 gal	30.8 gal.	+2,638%

Source: U.S. Department of Agriculture

Despite the spread of refined and synthetic foods around the world, cooked whole grains, beans, and vegetables continue to be the principal foods in many cultures today. For example, corn tortillas and black beans are the staple foods in Central America, rice and soybean products are eaten throughout Southeast Asia, and whole and cracked wheat and chickpeas are staples in the Middle East. These regions have the lowest cancer rates in the world.

Harmony with the Ecological Order

It is advisable to base our diet primarily on foods produced in the same general area in which we live. For example, a traditional people like the Eskimo base their diet mostly on animal products, and this is appropriate in a polar climate. However, in India and other more tropical regions, a diet based almost entirely on grains and other vegetable foods is more conducive to health. When we begin to eat foods that have been imported from regions with different climatic conditions, however, we lose our natural immunity to diseases in our own local environment and a condition of chronic imbalance results. In recent decades, advances in refrigeration, transportation, and other technology have made it possible for millions of people in temperate zones to consume large quantities of pineapples, bananas, grapefruits, avocados, and other tropical and subtropical products. Similarly, people in southern latitudes are now consuming significant amounts of milk, cheese, ice cream, and other dairy products and frozen foods that were originally eaten in more northerly or arctic regions. Since 1948, for example, when frozen orange juice became available, the intake of frozen citrus drinks in the United States soared 11,600 percent. The violation of ecological eating habits contributes to biological degeneration and the development of serious disease.

Harmony with the Changing Seasons

A habit like eating ice cream in a heated apartment while snow is falling outside is obviously not in harmony with the seasonal order, nor is charcoal-broiling steaks in the heat of summer. It is better to adjust naturally the selection and preparation of daily foods to harmonize with the changing seasons. For example, in colder weather we can apply longer cooking times, while minimizing the intake of raw salad or fruit. In the summer, lightly cooked dishes are more appropriate while the intake of animal food and heavily cooked items can be minimized.

Harmony with Individual Differences

Personal differences need to be considered in the selection and preparation of our daily foods, with variations according to age, sex, type of activity, occupation, original physiological constitution, present condition of health, and other factors. As individuals we are constantly developing physically, mentally, and spiritually, and our day-to-day eating naturally changes to reflect this growth. The following nutritional considerations are recommended to help us select a balanced diet:

1. **Water:** It is preferable to use clean natural water for cooking and drinking. Spring or well water is recommended for regular use. It is best to avoid chemically treated municipal water or distilled water.

2. **Carbohydrates:** It is advisable to eat carbohydrates primarily in the form of polysaccharide glucose, such as that found in cereal grains, vegetables, and beans, while minimizing or avoiding the intake of monosaccharide or disaccharide sugars, such as those in fruit, honey, dairy foods, refined sugar, and other sweeteners.

3. **Protein:** Protein from such vegetable sources as whole grains and bean products is more easily assimilated by the body than protein from animal sources. When we examine the dietary patterns of people living in Hunza in Pakistan and Vilcabamba in Ecuador, who are noted for their health, vitality, and longevity, we find that they rely primarily on vegetable sources for protein. In a study recently published by *National Geographic,* the average daily caloric intake of a group of men in Hunza was found to be 1,923 calories, with 50 grams of protein, 35 grams of fat, and 354 grams of carbohydrate. In Vilcabamba, the average daily caloric intake was found to be 1,200 calories, with 35 to 38 grams of protein, 12 to 19 grams of fat, and 200 to 260 grams of carbohydrate. In both cases, protein was obtained principally from vegetable sources. Cancer, it should be noted, is virtually unknown in both these regions. In comparison, the average American consumes 3,300 calories per day, with 100 grams of protein, 157 grams of fat, and 380 grams of carbohydrate.

4. **Fat:** It is better to avoid the hard, saturated fats found in most types of meat and dairy products as well as the polyunsaturated fats found in margarine and hydrogenated cooking oils. Fat currently makes up about 40 percent of the modern diet and in medical studies is the nutrient most associated with degenerative illnesses, including heart disease and cancer. Whole grains, beans,

nuts, and seeds contain fat in the ideal proportions for daily consumption. For cooking purposes, high-quality unrefined sesame or corn oil is recommended for regular use.

5. Salt: It is better to rely primarily on natural sea salt, which contains a variety of trace minerals, and to avoid refined table salt, which is almost 100 percent sodium chloride.

6. Vitamins: Vitamins exist naturally in whole foods and should be consumed as a part of the food together with other nutrients. Vitamin pills and other nutritional supplements became popular in recent decades to offset the deficiencies caused by modern food refining. However, when taken as a supplement to our regular food, vitamins produce a chaotic effect on our body's metabolism. In its report *Diet, Nutrition, and Cancer,* the National Academy of Sciences warned that some vitamins were toxic in high doses and advised that it was preferable to focus on whole foods rather than individual nutrients when planning our diet.

In a temperate, four-season climate, an optimum daily diet that will help protect against cancer and other serious illnesses consists of about 50 to 60 percent whole-cereal grains, 5 to 10 percent soup (especially soups made with a fermented vegetable base and sea-based minerals), 25 to 30 percent vegetables prepared in a variety of styles, and 5 to 10 percent beans and sea vegetables. Supplementary foods for occasional use include locally grown fruits, preferably cooked; fish and other seafood; and a variety of seeds and nuts. (A complete description of the Cancer Prevention Diet is presented in Chapter 5.)

AN ACTIVE DAILY LIFE

For many of us, modern life offers fewer physical and mental challenges than did life in the past. As a result, functions such as the active generation of caloric and electromagnetic energy, the circulation of blood and lymph, and the activity of the digestive, nervous, and reproductive systems often stagnate. However, a physically and mentally active life is essential for good health. The people living in Hunza and Vilcabamba remain active well into their eighties, nineties, and over a hundred. Their cultures have no concept of retirement, and their elders continue to farm, garden, teach, and walk long distances until the very end of their days. In contrast, modern life has become sedentary, soft, and comfortable. After age fifty-five or sixty-five many people decline and die from lack of meaningful work or recreation. Regular physical and mental exercise, throughout life, will contribute to overall health and happiness.

4

Diet and the Development of Cancer

To understand how cancer develops, use the analogy of a tree. A tree's structure is opposite to that of the human body. For example, the leaves of a tree have a more open structure and a green color, while the cells of the human body, which correspond to the leaves of a tree, have a more closed structure and are nourished by blood, which is red in color. A tree's sustenance comes from the nutrients absorbed through the external roots. The roots of the human body lie deep in the intestines in the region where nutrients are absorbed into the blood and lymph, from which they are then distributed to all of the body's cells. If the quality of nourishment is chronically poor in the soil or in the food that is consumed, the leaves of the tree or the cells of the body eventually lose their normal functional ability and begin to deteriorate. This condition results from the repeated intake of poor nutrients and does not arise suddenly. While it is developing, many other symptoms might arise in other parts of the tree trunk and branches or in the body.

Cancer develops over a period of time out of a chronically precancerous state. In my estimation, as many as 80 to 90 percent of Americans, Europeans, Japanese, and other modern people have some type of precancerous condition. The repeated overconsumption of excessive dietary factors causes a variety of adjustment mechanisms in the body, which progressively develop toward cancer. Since the body at all times seeks balance with the surrounding environment, the normal process is for this excess to be eliminated or stored when it exceeds the body's capacity for elimination. Eventually, the overaccumulation will be stored in the form of excessive layers of fat, cholesterol, and the formation of cysts and tumors. Let us consider the gradual stages in this process, particularly in their relation to the appearance of cancer.

NORMAL DISCHARGE

Normal elimination occurs through the processes of urination, bowel movement, respiration (exhaling carbon dioxide), and perspiration, in which excessive chemical compounds are broken down into simple compounds and ultimately into carbon dioxide and water for discharge from the body. Discharge also occurs through physical, mental, and emotional activity. Mental discharge occurs in the form of wave vibrations, while emotions such as anger indicate that a great amount of excess is being eliminated.

Women have several additional means through which excess is naturally discharged. These include menstruation, childbirth, and lactation. Women have a distinct advantage over men in more efficiently discharging excess and thereby maintaining a cleaner condition. They tend to adjust more harmoniously with their environment and usually live longer than men. To compensate for this disadvantage, men usually go out into society and expend energy through additional physical, mental, and social activities. All of these processes take place continually throughout life. If we take in only a moderate amount of excess, they will proceed smoothly. However, if the quantity of excess is large, these natural processes are not capable of discharging it, and various abnormal processes begin.

ABNORMAL DISCHARGE

Today practically everyone eats and drinks excessively, which often triggers a variety of abnormal discharge mechanisms in the body such as diarrhea, excessive sweating, overly frequent bowel movements, or excessive urination. Habits like scratching the head, tapping the feet, and frequent blinking of the eyes also represent abnormal discharges of imbalanced energy, as do strong emotions such as fear, anger, and anxiety. Periodically, excess is discharged through more acute or violent symptoms such as a fever, coughing, sneezing, shouting, screaming, trembling, and shivering, as well as wild thoughts and behavior.

CHRONIC DISCHARGE

Chronic discharges are the next stage in this process and often take the form of skin diseases. These are common in cases where the kidneys have lost their ability to properly cleanse the bloodstream. For example, freckles, dark spots, and similar skin markings indicate the chronic discharge of sugar and other refined carbohydrates, while white patches indicate the discharge of milk, cottage cheese, or other dairy products.

Hard, dry skin arises after the bloodstream fills with fat and oil, eventually causing blockage of the pores, hair follicles, and sweat glands. When these blockages prevent the flow of liquid toward the surface, the skin becomes dry. Many people believe that this condition results from a lack of oil, when in fact it is caused by the intake of too much fat and oil.

Skin cancers are more serious forms of skin disease. However, skin disorders are usually not very serious, since in most cases the discharge of toxins toward the surface of the body permits the internal organs and tissues to continue functioning smoothly. However, if our eating continues to be excessive and we cannot eliminate effectively, the body will start to accumulate this excess in other locations.

ACCUMULATION

If we continue to eat poorly, we eventually exhaust the body's ability to discharge. This can be serious if an underlying layer of fat has developed under the skin, which prevents discharge toward the surface of the body. Such a condition is caused by the repeated overconsumption of milk, cheese, eggs, meat, and other fatty, oily, or greasy foods. When this stage has been reached, internal deposits of mucus or fat begin to form, initially in areas that have some direct access to the outside and in the following regions.

Sinuses

The sinuses are a frequent site of mucous accumulation, and symptoms such as allergies, hay fever, and blocked sinuses often result. Hay fever and sneezing arise when dust or pollen stimulates the discharge of this excess, while calcified stones often form deep within the sinuses. Thick, heavy deposits of mucus in the sinuses diminish our mental clarity and alertness.

Inner Ear

The accumulation of mucus and fat in the inner ear interferes with the smooth functioning of the inner-ear mechanism and can lead to frequent pain, impaired hearing, and even deafness.

Lungs

Various forms of excess often accumulate in the lungs. Aside from the obvious symptoms of coughing and chest congestion, mucus often fills the alveoli or air sacs and breathing becomes more difficult. Occasionally, a coat of mucus in the bronchi can be loosened and discharged by coughing, but once the sacs are surrounded, it becomes more firmly lodged and can remain there for years. Then, if air pollutants or cigarette smoke enters the lungs, their heavier components are attracted to and remain in this sticky environment. In severe cases, these deposits can trigger the development of lung cancer. However, the underlying cause of this condition is the accumulation of sticky fat and mucus in the alveoli and in the blood and capillaries surrounding them.

Breasts

The accumulation of excess in this region often results in a hardening of the breasts and the formation of cysts. Excess usually accumulates here in the form of mucus and deposits of fatty acid, both of which take the form of a sticky or heavy liquid. These deposits develop into cysts in the same way that water solidifies into ice, a process that is accelerated by the intake of ice cream, cold milk, soft drinks, orange juice, and other foods that produce a cooling or freezing effect. Women who have breast-fed are less likely to develop breast cysts or cancer since this reduces excess accumulation in this region.

Intestines

In many cases, excess will begin accumulating in the lower part of the body as mucous and fat deposits coating the intestinal wall. This will often cause the intestines to expand or become less flexible, resulting in a bulging abdomen. A large number of people in the United States have this problem. Young people are often very stylish and attractive. However, after the age of thirty, and particularly between the ages of thirty-five and forty, a large number of Americans lose their youthful appearance and become overweight.

Kidneys

Deposits of fat and mucus may also accumulate in the kidneys. Problems arise when these elements clog the fine network of cells in the interior of these organs, causing them to accumulate water and become chronically swollen. Since elimination is hampered, fluid that cannot be discharged is often deposited in the legs, producing periodic swelling and weakness. If someone with this condition consumes a large quantity of foods that produce a chilling effect, the deposited fat and mucus will often crystallize into kidney stones.

Reproductive Organs

In men, the prostate gland is a frequent site of accumulation. As a result of continued consumption of excess or imbalanced food, the prostate often becomes enlarged and hard fat deposits or cysts often form within and around it. This is one of the principal causes of impotence. In women, excess may also accumulate within and around the sexual organs, leading to the formation of ovarian cysts, dermoid tumors, or the blockage of the Fallopian tubes. In some cases, mucus or fat in the ovaries or Fallopian tubes prevents the passage of the egg and sperm, resulting in an inability to conceive. Chronic vaginal discharge is one indication of accumulation in the reproductive region.

Although the symptoms that affect these inner organs may seem unrelated, they all stem from the same underlying cause. However, modern medicine often does not view them as related. For example, a person with hearing trouble or cataracts is often referred to an ear or eye specialist. However, cataracts are a symptom of a variety of related problems, such as mucous accumulation in the breasts, kidneys, and sexual organs.

STORAGE

In this stage, excess in various forms is stored within and around the deeper vital organs, including the heart and the liver. In the case of the circulatory system, excess often accumulates around and inside the heart as well as within the heart tissues. Accumulation may also occur both in and around the arteries. These fatty deposits, including cholesterol accumulation, replace the heart's ability to function properly and hamper the smooth passage of blood through the arteries. The end result is often a heart attack. The major causes of this problem are foods containing large amounts of hard, saturated fat. Many nutritionists and medical doctors are now aware of the relationship between the intake of saturated fats and cholesterol and cardiovascular disease, but they often overlook the effects of sugar and dairy products, both of which contribute greatly to the development of these illnesses.

Within the body, the proteins, carbohydrates, and fats that we consume often change into each other, depending on the amount of each consumed as well as the body's needs at a particular time. If we consume more of these than we need, the excess is normally discharged. However, the quantity of excess often exceeds the body's capacity to discharge it. When this happens, the excess is stored in the liver in the form of carbohydrate, in the muscles in the form of protein, or throughout the body in the form of fatty acids.

DEGENERATION OF THE BLOOD AND LYMPH

If the bloodstream is filled with fat and mucus, excess will begin to accumulate, as we have seen, in the organs. Since the lungs and kidneys are usually affected first, their functions of filtering and cleansing the blood become less efficient. The situation leads to further deterioration of the blood quality and also affects the lymphatic system. Operations such as tonsillectomies also contribute to the deterioration of the lymphatic system since they reduce the ability of this system to cleanse itself. Such operations eventually lead to frequent swelling and lymph-gland inflammation, producing a chronic deterioration of the quality of the blood, particularly the red and white blood cells.

TUMORS

When the red blood cells begin to lose their capacity to change into normal body cells, an organism cannot long survive. Poorly functioning intestines can also contribute to the degeneration of blood quality, since the qualities of blood cells and plasma originate largely in the small intestine. In many cases, the villi . of the small intestine are coated with fat and mucus, and the condition in the intestines is often acidic. A naturally healthy bloodstream will not be created in this type of environment.

Therefore, in order to prevent immediate collapse, the body localizes toxins at this stage in the form of a tumor. A tumor may be likened to a storage depot for the collection of degenerative cells from the bloodstream. As long as improper nourishment is taken in, the body will continue to isolate abnormal excess and toxins in specific areas, resulting in the continual growth of the cancer. When a particular location can no longer absorb toxic excess, the body must search for another place to localize it, and so the cancer spreads. This process continues until the cancer metastasizes throughout the body and the person eventually dies.

In summary, we may conclude that symptoms like dry skin, skin discharges, hardening of the breasts, prostate trouble, vaginal discharge, and ovarian cysts all represent potentially precancerous conditions. However, they need not develop toward cancer if we change our daily way of eating.

5

The Macrobiotic Cancer Prevention Diet

The following dietary recommendations have been formulated with universal human dietary traditions from both East and West in mind and have been further refined over several decades as a result of contemporary macrobiotic experience. When applied very carefully, these guidelines create a stabilized state of overall physical and mental balance. They may therefore be followed not only for the prevention of cancer, but also for the prevention of most other illnesses as well, such as cardiovascular disease. This approach may be followed by persons already in generally good health. For those people who already have cancer or a serious precancerous condition, adjustments need to be made depending on the specific case, and it is advisable to do so under the supervision of a qualified macrobiotic teacher or medical professional. These special adjustments are considered in full detail for each individual form of cancer in Part II. The following recommendations are for most of the temperate latitudes of the world. See Chapter 29, "General Dietary Recommendations," for an itemized list of recommended foods. For guidelines in tropical or semitropical climates, see Appendix II.

WHOLE GRAINS

Approximately 50 to 60 percent of our daily food (average 50 percent) should consist by volume of cooked whole-cereal grains. These include brown rice, whole wheat, millet, oats, barley, corn, rye, and buckwheat, and they can be prepared according to a variety of cooking styles. When preparing brown rice, it is best to use a pressure cooker made of stainless steel. Pressure-cooked rice is far superior to boiled rice for everyday use, since many nutrients are lost after boiling over a period of time. The usual pattern is to make freshly prepared pressure-cooked brown rice once a day, alternating between plain brown rice the first day, brown rice with about 10 to 20 percent millet the next day, brown rice with 10 to 20 percent barley the third day, brown rice with 10 to 20 percent aduki or other beans the following day, and then plain brown rice again.

In the case of wheat, whole wheat berries are rather tough and somewhat difficult to chew, so they are usually ground into flour, which is baked into bread. Bread should ideally be baked from freshly ground flour without the addition of yeast. In general, the majority of grain dishes should be eaten primarily in complete whole form rather than in cracked or processed form such as bulgar, corn grits, or rolled oats. Bread and flour products tend to be more difficult than whole grains to digest and, especially hard baked products, tend to be mucous-producing. Next to grain in whole form, chapatis, tortillas, and other traditional flat breads are most highly recommended, as well as sourdough wheat or rye, and bread is enjoyed two or three times a week. Grains may also be eaten several times a week in the form of pasta or noodles, especially buckwheat (soba) and whole wheat (udon) noodles. Grain products such as seitan (also known as wheat meat or gluten) may be consumed a few times a week as a source of protein.

SOUP

About 5 to 10 percent (one or two cups or bowls) of daily intake may be in the form of soup. Soup broth can be made with miso or shoyu (natural soy sauce), which are prepared from naturally fermented soybeans, sea salt, and grains, to which several varieties of land and sea vegetables, especially wakame or kombu (kelp), green vegetables, and occasionally shiitake mushroom, may be added during cooking. The taste of miso or shoyu should be mild, not too salty or too bland. Barley miso, rise miso, or all-soybean miso (hatcho miso), aged naturally two to three years, is recommended for regular use. Soups made with grains, beans, or vegetables can also be served from time to time. For instance, delicious seasonal varieties can be made, such as corn soup in the summer or squash soup in the fall.

VEGETABLE DISHES

About 25 to 30 percent of our daily food should be fresh vegetable dishes, which can be prepared in a wide variety of cooking styles: sautéing, steaming, boiling, blanching, deep-frying, marinating, and pressed and boiled salads. Among root and stem vegetables, carrots, onions, daikon (white radishes), turnips, red radishes, burdock, lotus root, rutabagas, and parsnips are excellent. When preparing root vegetables, cook both the root and leaf portions so as to achieve a proper balance of nutrients by using the whole food. Among vegetables from the ground, cabbage, cauliflower, broccoli, Brussels sprouts, Chinese cabbage, acorn squash, butternut squash, buttercup squash, and pumpkin are quite nutritious and may be used daily. Among green and white leafy vegetables, watercress, kale, parsley, leeks, scallions, dandelions, collard greens, bok choy, carrot tops, daikon greens, turnip greens, and mustard greens are fine for regular use. Vegetables for occasional use include cucumbers, lettuce, string beans, celery, sprouts, yellow squash, peas, red cabbage, mushrooms (various, including shiitake), kohlrabi, and others. In general, up to one-third of vegetable intake may be eaten raw in the form of fresh salad or traditionally prepared pickles. However, it is better to avoid mayonnaise and commercial salad dressings. Vegetables that originated historically in tropical or semitropical environments, such as eggplants, potatoes, tomatoes, asparagus, spinach, sweet potatoes, yams, avocados, green and red peppers, and other varieties, tend to produce acid and should be avoided or minimized unless you live in a hot and humid climate.

BEANS AND SEA VEGETABLES

From 5 to 10 percent of daily intake may be eaten in the form of cooked beans and sea vegetables. Beans for daily use are aduki (small red) beans, chickpeas, lentils, and black soybeans. Other beans may be used occasionally, two to three times a month: yellow soybeans, pinto, white, black turtle, navy, kidney, and lima beans, split peas, black-eyed peas, and others. Soybean products such as tofu, tempeh, and natto may be used daily or regularly in moderation and be considered part of the daily volume for this category. Sea vegetables are rich in minerals and should be used in small volume on a daily basis in soups, cooked with vegetables or beans, or prepared as a side dish. Wakame, kombu, and nori are usually used daily, while all other seaweeds, including arame and hijiki, may be used occasionally. These dishes may be seasoned with a moderate amount of shoyu, sea salt, or a grain-based vinegar, such as brown rice vinegar.

SUPPLEMENTARY FOODS

Persons in usually good health may wish to include some of the following additional supplementary foods in their diet.

Animal Food

A small volume of white-meat fish or seafood may be eaten a few times per week. White-meat fish such as cod and haddock contains less fat than red-meat or blue-skin varieties. Saltwater fish also usually have fewer pollutants in their systems than freshwater varieties. Whole small dried fish (iriko), which can be consumed entirely including bones, may also be used occasionally as a side dish with vegetables, in soup, or as a seasoning. Avoid or drastically limit all other animal products, including beef, lamb, pork, veal, chicken, turkey, duck, goose, wild game, and eggs. Avoid or drastically limit all dairy foods, including cheese, butter, milk, skim milk, buttermilk, yogurt, ice cream, cream, sour cream, whipped cream, margarine, and kefir.

Fruit

Fresh fruit may be eaten a few times a week—preferably cooked or naturally dried—as a supplement or dessert, provided the fruits grow in the local climatic zone. Fresh fruits can also be consumed in moderate volume occasionally during their growing season. In temperate areas these include apples, strawberries, cherries, peaches, pears, plums, grapes, apricots, prunes, blueberries, blackberries, raspberries, cantaloupe, honeydew melon, watermelon, tangerines, oranges, and grapefruit. In these climates, avoid or curtail tropical or semitropical fruits such as bananas, pineapples, mangoes, papayas, figs, dates, coconut, and kiwis. In the areas in which they grow, these fruits may be eaten in small volume. Fruit juice is generally too concentrated for regular use (e.g., ten apples go into one glass of apple juice). However, occasional consumption in very hot weather is allowable, as is consumption of apple cider, preferably warmed, in the fall. Dried fruit may be eaten on occasion so long as it is from the same or a similar climatic region.

Snacks

Seeds and nuts that have been lightly roasted and sometimes seasoned with sea salt or shoyu while roasting may be enjoyed occasionally as snacks. Suitable seeds and nuts include sesame seeds, sunflower seeds, pumpkin seeds, almonds, walnuts, pecans, filberts, and peanuts. It is preferable not to overconsume nuts and nut butters, as they are difficult to digest and are high in fat and oil. Other snacks may include mochi (pounded sweet rice), noodles, rice balls, vegetable sushi, rice cakes, puffed grain cereals, popcorn (homemade and unbuttered), and roasted beans and grains.

Desserts

Desserts may be eaten in moderate volume two or three times a week and may include cookies, pudding, cake, pie, and other sweet dishes prepared with natural ingredients. Often desserts can be prepared from apples, fall and winter squash, pumpkin, aduki beans, or dried fruit and other naturally sweet foods without adding a sweetener. However, for dishes that need one, recommended sweeteners include rice syrup, barley malt, amasake (a fermented sweet rice beverage), chestnuts, apple juice and cider, and dried fruits such as raisins. Avoid white sugar, brown sugar, raw sugar, turbinado sugar, molasses, honey, corn syrup, maple syrup, chocolate, carob, fructose, saccharine, and other concentrated or artificial sweeteners. For custards, whipped toppings, and frosting, plant-quality ingredients such as kudzu (also known as kuzu) root, agar-agar, tofu, or tahini (toasted sesame butter) should be used instead of eggs, cream, milk, and similar animal products. A delicious sea vegetable gelatin made of agar-agar, called kanten, can be seasoned with fruit, apple juice, and other natural sweeteners.

BEVERAGES

Recommended daily beverages include roasted bancha twig tea (also known as kukicha), roasted brown rice tea, roasted barley tea, and spring or well water. Occasional-use beverages include grain coffee (made without molasses, figs, etc.), dandelion tea, kombu tea, umeboshi tea, mu tea, carrot juice, celery juice, and sweet vegetable drink. Infrequent-use beverages include green tea, vegetable juice, fruit juice, beer, sake (hot or cool), and soy milk (with kombu). Any traditional tea that does not have an aromatic fragrance or a stimulant effect may also be used. However, coffee, black tea, and aromatic herbal teas such as peppermint, rose hips, and chamomile should be avoided. Daily foods and beverages should preferably be prepared or cooked with spring or well water.

Avoid municipal tap water that may be chlorinated or chemicalized, distilled water, cold drinks (served with ice cubes), mineral water, and all bubbling (carbonated) waters, sugared and soft drinks, and hard liquor.

ADDITIONAL DIETARY SUGGESTIONS

Oil

For daily use, only unrefined sesame, corn, or mustard seed oil in moderate amounts is recommended. Oil should be used in cooking and not eaten raw at the table as in salad dressings. Other unrefined vegetable oils, such as safflower, sunflower, soy, and olive, may be used occasionally. Avoid all chemically processed vegetable oils, butter, lard, shortening, palm oil, coconut oil, and egg or soy margarine.

Salt

Naturally processed, mineral-rich sea salt and traditional, nonchemicalized miso and shoyu may be used as seasonings. Daily meals, however, should not have an overly salty flavor, and seasonings should generally be added during cooking and not at the table except for condiments and garnishes. Avoid commercial table salt (to which additives and sugar are usually added) and gray sea salt or other sea salt excessively high in minerals. (Free-flowing white sea salt is usually suitable.)

Other Seasonings

In addition to oil and salt, miso, and shoyu, other seasonings may be used in cooking and before serving. The seasonings are all vegetable-quality, naturally processed. Suitable for occasional use are ginger, horseradish, mirin (fermented sweet brown rice sweetener), rice vinegar, umeboshi vinegar, umeboshi plum, umeboshi paste, garlic, lemon, orange, mustard, and black or red pepper. Commercial seasonings, spices, herbs, and other sugary, hot, pungent, aromatic seasonings, including all spices and herbs, are avoided.

Pickles

A small volume of homemade pickles may be eaten each day to aid in digestion. In macrobiotic food preparation, this naturally fermented type of food is made with a variety of root and round vegetables, such as daikon or radishes, turnips, carrots, cabbage, and cauliflower, and preserved in sea salt, rice or wheat bran, shoyu, umeboshi, or miso. Spices, sugar, and vinegar are avoided. Short-time, lighter pickles are recommended in warmer weather or for persons who need to reduce their salt intake. Long-time, saltier pickles can be eaten during colder weather or by those who wish to strengthen their condition. Different jars, crocks, and kegs can be used in pickle preparation, and aging varies from several hours to weeks, months, and even years.

Condiments

Condiments should be available on the table for daily use if desired. They allow family members to individually adjust taste and seasoning. Condiments for daily use include gomashio (toasted sesame seed salt), made usually from 16 to 18 parts roasted sesame seeds to 1 part roasted sea salt, half-ground together in a small earthenware bowl called a suribachi; roasted kombu or wakame powder, made from baking these sea vegetables in the oven until black and crushing in a suribachi and sometimes adding toasted sesame seeds and storing in a small container or jar; umeboshi plums, small salt plums that have been dried and pickled for many months with sea salt and flavored with shiso (beef-steak) leaves; tekka, a combination of carrot, burdock, and lotus root that has been finely chopped and sautéed in sesame oil and miso for many hours; shoyu, which is traditionally processed natural soy sauce; and green nori flakes. Some of these, such as gomashio and the sea vegetable powders, should be prepared fresh in the home, while others, such as umeboshi plums and tekka, are available ready-made in natural foods stores. Other condiments may be used from time to time.

Garnishes

To balance various dishes at the table and make the meal more attractive, garnishes are frequently prepared. These include grated daikon, grated radish, grated horseradish, chopped scallions, grated ginger, green mustard pâté, freshly ground pepper, lemon pieces, red pepper, and others.

WAY OF EATING

You may eat regularly two to three times per day, as much as is comfortable, provided the proportion of each category of food is generally correct and in daily consumption each mouthful is thoroughly chewed. Proper chewing is essential to digestion and it is recommended that each mouthful of food be chewed fifty times or more or until it becomes liquid in form. Eat when you are hungry, but it is best to leave the table feeling satisfied but not full. Similarly, drink only when thirsty. Avoid eating for three hours before sleeping, as this causes stagnation in the intestines and throughout the body. Before and after each meal, express your gratitude verbally or silently to nature, the universe, or God who created the food and reflect on the health and happiness it is dedicated to achieving. This acknowledgment may take the form of grace, prayer, chanting, or a moment of silence. Express your thanks to parents, grandparents, and past generations who nourished us and whose dream we embody, to the vegetables or animals who gave their lives so we may live, and to the farmer, shopkeeper, and cook who contributed their energies to making the food available.

Eating less is also important. In 1991 researchers at Tufts University re-ported that mice on a very low calorie diet lived 29 percent longer than fully fed mice and had few tumors and other disorders. In studies designed to identify the changes that occur with aging, mice fed a diet containing 40 percent less calories enjoyed consistently better health and longer life. "What stunned us in this study was that every single type of tumor and nearly every kind of lesion were delayed," noted Richard Sprott, associate director for the National Institute on Aging's Biology of Aging program.

OBTAINING NATURAL FOODS

In selecting your foods it is important to obtain the freshest and highest-quality natural foods. Of course, growing your own grains and vegetables is ideal, and you may want to make your own miso, tofu, or seitan at home. For many people, however, especially those living in the city, the local natural foods, health food, or grocery and produce store will be the primary source of their daily food. Applied to food, the word *natural* means whole and unprocessed or processed by natural methods. The term *organic*, when further applied to natural foods, is understood to mean food that is grown without the use of chemical fertilizers, herbicides, pesticides, or other artificial sprays. Since it is fairly difficult to distinguish organic foods from nonorganic except by taste, you may need to rely on the reputation of the local store or the distributor. Many suppliers have been certified by an organic growers' association, which makes on-site inspections, performs lab tests on soil and product samples, and offers educational guidance to farmers and consumers.

The harmful effects of chemical farming on human health as well as on the topsoil and the environment have been well documented. As long ago as the end of the nineteenth century, Dr. Julius Hensel, a German agricultural chemist, warned that the introduction of synthetic fertilizers, insecticides, the forced fattening of livestock, and other modern practices were resulting in the degeneration of the human blood and lymph and giving rise to a host of degenerative diseases. In 1893, he wrote in his book *Bread from Stones:*

> Agriculture has entered into the sign of cancer. . . . [We] cannot be indifferent [to] what kind of crops we raise for our nourishment and with what substances our fields are fertilized. It cannot be all sufficient that great quantities are harvested, but the great quantity must also be of *good quality*. It is indisputable that by merely fertilizing with marl, i.e., with carbonate of lime, such a large yield may be gained as to make a man inclined to always content himself with marl, but with such a one-sided fertilization slowly but surely evil effects of various kinds will develop; these have given rise to the axiom of experience: "Manuring with lime makes rich fathers but poor sons." . . . As our present fine flour, freed from bran, is furnished almost entirely devoid of [nutrients], we need not wonder at the great number of modern maladies.

Organic foods are not always available, nor can they always be afforded, because of their higher price. In this case, the next best available produce should be obtained and thoroughly cleaned and properly cooked to eliminate potentially harmful chemicals. For better health, it is also wise to avoid all industrially mass-produced foods, including instant foods, canned foods, frozen foods, refined grains or flour, sprayed foods, dyed foods, irradiated foods, and all foods made with chemicals, additives, preservatives, stabilizers, emulsifiers, and artificial coloring.

STUDIES ON KEY FOODS IN THE MACROBIOTIC DIET

Over the last twenty years, modern society has gradually become aware of the limits of chemical agriculture and food technology. Recent medical studies have shown that most of the foods in the macrobiotic dietary approach protect against cancer and other degenerative diseases. In Part II, we summarize several hundred of these findings and classify them under specific forms of malignancy. However, as we have seen, cancer is not an isolated phenomenon, but a disease of the whole body. These foods will substantially help reduce the risk of cancer in general. Briefly, let us look at the major scientific and medical findings as they apply to the basic categories of food in the Cancer Prevention Diet.

1. **Whole Grains:** A wide variety of epidemiological, laboratory, and case-control studies show that as part of a balanced diet whole grains, high in fiber and bran, protect against nearly all forms of cancer. The U.S. Senate's report *Dietary Goals,* the Surgeon-General's reports, the National Academy of Sciences' report *Diet, Nutrition, and Cancer,* the Food Guide Pyramid, and many other sources all call for substantial increases in the daily consumption of whole grains, such as brown rice, millet, barley, oats, and whole wheat. The American Cancer Society has begun dietary intervention studies on patients at high risk for colon and breast cancer emphasizing whole grains and other high-fiber foods.

2. **Soup:** A ten-year study completed in 1981 by the National Cancer Center of Japan reported that people who ate miso soup daily were 33 percent less likely to contract stomach cancer than those who never ate miso (see Table 6). The study also found that miso was effective in preventing cancer at all other sites and helped protect against heart and liver disease. Soy sauce (shoyu) is also used frequently in soups and other dishes in macrobiotic cooking. A 1991 study by researchers at the University of Wisconsin found that in laboratory experiments, mice fed a diet that included soy sauce contracted 26 percent less stomach cancer, and the soy-supplemented mice averaged about one-quarter the number of tumors as the control group. Soy sauce "exhibited a pronounced anticarcinogenic effect," the researchers concluded.

3. **Vegetables:** A wide range of international population studies show that regular consumption of vegetables high in beta-carotene, particularly dark green and dark yellow and orange vegetables such as broccoli, Brussels sprouts, carrots, cabbage, kale, and collards, protect against cancer. The National Cancer Institute, the American Cancer Society, and other organizations highly recommend daily consumption of these vegetables, which have long been part of the standard macrobiotic diet. In addition, foods high in vitamins C and E have been shown to lower the risk of malignancy. These vitamins are found in natural abundance in green leafy vegetables, some citrus fruits, and whole grains, and this is the form in which they are ideally consumed.

TABLE 6. RELATION OF MISO INTAKE, CANCER, AND DISEASE

	MISO SOUP CONSUMPTION			
*Cause of Death**	*Daily*	*Occasionally*	*Rarely*	*Never*
Stomach Cancer	Baseline	Up 18%	Up 34%	Up 48%
Cancer at All Sites	Baseline	Up 4%	Up 12%	Up 19%
Coronary Heart Disease	Baseline	Up 7%	Up 10%	Up 43%
High Blood Pressure	Baseline	Up 29%	Up 11%	Up 453%
Cerebrovascular Disease	Baseline	Down 11%	Down 13%	Up 29%
Liver Cirrhosis	Baseline	Up 25%	Up 25%	Up 57%
Peptic Ulcer	Baseline	Up 17%	Up 41%	Up 52%
All Causes of Death	Baseline	Up 2%	Up 6%	Up 33%

* Association of age-sex standardized rate ratio for major causes of death, 1966–78.
Source: *Nutrition and Cancer*, 1982

One of the most promising foods to reduce the risk of cancer is shiitake mushroom, a staple of Oriental cooking that is now grown and sold widely in this country. Medical studies in the laboratory found that shiitakes had a strong antitumor effect in induced cancers and no toxic side effects. In macrobiotic cooking and home cares, shiitake mushrooms, especially the dried variety, are used to help reduce and eliminate fat deposits that have accumulated in the body.

"The dietary changes now under way appear to be reducing our dependence on foods from animal source," the National Academy of Sciences' panel commented in its comprehensive report on cancer. "It is likely that there will be continued reduction in fats from animal sources and an increasing dependence on vegetable and other plant products for protein supplies. Hence, diets may contain increasing amounts of vegetable products, some of which may be protective against cancer."

4. Beans and Bean Products: Epidemiological studies indicate that regular consumption of beans, pulses, and bean products reduces the risk of cancer. Beans have been shown to lower bile acid production by up to 30 percent. Bile acids are necessary for proper fat digestion but in excess have been associated with causing cancer, especially in the large intestine. Beans also contain fiber, which is protective in the colon and elsewhere. Soybeans and soy products, a major source of protein in the macrobiotic diet, have been singled out as especially effective in reducing tumors. Soybeans contain protease inhibitors, isoflavanoids, lignons, and other ingredients that have been shown to help prevent the development of breast, stomach, and skin tumors.

In Japan, the incidence of breast cancer is about one-fifth that in the United States. To test the hypothesis that soyfoods helped protect against this disease, researchers at the University of Alabama initated feeding trials with rats and found that animals fed miso, natto, soy sauce (shoyu), and other traditionally fermented soybean foods had fewer induced tumors, more benign tumors, and a slower growth rate of malignancy than the control group. "This data suggests that miso consumption may be a factor producing a lower breast cancer incidence in Japanese women," the researchers concluded. "Organic compounds found in fermented soybean-based foods may exert a chemoprotective effect." In another study, researchers found that people who regularly ate tofu were at less risk for stomach cancer than those who did not. Miso is also protective against leukemia, lymphoma, bone cancer, and other cancers related to radiation exposure (see next section, on sea vegetables).

5. Sea Vegetables: Kombu, wakame, nori, and other edible seaweeds are a small but important part of the daily macrobiotic diet. In Japan, a macrobiotic doctor in Nagasaki who survived the atomic bombing in August 1945 put all of his surviving patients on a strict diet of brown rice, miso soup, sea vegetables, and sea salt. In contrast to patients at other hospitals and medical centers who died from radiation sickness, all his patients and staff were saved. This experience (and others in Hiroshima) inspired scientists to study the mechanism by which certain foods protect against cancer. Beginning in the 1960s, scientists at McGill University in Montreal reported that a substance in kelp and other common sea vegetables could reduce the amount of radioactive strontium absorbed through the intestine by 50 to 80 percent. Japanese scientists subsequently reported that adding seaweed to the diet resulted in the complete regression of induced sarcomas in more than half of the mice tested (see Table 7). Similar experiments on mice with leukemia showed promising results. At the University of Hiroshima, mice fed miso were found to be five times more resistant to radiation-induced tumors than controls.

In the last ten years, there has been increasing study of the protective effect of sea vegetables on breast cancer. At Harvard School of Public Health, feeding trials were initiated in which it was found that mice fed kombu developed induced breast cancer later than controls. "Seaweed has shown consistent anti-tumor activity in several in vivo animal tests," the researcher concluded. "In extrapolating these results to the Japanese population, seaweed may be an important factor in explaining the low rates of certain cancers in Japan." Cancer researchers in Japan reported similar findings.

Studies on the Macrobiotic Approach to Cancer

During the last ten years, the first scientific and medical studies of the macrobiotic approach to cancer began.

1. Macrobiotics and Breast Cancer: Researchers at New England Medical Center in Boston reported in 1981 that women on macrobiotic and vegetarian diets were at less risk of developing breast cancer than other women. They found that the macrobiotic women processed estrogen more efficiently and

TABLE 7. ANTITUMOR EFFECT OF SEAWEEDS ON SARCOMAS IN MICE

Sample	Dose (mg/kg)	Average tumor weight (g.)	Inhibition ratio	Complete regression	Mortality
Sargassum fulvellum	100 × 10	0.18	89.3%	7/9	1/10
Control		1.67		0/10	0/10
Laminaria angustata	100 × 5	0.08	94.8%	6/9	1/10
Control		1.59		0/10	0/10
Laminaria angustata var. longissima	100 × 5	0.21	92.3%	5/9	1/10
Control		2.71		0/7	0/7
Laminaria japonica	100 × 5	1.40	13.6%	2/9	1/10
Control		1.62		0/9	1/10

Source: *Japanese Journal of Experimental Medicine*, 1974

eliminated it more quickly from their body. The study involved forty-five pre- and postmenopausal women, about half of whom were macrobiotic and about half eating the standard modern diet. The women consumed the same number of total calories. Although the macrobiotic women took in only one-third as much animal protein and animal fat, they excreted two to three times as much estrogen, a substance that has been associated in high levels with the development of breast cancer. Results were published in *Cancer Research*, a leading research journal.

2. Macrobiotics and Pancreatic Cancer: In a study of twenty-four patients with pancreatic cancer who adopted a macrobiotic diet, Tulane University researchers found that their mean length of survival was 17.3 months, compared with 6.0 months for matched controls from a national tumor registry diagnosed during the same time period (1984–85). The one-year survival rate was 54.2 percent in the macrobiotic patients versus 10.0 percent in the controls. All comparisons were statistically significant.

3. Macrobiotics and Advanced Malignancy: In a study of patients with advanced malignancies who followed a macrobiotic way of eating, Vivien Newbold, M.D., a Philadelphia physician, documented six cases of remission. The patients had pancreatic cancer with metastases to the liver; malignant melanoma; malignant astrocytoma (central nervous system tumor); endometrial stormal sarcoma (uterine tumor); adenocarcinoma of the colon; and inoperable intraabdominal leimyosarcoma (bone cancer). Review of CAT scans and other medical tests revealed no evidence of tumors after adherence to the macrobiotic diet. The cases were all reviewed independently and the diagnoses confirmed by the pathology and radiology departments of Holy Redeemer Hospital in Meadowbrook, Pennsylvania. In a review of the study, Congressional investigators recommended further research on the macrobiotic approach to cancer: "If cases such as Newbold's were presented in the medical literature, it might help stimulate interest among clinical investigators in conducting controlled, prospective trials of macrobiotic regimens, which could provide valid data on effectiveness."

4. Macrobiotics and Cancer Risk Factors: In 1983 J. P. Deslypere, M.D., a researcher at the Academic Hospital of the Ghent University in Belgium, conducted medical tests, especially blood work, on twenty men eating macrobiotically. "In the field of cardiovascular and cancer risk factors this kind of blood is very favorable," he reported. "It's ideal, we couldn't do better, that's what we're dreaming of. It's really fantastic, like children, whose blood vessels are still completely open and whole. This is a very important matter, deserving our full attention."

5. Macrobiotics and General Health: In 1986 Dr. Peter Gruner, director of oncology at St. Mary's Hospital in Montreal, launched a study of approximately thirty individuals on macrobiotic diets to find if there were significant differences between their levels of health and that of the general population. Gruner subjected the participants, who had been practicing a macrobiotic diet for anywhere from nine months to fourteen years, to a battery of physiological tests and found them to be in excellent health.

The Kushi Foundation cooperated in many of these studies. Others are in process. A team of researchers at medical schools and hospitals in Boston, headed by Dr. Robert Lerman, director of clinical nutrition at University Hospital, announced plans to evaluate several hundred cancer patients who had tried the macrobiotic approach and match them with controls from the Eastern Cooperative Oncology Group tumor registry at the Dana Farber Cancer Center in Boston. At Tulane University results of a study on prostate cancer and macrobiotics are being prepared for publication, and at the University of Michigan the macrobiotic approach to breast cancer is under review.

Over the last decade, the medical profession has begun to inquire into the philosophy behind macrobiotics. In its 1987 *Family Medical Guide*, the American Medical Association noted:

In the macrobiotic diet foods fall into two groups, known as yin and yang (based on an Eastern principle of opposites), depending on where they have been grown, their texture, color, and composition. The general principle behind this diet is that foods biologically furthest away from us are better for us. Cereals, therefore, form the basis of the diet and fish is preferred to meat. Although fresh foods free of additives are preferred, no food is actually prohibited, in the belief that a craving for any food may reflect a genuine bodily need. In general, the macrobiotic diet is a healthful way of eating.

In 1991 the American Health Foundation announced plans for a major nutritional and metabolic study on persons who had been practicing macrobiotics for ten years or more.

For complete references to the studies mentioned in this chapter, please see the individual entries in Part II. For a comprehensive summary of 185 scientific and medical studies on the macrobiotic diet and holistic approaches to health in general, please see Alex Jack, *Let Food Be Thy Medicine* (Becket, MA: One Peaceful World Press, 1991).

SWITCHING TO NATURAL FOODS

Over the last decade, hundreds of thousands of people in the United States, Canada, Europe, Latin America, the Middle East, Australia, and the Far East have adopted the Cancer Prevention Diet and have found it nourishing, satisfying, and delicious. Most people find that soon after changing to whole unprocessed foods, their natural sense of taste returns. After years of eating refined foods and artifically flavored products, our taste buds begin to atrophy and we forget the rich flavors, subtle aromas, and variety of textures

TABLE 8. CANCER-INHIBITING SUBSTANCES IN BASIC MACROBIOTIC FOODS

Food	Cancer-inhibiting Factors
Whole grains	Fiber, protease inhibitors, vitamin E
Beans	Fiber, protease inhibitors, vitamin E
Miso, tofu, tempeh, and other soyfoods	Isoflavones, protease inhibitors, phytosterols, saponins, phytoestrogens
Green leafy vegetables	Beta-carotene and other carotenoid pigments, chlorophyll, fiber, vitamins A, C, and E
Orange-yellow vegetables	Beta-carotene and other carotenoid pigments, fiber, vitamins A and C
Cruciferous vegetables	Indoles, dithiolthiones, glucosinolates, carotenoids, chlorophyll, fiber, vitamins A, C, and E
Sea vegetables	Fiber, chlorophyll, fucoidan, vitamin C

offered by grains and vegetables. Changing to natural foods ultimately results not only in improved health but also in recovery of our appetite for life itself.

In making the transition from a refined modern diet, it is important to proceed gradually and not try to make the change all at once. Meat and poultry are relatively easy to give up, and most people discover that they have little or no desire to consume them after a few weeks. However, if cravings occur, seitan (wheat meat) or tempeh (soy meat) may be consumed more frequently in such forms as a grain- or soyburger. The wheat or soy meat tastes and looks like hamburger and many people cannot tell the difference.

Sugar and sweets are usually more difficult to give up than meat. A gradual transition to more natural sweeteners should be made to allow the body to adjust itself to a change in blood sugar levels. First, honey or maple syrup may be substituted for sugar. When balance begins to be restored, over a period of several weeks to several months, the change to the comparatively milder rice syrup, barley malt, or other grain-based sweetener can be easily made. When full health is restored, a single mouthful of food containing sugar, honey, or maple syrup will usually trigger an instant headache or discomfort as the body's natural defense system signals the ingestion of highly imbalanced food. Modern people, however, have consumed so much sugar and sweets over the years that their bodies have become dulled to these effects.

TABLE 9. CANCER, DIET, AND OTHER FACTORS

CANCER	HIGH RISK Primary Factors	Contributing Factors	LOW RISK Protective Factors
Breast	milk, cheese, butter, and other dairy, fat, sugar, oil, white flour, low fiber	meat, eggs, poultry, spices, soft drinks, drugs, medications, X rays, mammograms, hair dyes, synthetic clothing, electromagnetic fields	whole grains, beans, miso, shoyu, tempeh, tofu, leafy green and white vegetables, sea vegetables, breastfeeding
Lung	meat, eggs, poultry, cheese, dairy, sugar, oil, white flour	spices, fruit, stimulants, drugs, smoking, secondhand smoke, air pollution, asbestos	whole grains, leafy green and yellow vegetables, beans, sea vegetables, fresh air
Colon and rectum	beef, pork, lamb, and other meat, eggs, hard fats, poultry, white flour	sugar, dairy, oil, spices, soft drinks, beer, chemicals, drugs, medications, sedentary jobs and lifestyle	whole grains, fiber, beans and lentils, leafy green vegetables, sea vegetables, thorough chewing, exercise

CANCER	HIGH RISK Primary Factors	Contributing Factors	LOW RISK Protective Factors
Oral and upper digestive	oil, fat, sugar, dairy, spices, chemicals, soft drinks, refined flour and white rice, alcohol	animal food, especially cured meats, ham, bacon; alcohol; tobacco; radiation	whole grains, lentils and beans, green and yellow vegetables, sea vegetables
Stomach	white rice, white flour, oil, vinegar, MSG, stimulants, alcohol	animal food, dairy, industrial pollutants	whole grains, beans, miso, shoyu, leafy green and white vegetables, sea vegetables, ginger
Liver	chicken, eggs, hard fat, cheese, animal protein, oil, white flour	sugar, spices, dairy, alcohol, pesticides, birth-control pills, drugs, medications	whole grains, beans, vegetables, sea vegetables, shiitake mushrooms
Kidney and bladder	fats, oil, meat, dairy, eggs, sugar	fruit, juices, spices, soft drinks, stimulants, chemicals, drugs, medications, coffee, chlorinated water, artificial sweeteners, air pollution	whole grains, lentils and beans, green and yellow vegetables, sea vegetables, spring water
Pancreatic	meat, eggs, poultry, cheese, fat, oil, sugar	milk and other dairy, white flour, spices, coffee, tobacco, radiation	whole grains, beans, green and yellow vegetables, sea vegetables, shiitake mushrooms
Female Reproductive (ovary, uterus, cervix)	meat, hard fat, eggs, animal protein, dairy, oil	sugar, white flour, fruit, juices, stimulants, chemicals, birth-control pills, medications, DES (diethylstilbestrol)	whole grains, beans, green and yellow vegetables, shiitake mushrooms
Male Reproductive (prostate, testicular)	hard fats, meat, eggs, cheese, milk	oil, dairy, sugar, white flour, fruit, coffee, chemicals, drugs, medications, surgery and radiation	whole grains, beans, green and yellow vegetables, sea vegetables, shiitake mushrooms

CANCER	HIGH RISK Primary Factors	Contributing Factors	LOW RISK Protective Factors
Skin	fat, oil, dairy, white flour, sugar, fruit, juices, spices, soft drinks, chemicals	animal food, sunlight, industrial pollutants, fluorescent lights, halogen lights, electromagnetic fields	whole grains, beans, miso, shoyu, vegetables, sea vegetables
Melanoma	meat, sugar, poultry, eggs, cheese and other dairy, oil, white flour	fruit, soft drinks, spices, stimulants, chemicals, medications, PCBs, fluorescent lights	whole grains, beans, green and yellow vegetables, sea vegetables
Bone	chicken, eggs, hard fat, salted and baked food	sugar, dairy, stimulants, radiation and electromagnetic fields, pesticides	whole grains, beans, green and yellow vegetables, sea vegetables, shiitake mushrooms, sea salt
Leukemia	oil, fat, sugar, soft drinks, stimulants, chemicals	animal food, fruit, spices, pesticides, radiation, X rays, industrial pollutants, electromagnetic fields	whole grains, miso, shoyu, beans, vegetables, sea vegetables, sea salt
Lymphatic	milk and other dairy, sugar, oil, fat, soft drinks, chemicals	animal food, spices, pesticides, benzene, radiation, X rays, tonsillectomies	whole grains, pulses, beans, green and yellow vegetables, seeds, sea vegetables
Brain (inner regions)	meat, dairy, poultry, eggs, oily fish	sugar, oil, fruit, juices, spices, stimulants, drugs, medications, pesticides	whole grains, beans, green and yellow vegetables, sea vegetables
Brain (outer regions)	oil, fat, sugar, dairy, spices, soft drinks, chemicals, medications, drugs	animal food, vinyl chloride and other plastics, synthetic clothing, electromagnetic fields	whole grains, beans, green and yellow vegetables, sea vegetables

CANCER	HIGH RISK Primary Factors	Contributing Factors	LOW RISK Protective Factors
Children's (leukemia, lymphoma, brain, bone, kidney)	milk and other dairy, eggs, meat, sugar, sweets	cold foods, spices, herbs, stimulants, tropical foods, pesticides, tonsillectomies, chemicals, radiation, electromagnetic fields	whole grains, beans, miso, shoyu, green and yellow vegetables, sea vegetables, breast-feeding
Radiation- and environmentally related (leukemia, lymphoma, brain, bone)	dairy, eggs, meat, sugar, sweets, white flour, and other acidic foods	electromagnetic fields from power lines, nuclear power plants, computers, television, hair dryers, electric blankets, radar guns, and other appliances; X rays; fluorescent lights; electric occupations; electric or microwave cooking	whole grains, beans, miso, shoyu, natto, tempeh; kombu, wakame, kelp, and other sea vegetables; sea salt
AIDS-related (Kaposi's sarcoma and others)	dairy, sugar, sweets, fruit and juices, refined flour, tropical foods, oily and fatty foods	animal food, soft drinks, carbonated water, wine, alcohol, additives, chemicals, medication, drugs, infant formula, tonsillectomies	whole grains, beans, miso, shoyu, natto, tempeh; kombu, wakame, kelp, and other sea vegetables; sea salt, breast-feeding

For psychological reasons, the third category of foods, dairy products, is the most difficult for people to give up. In many cases, dairy food was the original food of infants and children for several generations of mothers who avoided breast-feeding. We all have a strong emotional attachment to the food on which we were initially raised. In the case of cow's milk and other dairy products, it often takes a long time for modern people, including otherwise nutritionally aware individuals, to overcome this unconscious dependency. Soyfoods and other bean products, which have little saturated fat and no cholesterol, provide an excellent alternative to dairy products. In the natural foods kitchen, a wide variety of foods that have a taste and texture similar to dairy products can be prepared for those in transition, including soy milk, soy ice cream, soy yogurt, tofu cheese, and tofu cheesecake.

Depending upon their condition, cancer patients and other people with serious illnesses may not have time to make this gradual transition and need to adopt a stricter, more medicinal form of the diet immediately. Information on how to accomplish this is presented in subsequent chapters of Part I and in Part II. In order to make a successful change in your way of eating, proper cooking is essential. Everyone, well or sick, is strongly encouraged to learn how to cook from qualified macrobiotic instructors. Until you have actually tasted the full range of macrobiotically prepared foods and seen how they are prepared, you may not fully appreciate the depth and scope of the diet or have a standard against which to measure your own cooking. Cooking is the supreme art and cookbooks, including this one, can only provide general guidance. You will save yourself endless confusion and mistakes by receiving introductory cooking instruction. Once you have mastered the fundamentals, then you can improvise and experiment on your own and ultimately learn to cook with only your intuitive sense of balance as your guide.

6

Yin and Yang in the Development of Cancer

Everything in the universe is eternally changing, and this change proceeds according to the infinite order of the universe. This order of the universe has been discovered, understood, and expressed at different times and at varying places throughout human history, forming the universal and common basis for all great spiritual, philosophical, scientific, medical, and social traditions. The way to practice this universal and eternal order in daily life was taught by Lao-tzu, Confucius, Buddha, Moses, Jesus, Muhammad, and other great teachers in ancient times, and has been rediscovered, reapplied, and taught repeatedly in many lands and cultures over the past twenty centuries.

From observation of our day-to-day thought and activity, we can see that everything is in motion. Everything changes: Electrons spin around a central nucleus in the atom; the Earth rotates on its axis while orbiting the sun; the solar system is revolving around the galaxy; and galaxies are moving away from each other with enormous velocity as the universe continues to expand. Within this unceasing movement, however, an order or pattern is discernible. Opposites attract each other to achieve harmony; the similar repel each other to avoid disharmony. One tendency changes into its opposite, which shall return to the previous state. Thus summer changes into winter; youth changes into old age; action changes into rest; the mountain changes into the valley; day changes into night; hate changes into love; the poor change into the rich; civilization rises and falls; life appears and disappears; land changes into ocean; matter changes into energy; space changes into time. These cycles occur everywhere throughout nature and the universe.

Several thousand years ago in China, the universal process of change was called the Tao. Understanding the dynamic nature of reality formed the basis for the *I Ching* or *Book of Changes*, which was studied by thousands of people, including Confucius and Lao-tzu. These two philosophers based their teachings on the underlying principle of yin and yang—the universal laws of harmony and relativity. Thus in most complete translations of the *I Ching*, such as the Wilhelm/Baynes edition, we find the Book of Commentaries, which was added by Confucius, in which he recorded his interpretation of the order of change. Lao-tzu wrote his own interpretation in the *Tao Te Ching*, the central verses of which read:

> Tao gave birth to One,
> One gave birth to Two,
> Two gave birth to Three,
> Three gave birth to all the myriad things.
> All the myriad things carry the Yin on their backs
>   and the Yang in their embrace,
> Deriving their vital harmony from the proper blending
>   of the two vital Breaths.

We find the same underlying principles in other Eastern philosophies. For instance, in Hinduism we find Brahman, or the Absolute, differentiating into Shiva and Parvati, the god and goddess whose cosmic dance animates and gives rise to all phenomena in the universe. The same concept is expressed in Shinto in the *Kojiki* or Book of Ancient Matters. In this version of the creation story, Ame-no-minakanushi, or Infinity, gives birth to Takami-musabi and Kami-musubi, or the gods of centrifugality and centripetality, and from these two deities the entire phenomenal universe arose. In Buddhism, the world of change is called *samsara* and is viewed as a revolving wheel turned by the forces of sorrow and compassion. The traditions and legends of most ancient societies, especially myths about twin brothers or brother and sister, all point to the same idea.

In the West, the unifying principle has also been expressed under a multitude of names and forms. In ancient Greece, the philosopher Empedocles held that the universe is the eternal playground of two forces, which he called Love and Strife. Although only fragments of his work survive, we find one passage that reminds us very much of the Tao Te Ching, which was composed about the same era:

> I shall speak a double truth; at times
> one alone comes into being;
> at other times, out of one several things grow.
> Double is the birth of mortal things and double
>   demise . . .
> They [Love and Strife] are for ever themselves,
>   but running
> through each other they become at times different,
>   yet are for ever
> and ever the same.

In the Old Testament, the rhythmic alternation of complementary energies is often expressed in terms of light and darkness and symbolized in the six-pointed Star of David, showing the balanced intersection of ascending and descending triangles. In the New Testament, we find evidence of an underlying teaching about two interrelated opposites in the story of the Sermon on the Mount, where Jesus feeds the multitude with loaves of barley bread and two small fishes. The fishes can be seen to symbolize the two fundamental energies of the universe whose understanding satisfies our spiritual hunger and confers eternal life. In the recently discovered Gospel according to Thomas, we find further elaboration upon this theme. In this text, Jesus says to his disciples, "If they ask you, 'What is the sign of your Father in you,' say to them: 'It is movement and rest.' "

In more recent times, the unifying principle has been studied and applied, directly and indirectly, by many great philosophers and scientists. In 1790 the English essayist Walking John Stuart observed, "Discover that moral and physical motion have the same double force, centripetal and centrifugal, and that, as the celestial bodies are detained in tranquil orbits . . . so moral bodies . . . move . . . in the orbit of society." In Ralph Waldo Emerson's writings, we find further development of this idea. For example, in his essay "History" he wrote: "As the air I breathe is drawn from the great repositories of nature, as the light on my book is yielded by a star a hundred millions of miles distant, as the poise of my body depends on the equilibrium of centrifugal and centripetal forces, so the hours should be instructed by the ages and the ages explained by the hours. Of the universal mind each individual man is one more incarnation."

Meanwhile, in Europe the German philosopher Hegel postulated that human affairs develop from a phase of unity, which he termed thesis, through a period of disunity, or antithesis, and on to a higher plane of reintegration, or synthesis. Hegel's principle of dialectics was, of course, later studied by Karl Marx and formed the basis of his philosophical speculations in the sphere of politics and economics. Unfortunately, Marx's system remained largely abstract and he did not apply dialectics to health and many other aspects of daily life. As a result of chronic illness, he was unable to complete *Das Kapital*, and his wife, daughter, and associate, Friedrich Engels, died of cancer.

In the twentieth century, Albert Einstein, among many other scientific thinkers, sensed the complementary antagonism between the visible world of matter and the invisible world of vibration, or energy. Based on this insight, he formulated the universal theory of relativity, in which he stated that energy is constantly changing into matter and matter is continuously becoming energy. The present generation of scientists has discovered the nondual nature of reality under the electron microscope in the double helical structure of DNA. The coiled spirals of chromosomes in the nucleus remind us of the ancient caduceus, the intertwined snake or snakes that have long served as the symbol of Hermes, the god of healing, and the medical profession.

In the social sciences, historian Arnold Toynbee based his study of civilization on the alternating movement of two forces, which he called challenge and response. In one of the early chapters of his multivolume *Study of History*, we read:

Of the various symbols in which different observers in different societies have expressed the alternation between a static condition and a dynamic activity in the rhythm of the Universe, Yin and Yang are the most apt, because they convey the measure of the rhythm directly and not through some metaphor derived from psychology or mechanics or mathematics. We will therefore use these Sinic [Chinese] symbols in this study henceforward.

By whatever name we call them, yin and yang govern all phenomena and produce either an outward or inward movement or tendency. Yin, or outward centrifugal movement, results in expansion, while yang, or inward centripetal movement, produces contraction. We can see these universal tendencies in the human body as the alternating expansion and contraction of the heart and lungs, for example, or in the stomach and intestines during the natural process of digestion. In the areas of astronomy and geophysics, these two forces are manifested as a downward, centripetal, or yang force generated inward to the center of the Earth by the sun, the stars, and far distant galaxies; and an upward, centrifugal, or yin force generated outward due to the rotation of the Earth. All phenomena on the Earth are created and maintained in balance by these two forces, which ancient people universally referred to as the forces of Heaven and Earth.

The classifications shown in Table 10 of the antagonistic and complemental tendencies, yin and yang, show practical examples of these relative forces.

CLASSIFYING FOODS INTO YIN AND YANG

As we saw in an earlier chapter, food is the mode of evolution, the way one species transforms into another. To eat is to take in the whole environment: sunlight, soil, water, and air. The classification of foods into categories of yin and yang is essential for the development of a balanced diet. Different factors in the growth and structure of foods indicate whether the food is predominantly yin or yang:

YIN Energy Creates:
Growth in a hot climate
Foods containing more water
Fruits and leaves
Growth upward high above the ground
Sour, bitter, sharply sweet, hot, and aromatic foods

YANG Energy Creates:
Growth in a cold climate
Drier foods
Stems, roots, and seeds
Growth downward below ground
Salty, plainly sweet, and pungent foods

To classify foods we must see the predominant factors, since all foods have both yin and yang qualities. One of the most accurate methods of classification is to observe the cycle of growth in food plants. During the winter, the climate is colder (yin); at this time of year the vegetal energy descends into the root system. Leaves wither and die as the sap descends to the roots and the vitality of the plant becomes more condensed. Plants used for food and grown in the late autumn and winter are drier and more concentrated. They can be kept for a long time without spoiling. Examples of these plants are carrots, parsnips, turnips, and cabbages. During the spring and early summer, the vegetal energy ascends and new greens appear as the weather becomes hotter (yang). These plants are more yin in nature. Summer vegetables are more watery and perish

TABLE 10. EXAMPLES OF YIN AND YANG

Attribute	YIN ∇* Centrifugal Force	YANG Δ* Centripetal Force
Tendency	Expansion	Contraction
Function	Diffusion Dispersion Separation Decomposition	Fusion Assimilation Gathering Organization
Movement	More inactive, slower	More active, faster
Vibration	Shorter wave and higher frequency	Longer wave and lower frequency
Direction	Ascent and vertical	Descent and horizontal
Position	More outward and peripheral	More inward and central
Weight	Lighter	Heavier
Temperature	Colder	Hotter
Light	Darker	Brighter
Humidity	Wetter	Drier
Density	Thinner	Thicker
Size	Larger	Smaller
Shape	More expansive and fragile	More contractive and harder
Form	Longer	Shorter
Texture	Softer	Harder
Atomic particle	Electron	Proton
Elements	N, O, P, Ca, etc.	H, C, Na, As, Mg, etc.
Environment	Vibration . . . Air . . . Water . . . Earth	
Climatic effects	Tropical climate	Colder climate
Biological	More vegetable quality	More animal quality
Sex	Female	Male

TABLE 10. *(Con't.)*

	YIN ∇*	YANG Δ*
Attribute	*Centrifugal Force*	*Centripetal Force*
Organ structure	More hollow and expansive	More compacted and condensed
Nerves	More peripheral, orthosympathetic	More central, parasympathetic
Attitude, emotion	More gentle, negative, defensive	More active, positive, aggressive
Work	More psychological and mental	More physical and social
Consciousness	More universal	More specific
Mental function	Dealing more with the future	Dealing more with the past
Culture	More spiritually oriented	More materially oriented
Dimension	Space	Time

* For convenience, the symbols ∇ for Yin and Δ for Yang are used

quickly. They provide a cooling effect, which is needed in warm months. In late summer, the vegetal energy has reached its zenith and the fruits become ripe. They are very watery and sweet and develop higher above the ground.

This yearly cycle shows the alternation between predominating yin and yang energies as the seasons turn. This same cycle can be applied to the part of the world in which a food originates. Foods that find their origin in hot tropical climates where the vegetation is lush and abundant are more yin, while foods originating in northern or colder climates are more yang. We can also generally classify plants according to color, although there are often exceptions, from the more yin colors (violet, indigo, green, and white) through the more yang colors (yellow, brown, and red). In addition, we should also consider the ratio of various chemical components such as sodium, which is yang or contractive, to potassium, which is yin or expansive, in determining the yin/yang qualities of vegetables and other foods.

In the practice of daily diet, we need to exercise proper selection of the kinds, quality, and volume of both vegetable and animal food. With some minor exceptions, most vegetable food is more yin than animal food because of the following factors:

1. Vegetable species are fixed or stationary, growing in one place, while animal species are independently mobile, able to cover a large space by their activity.

2. Vegetable species universally manifest their structure in an expanding form, the major portion growing from the ground upward toward the sky or spreading over the ground laterally. On the other hand, animal species generally form compact and separate unities. Vegetables have more expanded forms, such as branches and leaves, growing outward, while animal bodies are formed in a more inward direction, with compact organs and cells.

3. The body temperatures of plants are cooler than those of some species of animals and generally they inhale carbon dioxide and exhale oxygen. Animal species generally inhale oxygen and exhale carbon dioxide. Vegetables are mainly represented by the color green, chlorophyll, while animals are manifested in the color red, hemoglobin. Their chemical structures resemble each other, yet their nuclei are, respectively, magnesium in the case of chlorophyll and iron in the case of hemoglobin.

Although vegetable species are more yin than animal species, there are different degrees even among the same species, and we can distinguish which vegetables are relatively more yin and which are yang. As a general principle, when we use plant foods in the warmer season of the year or in a warmer environment, it is safer to balance these yang factors with vegetables from the yin category. Conversely, when selecting plants in the colder season of the year or in colder regions, we can offset these yin environmental factors with a diet high in vegetable food from the yang category. Food can also be made more yang by increasing the length of cooking as well as increasing other factors such as heat, pressure, and salt.

Thus we are able to classify, from yin to yang to yin, the entire scope of food as well as classify within each category. Generally speaking, animal food is extremely yang; fruits, dairy food, sugar, and spices are extremely yin; and grains, beans, and vegetables are more centered and fall in the middle of the spectrum. Within the category of extreme yang foods, we can further classify from most yang to less yang the following: salt, eggs, meat, poultry, salty cheeses, and fish. In the category of extreme yin, from less yin to most yin, we find milk and other dairy products; tropical vegetables and fruits; coffee and tea; alcohol; spices; honey, sugar, soft drinks, and other sweetened foods; all food prepared with chemicals or artificial additives; marijuana, cocaine, and other drugs; and most medications. In the center of the spectrum, relative to each other, cereal grains are more yang, followed by beans, seeds, root vegetables, leafy round vegetables, leafy expanded vegetables, nuts, and fruits grown in a temperate climate.

Since we need to maintain a continually dynamic balance and harmony between yin and yang in order to adapt to our immediate environment, when we eat foods from one extreme we are naturally attracted to the other. For example, a diet consisting of large quantities of meats, eggs, and other animal foods, which are very yang, requires a correspondingly large intake of products in the extreme yin category such as tropical fruits, sugar, alcohol, spices, and, in some cases, drugs. However, a diet based on such extremes is very difficult to balance, and often results in sickness, which is nothing but imbalance caused by excess of one of the two factors, or both.

Among our foods, the cereal grains are unique. As both seed and fruit, they combine the beginning and end of the vegetal cycle and provide the most balanced food for human consumption. It is for this evolutionary reason, as well as their well-balanced nutritional contents and the great ability of cereals to combine well with other vegetables, that whole grains formed the principal food in all previous civilizations and cancer-free societies.

CLASSIFYING DISEASES INTO YIN AND YANG

The principle of yin and yang can also be used to understand the structure of the body and the origin and development of disease. In the human body, for example, the two branches of the autonomic nervous system—the orthosympathetic and parasympathetic—work in an antagonistic, yet complementary, manner to control the body's automatic functions. The endocrine system functions in a similar way. The pancreas, for example, secretes insulin, which controls the blood sugar level, and also secretes anti-insulin, which causes the level to rise.

Among sicknesses, some are caused by an overly expanding tendency; others result from an overly contracting tendency, while others result from an excessive combination of both. An example of a more yang sickness is a headache caused when the tissues and cells of the brain contract and press against each other, resulting in pain, while a more yin headache arises when the tissues and cells press against each other as a result of swelling or expansion. Therefore, similar symptoms can arise from opposite causes.

Cancer is characterized by a rapid increase in the number of cells and in this respect is a more expansive or yin phenomenon. However, the cause of cancer is more complex. As everyone knows, cancer can appear almost anywhere in the body. Skin, brain, liver, uterine, colon, lung, and bone cancer are just a few of the more common types. Each type has a slightly different cause.

To better understand this, let us consider the difference between prostate and breast cancer, both of which are increasing in incidence. Recently, female hormones have been used to control prostate cancer temporarily. At the same time, a male hormone has been found to have a similar controlling effect with breast cancer. Suppose, however, that female hormones were given to women with breast cancer. This would cause their cancers to develop more rapidly, while male hormones would accelerate the growth of prostate cancer. Therefore, women who have taken birth-control pills containing estrogen have a higher risk of developing breast cancer.

As we can see in the above example, breast and prostate cancer have opposite causes. Since more yin female hormones help neutralize prostate cancer, we can assume that this condition is caused by an excess of yang factors. Since breast cancer can be temporarily neutralized by more yang male hormones, this disorder has an opposite, or more yin, cause. In general, there are two types of cancer, which we can classify according to cause. The first results from excess consumption of foods in the extreme yang category, including eggs, meat, fish, poultry, condensed types of dairy food such as cheese, other salty foods, and baked flour products. The second type of cancer is caused by excessive intake of foods in the extreme yin category, including soft drinks, sugar, milk and ice cream, citrus fruit, stimulants, chemicals, refined flour, spices, and foods containing chemicals and artificial additives.

In general, if the cancer appears in the deeper or lower parts of the body or involves the more compact organs, it is caused by the overconsumption of yang foods. Yin cancers usually develop at the peripheral or upper parts of the body or in the more hollow, expanded organs. However, this classification is not absolute. Although cancer arises as the result of a predominance of one factor or another, the opposite factor is also involved, though to a lesser degree. For example, cancers resulting from the overconsumption of yang foods also require an intake of extreme yin, since this provides the stimulus for tumor growth.

Thus, among the Eskimos, whose diet largely consists of meat and fish, cancer was unknown until sugar and other refined products of modern civilization were introduced. The inclusion of these extremely yin items provided the necessary stimulus for their normally very yang diet to lead to the formation of a variety of malignant tumors.

Also, regions within each organ of the body have a more yin or more yang nature. For example, the stomach as a whole is classified as a yin organ because it is relatively hollow and expanded in comparison, say, to the pancreas, which is tight and compact. However, the stomach can be divided into the more expanded upper region, which secretes a strong acid (more yin), and the more compact lower region, which secretes a much weaker acid (less yin). The upper portion of the stomach known as the body is more yin, while the lower pylorus is more yang in structure. Cancers that appear in the upper stomach region result from the intake of foods such as sugar, MSG, white rice, white flour, and other extremely yin products; while those tumors that develop in the pylorus result from the overconsumption of meat, eggs, fish, and other extremely yang products combined together with yin substances. Since these more yin foods are consumed widely in Japan, the people in that nation have a very high incidence of stomach cancer. Cancers of the large intestine, rectum, prostate, and ovaries, resulting from the intake of more yang foods including saturated fat, are predominant in the United States, where more red meat and other animal foods are consumed. Other cancers, such as those of the lung, kidney, bladder, and more centrally located organs, are usually caused by a combination of extreme yin and extreme yang foods, though more yang foods are the primary cause. Table 11 shows common varieties of cancer and their general classification according to yin and yang. It should be kept in mind that different parts of each organ—e.g., the upper or lower part, the expanded or condensed part, the peripheral or central part, the ascending or descending part—differ respectively in their degree of yin and yang owing to various combinations of yin foods and yang foods.

To help offset the development of cancer, it is important to center the diet and avoid foods from both the extreme yin and yang categories. A more centrally balanced diet based on foods such as whole-cereal grains, beans, and cooked vegetables can help protect against and relieve cancers caused by either more yin or yang factors. This does not mean, however, that the same dietary program should be adopted in every case. For a person in good health, the Cancer Prevention Diet allows a wide variety of foods and cooking styles to be

TABLE 11. GENERAL YIN AND YANG CLASSIFICATION OF CANCER SITES

More Yin Cause	More Yang Cause	Yin and Yang Combined
Breast	Colon	Lung
Stomach (upper region)	Prostate	Bladder/kidney
Skin	Rectum	Uterus
Mouth (except tongue)	Ovary	Liver
Esophagus	Bone	Spleen
Leukemia	Pancreas	Melanoma
Hodgkin's disease	Brain (inner regions)	Tongue
Brain (outer regions)		Stomach (lower region)

selected according to a variety of factors, including personal needs and enjoyment. For persons with cancer or a serious precancerous condition, a stricter diet needs to be followed at first until vitality is restored and gradually more and more foods can be added for variety.

7

Relieving Cancer Naturally

In treating illness with dietary methods, it is important that the sickness be properly classified as predominantly yin or yang, or sometimes as a combination of both extremes. This is especially true with a life-threatening disease such as cancer. Once the determination is made, dietary recommendations can be more specifically aimed at alleviating the particular condition of excess.

Location of the tumor in the body generally determines whether a cancer is more yin or yang. However, in some cases, as we have seen, cancer in a specific organ can take either a yin or a yang form. In the case of a predominantly yang cancer, the general Cancer Prevention Diet should be followed, slightly modified so as to accentuate more yin factors. The reverse is true in the case of more yin cancers. The standard diet should be followed and partially adjusted to emphasize more yang factors. For cancers caused by both extremes, a central way of eating is recommended. In all cases, however, all overly expansive and contractive food should be strictly avoided, as these items initially caused the cancer to appear.

By centering the diet and, if necessary, making nutritional adjustments emphasizing the complementary opposite quality, healthy balance can be restored. This commonsense method underlies traditional healing and medicine in both East and West. For example, in Hippocrates' *The Nature of Man*, we read:

> Diseases caused by overeating are cured by fasting, those caused by starvation are cured by feeding up. Diseases caused by exertion are cured by rest; those caused by indolence are cured by exertion. To put it briefly: the physician should treat disease by the principle of opposition to the cause of the disease according to its form, its seasonal and age incidence, countering tenseness by relaxation, and vice versa. This will bring the patient most relief and seems to me to be the principle of healing.

In treating illness, the Hippocratic writings employ a variety of polarities and relativities to describe the organs of the body, the different foods that relieve illnesses, and varying human constitutions and conditions. These include strong/weak, fierce/tame, and elongated/hollow.

Over the last 2,500 years, the unifying principle has gradually disappeared from the Western scientific and medical vocabulary as ever smaller fragments of reality have been discovered under the magnifying glass and the microscope. Diseases are no longer looked at as wholes or parts of larger systems, but are broken down into cellular components. Instead of seeing sickness as a form of healthy adjustment, modern medicine sees health and disease as deadly enemies to one another. Instead of seeing that disease develops in one of two fundamentally different directions, modern medicine categorizes sickness into thousands of unrelated subgroupings and symptoms.

A failure to understand the distinction between the general tendencies of yin and yang illnesses explains why some people experience serious side effects from certain medications and others do not. It also explains why so many nutritional therapies and popular health diets produce mixed results or fail entirely. Vitamin C, for instance, is a yin substance that can benefit people with a cold caused by overconsumption of contractive yang foods. However, vitamin C taken in supplement form rather than in daily whole foods can further weaken persons with a cold caused by intake of excessive yin because it contributes further expansive energy to their system.

Across-the-board recommendations to take vitamin X, drug Y, or food Z to prevent or relieve cancer do not take into account the two opposite forms that illness may take. Nor do they always make room for differing human constitutions and conditions and varying geographical, social, and personal factors. Modern science is justified in rejecting alternative cancer remedies that ignore these variables. On the other hand, holistic medicine is correct in questioning modern science for focusing on quantity rather than quality. Eating whole foods containing vitamin C, such as broccoli, produces a different effect on the body than taking vitamin C pills, even though the actual amount of the nutrient may be the same.

DIETARY CONSIDERATIONS

On the whole, dietary suggestions should be directed primarily toward restoring the individual's excessively yin or yang condition to one that is less extreme. Signs of an overly yin condition include passivity, negativity, and shyness, while signs of an overly yang condition include hyperactivity, aggression, and loudness (see Table 12). Once a more natural, balanced condition has been established and stabilized, the person's body will no longer need to accumulate toxic excess in the form of cancer. If we keep this holistic view in mind, we can avoid being caught up in an endless maze of symptoms.

If there is any uncertainty about whether the cause of a cancer is more yin or yang, we can safely recommend the central Cancer Prevention Diet, which minimizes both tendencies.

Since cancer is a disease of excess, someone with cancer should be careful not to overeat. To prevent this, two important practices are advised. The first is to chew very well, at least 50 and preferably 100 times per mouthful, until the food becomes liquefied. A person may eat as much food as he or she wants, provided it is well chewed and thoroughly mixed with saliva. Proper chewing releases an important enzyme in the mouth, which is essential for digestion.

TABLE 12. SELF-EVALUATION OF HEALTH CONDITION

Too Yin	*Too Yang*
Passive	Aggressive
Overly relaxed	Overactive
Depressed, sad	Angry, irritable
Negative, retreating	Attacking, intolerant
Self-pity	Self-pride
Voice too soft, timid	Voice too loud, tense
Loose muscles	Tense muscles
Moist skin	Dry skin

The second point of caution is not to eat for at least three hours before going to bed. Food eaten during that time often becomes surplus and will serve to accelerate indigestion, gas, mucous and fat formation, and enhance the development of cancer. Regarding liquid intake, the individual should drink moderately and only when thirsty.

For both yin and yang cancers, all intake of fatty animal foods, including meat, eggs, poultry, and dairy food, and other oily, greasy foods (including those of vegetable quality) should be strictly avoided. A person with more yin cancer, however, may have a very small quantity of fish once or twice a week if he or she craves it. In such instances, cooking a small portion of dried fish in a soup may be appropriate. A person with yang cancer should stay away from all animal food, including fish, at least for the initial period of a few months. In both cases, nuts and nut butters should be avoided or limited because they are very oily and contain excess protein. It is also advisable for an individual with a more yin cancer to avoid or limit fruit and dessert completely. A person with a more yang cancer may occasionally have small amounts of cooked, dried, and, in some cases, fresh fruit, but only when craved.

The cooking of vegetables is slightly different for yin and yang cancers. In the case of yang cancer, one advisable method is to chop the vegetables while bringing water to a boil; add the vegetables to the boiling water for a few minutes or even one minute, then remove; a small amount of shoyu may be added for taste. Another method is to sauté the vegetables quickly for about two to three minutes on a high flame, adding a pinch of sea salt. These styles of cooking will preserve the crispness, freshness, and slightly more yin qualities of the vegetables. For yin cancer, vegetables should be cooked in a slower, longer, and more thorough manner, and shoyu or miso seasoning may be a little stronger. An emphasis on green leafy vegetables such as watercress or kale produces a slightly more yin effect; an emphasis on root vegetables such as carrots or turnips will produce a slightly more yang effect; an emphasis on round vegetables such as onions or acorn squash will result in a slightly more centered effect.

As for daily beverages, there are now several varieties of bancha tea available in natural foods and health food stores, including green tea, usual bancha tea, and bancha stem tea. Bancha stem tea is also commonly known as kukicha tea. All are produced from the same tea bush. Green tea is harvested in the summer and consists of the green leaves taken from the upper parts of the bush. However, some leaves are left on the plant until fall, at which time they become harder, drier, and darker in color. These leaves are used to produce the usual bancha tea. Bancha stem tea is made from the branches and stems of the plant, which are then dry-roasted. More yin green tea contains plenty of vitamin C and can be used to help offset the toxic effects resulting from the overconsumption of animal foods, while more yang bancha stem tea contains less vitamin C, but plenty of calcium and minerals. It is advisable for all cancer patients to use bancha stem tea (kukicha) as their usual beverage. However, persons with more yang cancers may occasionally use the green tea from time to time for a short duration only. Green tea is not recommended for persons with other types of cancer. Of course, dyed black tea and aromatic herbal teas, especially those that have been cultivated and processed chemically, are not recommended for use even by healthy persons.

Among some daily condiments such as gomashio (sesame salt) or umeboshi salt plums, slight adjustments in use may also need to be made depending upon the form of cancer. The specific dietary recommendations for each major form of cancer are listed in detail in Part II and recipes and sample menus are provided in Part III.

GUIDELINES FOLLOWING MEDICAL TREATMENT AND NUTRITIONAL SUPPLEMENTS

Based on medical advice, some people may choose to treat their cancer with surgery, chemotherapy, radiation treatment, hormone treatment, or vitamin or mineral supplementation, as well as observe the approach presented in this book. In other cases, some people may have had medical treatment or nutritional supplementation prior to starting macrobiotics. In such cases, the following general principles may be followed:

1. **Surgery:** In case of surgery, the standard dietary recommendations for each particular form of cancer listed in Part II may be followed, including the use of oil for sautéing, unyeasted whole-grain bread, and cooked fruits several times a week. Since surgery is usually weakening, kombu tea can be taken following the operation three to four times a week for about three weeks and then occasionally as needed. Ume-sho-kuzu drink may also be taken two to three times a week for about three weeks and then as needed in order to develop strength. As an external application, a kombu plaster may be prepared and placed over the scar to help the healing process.

2. **Chemotherapy:** Chemotherapy is very yangizing. Strong drugs are used to shrink or dissolve the tumor, and the body as a whole tends to lose moisture, dry out, and contract. To balance this treatment, it is important that the dietary guidelines encompass a variety of foods, including lighter cooking. Steamed greens and boiled salad should be prepared daily or often. To normalize white blood cell counts, fish can be taken twice a week. Carp and burdock soup (koi

koku), which is very good for this purpose, can be prepared and served three times over a ten-day period: one bowl a day for three days, then repeated a week later, followed by one more series of one bowl for three days after another week. Mochi is also strengthening and may be taken two to three times a week prepared in the usual way or added to soup.

Sweets are often craved following chemotherapy. Sweet vegetable drink may be taken daily or every other day during or following chemotherapy. Fresh carrot juice may be taken two to three times a week, and fruits can also be consumed two to three times a week, cooked, dried, or occasionally raw. Amasake and grain-based sweeteners such as barley malt or rice syrup may also be taken to satisfy a sweet craving.

3. Radiation: Radiation has a very yinnizing effect. It is especially important to avoid raw salad. Steamed greens and boiled salad may be prepared daily or often. Oil should be minimized during or following radiation treatment, though several times a week a small volume of oil may be brushed on the skillet in cooking following the guidelines in the chapters that follow. Sweet vegetables may be taken daily, though in small volume. For strength, ume-sho-kuzu drink may be prepared three times a week for about three weeks and then occasionally as needed.

A kombu plaster may be placed over the irradiated part of the body for ten days to two weeks to facilitate healing. As an alternative, a green chlorophyll plaster may be used instead.

4. Hormone Therapy: Hormone therapy can have either strong yin or yang effects depending upon the treatment. Some medications such as tamoxifen, used to treat breast cancer in women, give strong yang results. Others, including some estrogen treatments given to men with prostate cancer, are very yin.

There is no particular special drink, dish, or home care remedy recommended for counteracting the effects of hormone therapy. Generally, it is advisable to limit hormone treatment, usually taking it for not longer than six months. The amount of the dose can also be controlled. Moderate doses produce longer, more gradual effects than high doses aimed at immediate relief.

5. Supplements: Mineral supplements are usually recommended by the doctor according to the blood condition. If the blood is normally balanced, such supplements are not necessary. However, abnormal conditions sometimes arise in the course of illness, including anemia or lack of iron in the blood, prolonged or heavy bleeding, and others. In such cases, mineral supplements based on blood analyses and carried out under medical supervision may be needed. There is no special macrobiotic approach to adjusting or modifying the diet in cases of supplementation.

6. Vitamins: In the event of general fatigue or lack of vitality, the condition may temporarily be improved by use of vitamin supplements. However, their use should not be continued indefinitely. In general, we recommend that vitamins be consumed primarily in natural form in whole foods or (in the case of vitamin D) through outdoor activities in the sunshine. In some cases, however, vitamin or mineral supplements may be taken over a period of one month to several months until the general condition improves, together with proper lifestyle and dietary practice.

8

Exercise, Lifestyle, and the Power of the Mind

PHYSICAL ACTIVITY

In addition to dietary change, several other measures are important in cancer recovery. When we start to change our blood to a healthy quality by eating a more centrally balanced diet, we naturally become more physically active and begin to reduce our reliance upon technological comforts in our environment. Our natural defense mechanism is restored and our bodies adjust more easily to extremes of hot and cold, necessitating less dependence on central heating in winter and air-conditioning in summer. We appreciate, value, and continue to use some of the technological advances that modern civilization offers. However, we should reduce our reliance on the use of excessive mechanical or electronic conveniences that may hinder the smooth exchange of energy between ourselves and the natural environment. We especially try to avoid those features of modern life that may contribute to the development of sickness or make the recovery from sickness more difficult.

Stress Reduction

Stress has become a byword referring to all the pressures and strains of modern life, and stress reduction has become a big industry. The pace of life today is certainly faster and more contracted than in the past. However, most stress originates from the inside, rather than the outside. The declining health of people today makes it more difficult to carry out normal daily activities, and they can no longer cope with life. From the macrobiotic view, the problem of stress is largely one of no longer being able to exchange energy, or discharge energy, smoothly with the environment. If we continuously take in more energy than we need, especially high-caloric, high-fat, high-protein foods, blockages develop under the skin and around the organs and tissues. We no longer sweat properly. Our lungs, kidneys, liver, intestines, and other organs of discharge become overburdened as fat, mucus, and other excess accumulates. We carry stress inside, yet complain as if it were coming from outside. Our inside condition creates continuous pressure. Then each cell begins to pool or collect high energy. An explosion finally comes, which we call cell division. That we call cancer. If we are active, we can discharge more harmoniously. The sedentary modern way of life and lack of hardshp and difficulties is a contributing factor to degenerative disease. Ultimately, to reduce stress we must regulate and control the basic energy coming into our bodies in the form of daily food.

Among modern foods, salty foods, hard baked flour products, icy drinks, food that has been broiled, grilled, baked, or roasted, and some sour foods inhibit or suppress discharging. Among external conditions, cold temperature, dry air, smoking, and air pollution, especially the buildup of carbon dioxide, inhibit the discharge process. Conversely, among modern foods, sugar, fruit juice, coffee, tea, and other stimulants, alcohol, drugs, and other excessively yin products cause high dispersing energy and can lead to wild, erratic behavior. Hot temperature, high humidity, chemical pollution, electrical or microwave cooking, and exposure to artificial electromagnetic fields can also lead to rapid decomposing, disintegrating tendencies. Grains, beans, and vegetables from land and sea give more stable, balanced energy, and it is far safer to manage our health on this foundation.

Walking

To promote better circulation of the body's natural flow of energy, direct contact with the elements of nature is advisable. Walking outdoors on the grass, soil, or beach, preferably barefoot, is an excellent therapeutic measure. In my personal guidance sessions, I usually recommend that everyone take a half-hour walk each day, rain or shine. This helps the body adjust to seasonal change and builds up natural immunity. A recent study published in the *Journal of the American Medical Association* noted that people who exercise moderately, including a half-hour walk each day, live longer and have less risk of cancer and heart disease. Walking activates circulation, improves breathing, tones the muscles, and improves appetite. Walking increases oxygen in the blood and lymph, which stimulate cleansing and disposal of waste from body cells and tissues. Walking calms and clears the mind and helps reduce stress and tension.

Exercise

Modern life is basically sedentary, and a high percentage of people today are overweight. The average family watches TV seven hours a day. A sedentary lifestyle contributes to stagnation in the generation of caloric and electromagnetic energy, blood and lymph circulation, and digestive and nervous system functions. Regular exercise, including Do-in (Oriental self-massage), yoga, the martial arts, dancing, or sports, can be beneficial. A person should be as active as his or her health allows without becoming tired or overworked. Several recent scientific and medical studies have shown that people who exercise are healthier than those who are sedentary. The incidence of cardiovascular disease and other serious illnesses is often less for those who are physically active.

Daily Body Scrubbing

Scrubbing your body with a moist, hot towel is a marvelous way to relieve stress, reduce tension, and energize your daily life. It also activates circulation, softens deposits of hard fat below the skin, opens the pores, and allows excess to be actively discharged to the surface rather than accumulate around deeper vital organs. For maximum effect, you can scrub your body twice a day: once in the morning and again in the evening. See Chapter 35 for recommended procedure.

ARTIFICIAL ELECTROMAGNETIC ENERGY

The discoveries and inventions of modern science and technology have contributed substantial convenience and efficiency to our daily life. However, at the same time, many technological applications are hazardous to our health and well-being. Artificial electromagnetic energy in our environment changes the atmospheric charge surrounding us, producing various effects on our physical and mental condition. Often we may notice a general fatigue, mental irritability, and unnatural metabolism as the result of high-voltage lines, electrical appliances, and other communications equipment in our vicinity. Electricity particularly affects the nervous system.

Over the last ten years, research has begun to emerge showing that leukemia, lymphoma, brain cancer, and other tumors, as well as many other serious illnesses, are more frequent in those who live in close proximity to power lines, transformers, and electrical stations and those who use electric blankets, fluorescent lights, and other devices (see Table 13). Some modern medical tests are potentially harmful. For example, X rays and mammograms have been associated with enhancing the risk of breast cancer in some studies. The most advanced technology, including CAT scans and MRI (magnetic resonance imaging) scans, also exposes the patient to various kinds of radiation, and further studies will show whether they are safe or harmful.

TABLE 13. MODERN APPLIANCES AND RELATIVE RISK OF DISEASE*

High Risk	Medium Risk	Low Risk
Fluorescent lights	Desk lamps	Electric lights
Hair dryers, electric shavers	Washers, dryers	Irons
Computers	Televisions	Radios, stereos
Microwave ovens	Electric ovens, ranges	Refrigerators
Blenders, can openers, mixers	Dishwashers	Coffee makers
Electric blankets	Vacuum cleaners	Disposals
Power lines	Fans, heaters	

* Based on exposure to strength of the electromagnetic field
Sources: "Science Debates Health Hazards of Electromagnetic Fields," *New York Times,* July 11, 1989, and International Electricity Energy Exchange, 1985

ELECTRIC AND MICROWAVE COOKING

Cooking on an electric range or in a microwave oven contributes to undesirable effects on our digestion and nourishment and should be avoided. Electricity alternates at sixty cycles per second, emitting radiation that can cause biochemical changes and affect human health. Microwave vibrates at 2.45 million times per second, changing the molecular structure of the food. Overall, both electric and microwave cooking contribute to an overall weakening and loss of natural immunity. When people adopt a macrobiotic way of eating but do not experience an improvement in their condition, one of the first things I ask them is how they are cooking their food. In many cases, switching to gas heat produces an immediate benefit. If they are renting and their landlord will not install gas, or gas service is not available, I will recommend that they get a portable gas stove—with one, two, or four burners—to prepare their food. Inexpensive propane camping stoves are fine for this purpose. Wood heat is also recommended and, in fact, gives the most centered energy and most delicious food. However, wood heat is not usually practical in modern urban society, so gas—which gives a calm, balanced flame and energy—is the standard in most macrobiotic homes.

COMPUTERS

Over the last ten years, the personal computer entered millions of households as well as many businesses, shops, schools, and other institutions. Computers and VDTs (video display terminals) give off various kinds of artificial electromagnetic radiation, which are increasingly suspected to be harmful to human health and, like cigarette smoke, affect not only the user, but also others in the immediate vicinity. In 1990 an Environmental Protection Agency draft report recommended that ELF (extremely low frequency) radiation generated by ordinary personal computers be designated a possible human carcinogen. Exposure to ELF emissions has particularly been associated with leukemia, lymphoma, nervous system malignancies, and other cancers. For people with cancer, we advise that computers be avoided or exposure limited to one half hour per day. See Chapter 27 on radiation- and environmentally related cancer for further information.

TELEVISION

Television, too, has potentially harmful effects, especially color television. TVs contain a CRT (cathode ray tube) that zigzags 15,000 times a second down the screen, projecting a big electromagnetic field. Several decades ago, as a spoof, a British epidemiologist correlated television use with cardiovascular disease in a medical journal and found an almost exact correspondence between the rise in number of TV sets in use and serious illness. Since then, various studies have come out showing that television, like computers, may have small but incremental adverse effects on our health. For those with cancer, we advise that TV be avoided or limited to a half hour a day.

CLOTHING AND PERSONAL ACCESSORIES

Synthetic clothing, such as that made of nylon, polyester, and acrylic, impedes the regular flow of energy through the body. It is therefore advisable to begin to change to more natural materials such as cotton, especially for clothing that comes into direct contact with the skin. Cotton underwear, socks, and shirts are widely available, and as we gradually replace our wardrobe we begin to feel more comfortable in all-natural clothing. Synthetic sheets, blankets, and other furnishings should be avoided if possible. Metallic accessories, such as rings, pendants, and other jewelry, should be kept to a minimum, though it is fine to wear a wedding ring.

BODY CARE

Commercial soaps, deodorants, and other body care products may be harmful. Safe, simple products can be made at home using all-natural ingredients (see Aveline Kushi and Wendy Esko's new book, *Diet for Natural Beauty* [New York and Tokyo: Japan Publications, 1991]), or obtained at the natural foods store. Long hot baths or showers, which deplete the supply of minerals in the body, should be reduced.

AIR CIRCULATION

Free circulation of air and open sunshine should be encouraged in the home or place where the person is recovering. The addition of several green plants will also help stimulate deeper breathing and stronger metabolism. Plants are complementary to human beings. While humans breathe oxygen and give off carbon dioxide, plants take in carbon dioxide and give off oxygen. Recent scientific studies showed that nineteen common house plants, including the peace lily, gerbera daisy, English ivy, chrysanthemum, bamboo palm, and moss cane, increased oxygen content in the house and helped eliminate harmful chemicals from the air, including benzene, formaldehyde, and trichloroethylene. Green plants may also help protect against radon, a naturally occurring gas present in ground, surface water, and granite or other construction materials, which can accumulate indoors and has been associated with a higher risk for lung cancer.

HOME FURNISHINGS AND BUILDING MATERIALS

Synthetic home furnishings and artificial building materials may prevent healthy relaxation and cause a variety of health problems. These include furniture, appliances, building materials, paints and varnishes, and other items in our home environment that are made of artificial materials or contain potentially harmful chemicals. As our health is restored, we may want to gradually furnish our home with rugs, draperies, and other materials made of natural fabrics, with furnishings and structural parts made of wood, glass, metal, straw, or other natural substances. However, we should not become overly concerned about our immediate environment and try to replace everything at once. This is impractical and stressful. Slow and steady change, once again, is the general rule.

OCCUPATIONAL HAZARDS

People whose daily work involves chemicals, drugs, electronics, and other potentially harmful materials or who are exposed to artificial electromagnetic fields have a higher risk of cancer than others. This includes painters, printers, carpenters, chemists, textile workers, farmers, foundry workers, computer operators, and telephone repairmen.

Table 14 summarizes a holistic approach to cancer and serious illness.

OUTLOOK AND SPIRITUAL PRACTICE

Mental attitude is, of course, very important in maintaining our health and well-being. Everything in the universe is composed of energy, including the mind and the body. In fact, we may say that the mind is an expanded form of the body, and the body is a condensed form of the mind or spirit. Outlook and mental and spiritual practice take a variety of forms, including the following.

Developing Intuition

Deeper consciousness, or intuition, transcends ordinary levels of awareness and helps alert us to potential danger, sickness, or harm. It functions as an internal compass or inner guide that helps us make balance, or rebalance, with nature. Intuition inspires us to change our thinking and way of life, especially

TABLE 14. A HOLISTIC APPROACH TO CANCER

Way of Life	*Healthy*	*Degenerative*
Daily food	Whole	Processed
(primary factor)	Natural	Artificial
	Organic	Chemical
	Unrefined	Refined
	Balanced	Extreme
	Seasonal	Unseasonal
	Locally grown	Transcontinental
	Home-cooked	Precooked
Environment & lifestyle	Clean	Polluted
(contributing factor)	Orderly	Disorderly
	Active	Sedentary
	Real	Synthetic
Outlook	Peaceful	Complaining
(contributing factor)	Grateful	Arrogant
	Flexible	Rigid
	Cooperative	Competitive

self-destructive habits that have guided our behavior until now. It is the basis for self-reflection and change and emerges at times of crisis, including serious illness. Intuition is the unlearned, spontaneous awareness of the order of nature and the way to live in harmony with that changing order. It is the foundation for a long and healthy life on this planet. Intuition is the key to survival and realization and the foundation for self-reflection and change. The best way to develop our daily intuition is through our daily way of eating—eating very simply in harmony with the natural environment, being grateful for all difficulties including our sickness, and extending our love and care to everyone.

Self-reflection

A person with cancer needs to understand that while cancer and other sicknesses are a disease of modern civilization as a whole, he or she was largely responsible for the development of the disease, through his or her daily diet, environment, and lifestyle choices, way of thinking, and way of life. The person should be encouraged to reflect deeply, to examine those aspects of modern mentality that have produced the problem of cancer and a host of other unhappy situations. These reflections should include a review of the rich heritage of traditional wisdom developed by many cultures over thousands of years, an appreciation of the endless wonders of the natural world, including the body's marvelous self-protective and recuperative mechanisms, and a respect for the order of the universe that produces these phenomena.

The purpose of self-reflection is to review one's way of life, including way of eating, and take responsibility for one's condition. The purpose of self-reflection is also to resolve to take control in the future and change in a more positive direction. It is not aimed at producing guilt or guilty feelings. Once one has recognized one's past ignorance and foolishness, then just put it aside. There is no need to dwell on the past. The universe is very happy to hear your admission of past errors and resolution to continue now in a more healthful direction.

Prayer and Meditation

There are many prayers and meditations to calm the mind, dissolve negative thoughts and patterns of behavior, and heal the body. Several recent medical studies have shown that mental relaxation, emotional support, and awareness of being part of a larger community can improve health. Specifically, meditation helps to relax autonomic nerves, lowers blood pressure, and relieves stress on the heart and other internal organs. It can help us consciously control digestive, respiratory, and circulatory functions. In the case of cancer, meditation can help reduce tumor development in some cases by dissolving negative thoughts and images that disturb the smooth flow of healing energy in the chakras, meridians, and cells.

At the Kushi Institute, in my Spiritual Development Training Seminars, I teach palm healing, meditation, and other mental and physical exercises from around the world that have proved beneficial in helping people recover from sickness. It is important to understand, however, that these techniques and methods are all based on an understanding of yin and yang, or the flow of natural electromagnetic energy. When we eat, we are taking in the essence of those energies in the simplest, most balanced form. These energies can also be applied directly. However, these methods should serve as a complement to, not as a replacement, for fundamental dietary change.

All of us must realize that without food there is no life; without food we cannot create healthy blood; and without healthy blood, there is no cell formation, including the formation of healthy brain cells. The strength of our minds, emotions, and spirits is conditioned by the daily food we take, and these, in turn, reciprocally influence the health and vitality of our physical being. This relationship has often been misunderstood, however, and disease has been equated with sin and health with saintliness. To the eye of the universe, however, moral sanctity and religious practice do not necessarily protect from sickness or disability.

A number of years ago, my wife and I returned from giving seminars in Spain and Portugal. While in Spain, I saw many sick people who came to me for macrobiotic advice. One Catholic nun, about thirty-five years old, was among them. She attended my seminars, and when I saw her privately she explained that she was suffering from breast cancer. I asked her how many nuns were in her convent, and she replied that about three hundred were living there. I then asked how many had developed cancer, and she told me that sixty nuns had developed the disease and of these thirty had already died. Thirteen women had entered the convent when she did, and of this original group twelve had died from cancer and she was the only one left. In some instances, prayer may have prolonged the lives of these unfortunate women. However, only by changing the convent's daily way of eating would their lives be saved. Prayer and meditation alone are helpful, but if poor-quality food—the main cause of the problem—continues, there can never be complete recovery. Together, proper food—plus prayer and meditation—is very powerful.

Meditation offers a simple and practical method to quiet the mind, reduce stress and anxiety, and develop intuition. Please see Chapter 36 for one simple meditation that can be done at home.

Sound and Vibration

Sound and vibration carry energy. For thousands of years people have used words and music, including songs and chanting, to harmonize their inner and outer environment. In personal guidance sessions, I always tell people with cancer who come to see me to sing a happy song each day. It doesn't matter what the song is, so long as it is cheerful and positive. "You Are My Sunshine," "Row, Row, Row Your Boat,"—practically any simple song like this will raise your spirits, as well as harmonize your mental and physical condition. Of course, singing stimulates breathing, and the lungs, as we have seen, are one of the main avenues of discharge for the body as a whole. Excessive fat and mucus may accumulate or travel there, and singing will help them come out. Like everything else, sound and vibration are governed by yin and yang. Some sounds are more contractive, others more expansive. Sounds affect different organs and functions of the body differently. Some sounds energize and activate; others soothe and tranquilize. Correctly used, sound and vibration are powerful tools to help recover from sickness and maintain usual good health. Reading poetry or literature out loud for a few minutes each day is also very good exercise.

Creative Imaging or Visualization

Over the last decade, many people have turned to the use of creating imaging or visualization to help recover from cancer and other serious illnesses, and research is beginning to show the effectiveness of this approach. However, as in the case of prayer and meditation, by itself the power of visualization is limited. Combined with proper diet and way of life in general, it can be very effective (see Table 15).

It is important when we visualize that we do so in a peaceful, harmonious way. Some current visualization methods are based on negative images, including the same violent, conflicting model that gives rise to the disease. For example, some people come to me and ask my opinion about visualizing armies of white blood cells with laser beams going out to do battle and zap cancer cells. I tell them this kind of imagery is completely inappropriate for healing and reinforces the idea that we are not responsible for our health and sickness and that our body is a battlefield.

Cancer, as we have seen, is not an enemy, but a friend. It does not originate outside, but inside. It is not caused by evil forces that invade and attack us. Rather, cancer is the body's own self-defense mechanism to protect itself against long-time dietary and environmental abuse. Cancer cells are localizing toxins in our body, allowing it to continue functioning until fundamental changes in diet and lifestyle are made. Cancer cells are working in harmony with all other cells, including white and red blood cells. This is an example of the process of natural attraction and harmony that is found throughout the universe. The antibodies secreted by immune cells actually complement and make balance with cancer cells, viruses, or other potentially harmful substances. Antibodies have an opposite polarity to these cells and neutralize their extreme or excessive qualities, thus keeping the body in a state of healthy equilibrium. When we are in good health, the immune system functions efficiently and we remain free of sickness. When our overall condition deteriorates, the immune system loses the ability to neutralize these substances and we become sick.

Visualization should be calm and peaceful. Visualizing our blood cells doing battle with sickness creates stress and anxiety that interfere with the harmonious flow of energy throughout the body. In order to be healthy, we need to bring our view of life into alignment with natural order. Love, gratefulness, and acceptance are basic to health and to living in harmony with ourselves and others around us. During visualization, rather than struggle and combat, we should concentrate on images of overall mental and physical health, on the nourishing properties and energy (ki or electromagnetic energy) of daily food, and on the beneficial influences of the sun and moon, the stars, and the environment. At the cellular level, we can imagine tumors naturally regressing as healthy blood and lymph are produced. At the family level, we can imagine our families and friends supporting, nourishing, and encouraging us and eventually, guided by our example, making changes in their own way of life. Several peaceful visualizations like this are included in Chapter 36.

FACTORS THAT ENHANCE RECOVERY

Over the years, I have seen thousands of people with cancer. In my view, there are several factors that influence the chances of recovery.

Gratitude

There are some people who are genuinely grateful for their illness and what it has to teach them. They do not complain and blame others but look within themselves for the source of their troubles. They realize their past way of eating and living was imbalanced, and they are happy to make a fresh start and change. Such people often have a deep faith in something larger than themselves, such as God, nature, or the universe, and they experience the coming of macrobiotics into their lives as an expression of that faith. As their health improves, they grow closer to their original religious heritage, whether it is Catholicism, Judaism, Protestantism, or Buddhism, and their appreciation of other spiritual traditions deepens. After healing themselves, such people go on to help many others. Looking back on their illness, they often say that cancer was one of the best things that ever happened to them because of the changes it brought in their understanding of life and relations with others.

Deep Suffering

People who have experienced the full range of pain and fear and who truly want to be free from suffering readily embrace the diet. They have tried many

TABLE 15. THE PHYSIOLOGICAL BENEFITS OF EXERCISE AND MEDITATION

Walking/Light Exercise	*Meditation/Visualization*
Stimulates circulation	Relaxes the autonomic nerves
Improves breathing	Lowers blood pressure
Tones the muscles	Relieves stress on internal organs
Increases appetite	Improves control over digestive, respiratory, and circulatory functions
Clears the mind	
Dissolves stress	Dissolves negative thoughts and emotions
Increases bowel motility	Improves energy flow to chakras, meridians, tissues, and cells
Improves energy flow to chakras, meridians, tissues, and cells	

different symptomatic approaches and been disappointed. They are now ready to give up their defensive way of life, their stubbornness, and their rigidity to find freedom and regain their health. They have developed the ability to self-reflect and embarked on a personal search for truth. When they discover the unifying principle of yin and yang, they learn how to transmute sickness into health and sorrow into joy.

Will and Determination

People who have cancer but still retain their cheerfulness, humor, and will to live also have a high likelihood of success. These people usually have very strong native constitutions inherited from their parents, grandparents, and ancestors who ate grains and vegetables as a major portion of their diet. Even though such persons have spoiled their health in later life, they have reservoirs of strength. They also have a foundation of common sense and appreciation, which they have forgotten. They only need to be reminded.

In contrast, some people who have no desire to live are introduced to macrobiotics (or to some other approach, including medical treatment) often by some well-intentioned family member or friend. Such persons, who frequently ignore the advice they are given, have a very slight chance of recovery. We can continue to extend to them our love, sympathy, and prayers, but ultimately we must respect a person's decision to die.

Love and Care of Family and Friends

With the close cooperation and support of the patient's immediate family, a successful outcome is greatly enhanced. The person's family should clearly understand the situation and begin to eat in a similar manner, while extending their love and support to the person in every possible way.

The approach offered in this book provides a clear and hopeful direction. However, it is usually up to the immediate family members to help the person implement that direction and make day-to-day decisions about what to cook, when to give a compress, and how to handle the disagreements and crises that inevitably crop up. Family members or friends taking care of the person with cancer must also constantly self-reflect and consider whether their advice is sound. As we develop as teachers and healers, we will face many difficulties and frustrations. However, as our own way of eating improves and our intuition develops, we are able to help more and more people.

Proper Dietary Practice

In some cases, the macrobiotic dietary recommendations are not well understood or carefully practiced. For example, when I advise, "Eat 50 to 60 percent whole grains every day, prepare rice in a pressure cooker, and add a pinch of sea salt," most people indicate that they understand. However, upon returning home, some might cook with plenty of salt and others with no salt. They may use too much water or not enough. Rather than buying a pressure cooker for the price of about one hospital X ray, they steam or bake their rice.

Still others apply the conventional wisdom that if a little is good, a lot is better, and eat 100 percent instead of 50 percent grain. As a result, their condition becomes excessively contracted and soon they are consuming desserts, salads, fruit juice, and other excessively expansive foods to restore balance. Naturally, these practices hinder recovery.

Another mistake is to confuse the macrobiotic approach with other dietary or nutritional approaches and, "to be on the safe side," try to combine them all. Moreover, some people new to natural foods assume that everything that is sold in the health food store is safe to eat—or otherwise it wouldn't be sold there. These misconceptions must be overcome or the way of eating will become chaotic and disorderly.

The most successful people are those who take macrobiotic cooking classes and learn from the beginning how to prepare foods properly. Without actually seeing the foods cooked by an experienced cook and tasting them for oneself, there is no standard to judge one's own cooking. So in the beginning, we recommend that everyone take cooking classes: men and women, boys and girls, young and old.

Women—and sometimes men—who are experienced cooks sometimes think that they already know how to prepare natural foods and neglect to take macrobiotic cooking classes. This is a big mistake. No matter how wonderful their previous style of cooking, they must recognize that this was a major cause of their problem. People who have never cooked for themselves have less trouble adjusting. They have what is called in the Far East "Beginner's Mind." Like children, their minds are open, fresh, original, clear. That is the kind of spirit that succeeds.

It isn't necessary to spend a great deal of time attending classes. If you are able to learn at least ten or twenty basic dishes, you can go on to develop your own cooking style. When beginning the diet, seek the advice of friends with experience who live near you. Don't hesitate to show them dishes you have prepared and ask for their advice and suggestions.

Following are some of the most common mistakes people make when beginning the macrobiotic dietary approach:

1. Using too much salt, in the form of sea salt, miso, shoyu, umeboshi, and other seasonings and using too many condiments at the table.

2. Using poor-quality salt such as gray sea salt, miso that has not aged two or three years, shoyu that contains chemicals, real or genuine tamari (which can contribute to poor digestion) instead of shoyu, umeboshi that have been treated with chemicals, etc.

3. Using too much oil or poor-quality oil, such as refined vegetable oil, as opposed to unrefined vegetable oil, which retains its natural taste, aroma, and nutrients.

4. Not eating whole grain at every meal and taking too many grain products, such as oatmeal, rye flakes, bulgur, grits, etc.

5. Taking too much bread and other hard baked flour products, including crackers, cookies, muffins, and biscuits, which easily create mucus, intestinal stagnation, and hardness. Instead of a whole bowl of popcorn, take just a handful. Instead of a whole pack of rice cakes, take just a couple.

6. Taking too many sweets and desserts, including too much barley malt and rice syrup.

7. Not taking enough greens.

8. Taking too much liquid or using poor-quality water (too high or low in minerals) for cooking and drinking.

9. Eating in a disorderly way, eating before sleeping, and not chewing enough. Also, using an electric rather than gas range.

10. Lack of variety in cooking, which leads to binging and eating out.

Often difficulties in recovery have to do with one of these or other common mistakes, and when the mistake is corrected immediate improvement is experienced.

GETTING STARTED

Once the decision has been made to reverse the cancerous condition, by embracing a more balanced way of life, combining diet, physical activity, and mental or spiritual exercises, the person should forget about the sickness and live as happily, actively, and normally as possible.

More serious cases may require the use of external applications along with the proper way of eating. Food should be cooked to the normal texture and consistency, provided the person is able to chew and swallow. If the person has difficulty eating in this manner, it is advisable to mash the foods after they have been cooked. It may also be necessary to cook the food with more water than usual, to arrive at a softer, creamier consistency. Grains, vegetables, beans, and other foods can be cooked in this way and then mashed by hand in a traditional mortar called a suribachi. An electric blender should not be used because it can create a chaotic vibration in the food.

The most important home care techniques are the ginger compress, the taro potato plaster, the green vegetable plaster, and the buckwheat plaster. The methods for preparing these and their proper uses are given in Part III. Most conditions can be dealt with successfully without the use of such external treatments. Only 20 to 30 percent require these special methods. These external applications are also effective for the relief of a variety of precancerous conditions, benign tumors, and cysts, including fibroid tumors, ovarian cysts, and breast cysts.

Simple, safe, and effective solutions to the problem of cancer and other degenerative diseases already exist. These methods extend back to the common roots of traditional medicine in East and West, including home remedies and folk medicine, and are now being successfully practiced by hundreds of thousands of people around the world to improve their health. Whether we are able practically to implement these approaches as a society will determine whether modern civilization continues to degenerate biologically or whether we create a sound and healthy future for ourselves, our children, and all humanity.

9

Diagnosing Cancer Safely

Early detection of cancer and accurate classification into categories of yin and yang make adjusting the diet and lifestyle easier and contribute to a smoother recovery. One of the universal features of modern life is that we have lost the natural ability to diagnose and treat disease without recourse to complex, expensive, and often dangerous technology.

However, over the last several years, the limits of this approach to sickness, and to cancer in particular, have become more widely recognized. Mammograms have been implicated in causing leukemia, and other diagnostic X rays may also be hazardous. Cervical Pap smears sometimes show the presence of cancer where none exists, or vice versa. Tissue samples taken in biopsies are subject to contamination and distortion in the operating room and can be misjudged under the microscope. Surgical procedures to remove tumors have actually helped some cancers spread. Radiation therapy can damage healthy tissue and lead to acute or chronic secondary disorders. Chemotherapy can poison normal as well as toxic cells and cause a host of blood-deficiency diseases leading to massive infection.

Hormone treatments have resulted in impotence or sterility. Anesthetics and painkillers frequently weaken the body's immune system and make healing more difficult. Today's miracle cure for cancer, such as Interferon, turns out to be tomorrow's tumor promoter. Even the chemical solution in which surgical instruments are routinely cleaned and the plastic tubing for intravenous feeding have been implicated in medical tests as cancer-causing.

Despite the most optimistic predictions and interpretation of the statistics, the casualties in the war on cancer continue to mount. As a result of this dilemma, the concept of a cure for cancer has undergone a significant change during this century. In cancer treatment, cure no longer carries the usual dictionary definition of restoration to a healthy and sound condition, but signifies only that the patient is still alive five years from the time the tumor was originally treated. *Control* is a more appropriate word than *cure*, and over the last few decades the slight increase in the control rate has reflected advances in surgery, blood transfusions, and antibiotics more than breakthroughs in actual cancer treatment.

The challenge to modern cancer therapy was underscored in an address to a panel of the American Cancer Society by Dr. Hardin Jones, a professor of medical physics at the University of California in Berkeley and an expert on statistics and the effects of surgery, drugs, and radiation.

> My studies have proven conclusively that untested cancer victims actually live up to four times longer than treated individuals. For a typical type of cancer, people who refused treatment lived for an average 12½ years. Those who accepted surgery and other kinds of treatment lived an average of only three years. . . . I attribute this to the traumatic effect of surgery on the body's natural defense mechanism. The body has a natural defense against every type of cancer.

Dr. Hardin's conclusions echo Hippocrates' warning that cancer patients who are treated with incision die, but those who are not treated with the knife live a relatively long time. Three hundred years ago, on the eve of the scientific revolution, the French author Molière observed laconically, "If we leave Nature alone, she recovers gently from the disorder into which she has fallen. It is our anxiety, our impatience, which spoils all; and nearly all men die of their remedies, not of their diseases."

From reports such as Dr. Hardin's, some people have concluded that modern medicine is iatrogenic (disease-causing) and will no longer see a doctor or go to a hospital under any circumstances. However, this is to overlook the many positive advances in emergency treatment and in the control and relief of pain that have developed over the decades. In general, we recommend avoiding those features of modern medicine that treat symptoms rather than underlying causes and that are potentially harmful. However, under a few special circumstances, it may be necessary to take advantage of the lifesaving apparatus and techniques afforded by hospitals. For example, if a cancer patient can no longer eat and is rapidly losing weight, it may be necessary to supply intravenous glucose injections until body metabolism is stabilized. Meanwhile, soft grains and mashed vegetables can be prepared and given the patient in the hospital room as his or her appetite returns. Similarly, there may be emergency situations when surgery or radiation treatment is advisable, such as obstructions in the digestive system totally blocking ingestion of food of any kind.

The crisis of faith in modern medicine's ability to cure cancer reflects a deeper loss of awareness and judgment we all share regarding our health and well-being. Every day we hear about someone who is active and seemingly fit discovering in a routine medical examination that his body is riddled with tumors. How often we hear of someone who dies of a heart attack shortly after being given a clean bill of health by his or her doctor, or read in the newspapers about a tragic crime that has been committed by someone with a serious mental or emotional disorder that has escaped the attention of his or her family, neighbors, and coworkers. Our most sophisticated technology can reveal the chemical structure of our blood and brain tissue, but it cannot tell us very long in advance whether we are developing a serious physical, mental, or emotional ailment. It is increasingly acknowledged that cancer takes many years, perhaps decades, to develop. However, approximately 50 percent of tumors are not discovered until after they have spread from the primary site to other regions or organs of the body.

Clearly we need to supplement our health care with a medicine that is preventive in direction and humane and educational in application. The traditional medicine in China, Japan, and other countries of the Far East, as well as folk medicine and home cares, can contribute greatly to filling this need.

The *Yellow Emperor's Classic of Internal Medicine,* the *Caraka Samhita,* and other standard Oriental medical texts on the causes of disease stressed the relationship between an individual's health and his or her diet, activity, spiritual development, and total environment. No single aspect of human life was considered separate from another aspect. The biological, psychological, and spiritual were seen as interrelated aspects of the totality. The medical practitioner was an adviser and teacher who could point out the source of a potential sickness and give practical suggestions for changes in diet and lifestyle that could eliminate the problem before visible symptoms occurred.

Modern medicine diagnoses a disease principally by observing physical symptoms. The experienced macrobiotic counselor, however, can foresee the development of sickness before pain, fever, rash, or other symptoms surface. In former times, Oriental physicians were ordinarily paid by a family so long as the family members remained in good health. In case of sickness, the doctor received no stipend because he or she should have foreseen the ailment and prevented it through proper dietary adjustments. This was the traditional test of a good healer.

DIAGNOSIS BY PHYSIOGNOMY

The principal tool of macrobiotic diagnosis is physiognomy, which the *Oxford English Dictionary* defines as "the art of judging character and disposition from the features of the face or the form and lineaments of the body generally." The basic premise of physiognomy is that each of us represents a living encyclopedia of our entire physical, mental, emotional, and spiritual development. The strengths and weaknesses of our parents, the environment we grew up in, and the food we have eaten are all expressed in our present condition. Our posture, the color of our skin, the tone of our voice, and other traits are external manifestations of our blood quality, inner organs, nervous system, and skeletal structure. These, in turn, are the result of our heredity, diet, environment, daily activity, thoughts, and feelings.

The secret of diagnostic skill is to recognize the signs of a particular set of changes before they become serious—to see visual clues on the face or in the eyes that stones are developing in the kidneys, that the heart is expanding, or that a cancer is developing—even before these symptoms bring pain or discomfort. This type of diagnosis depends completely on the practitioner developing his or her own sensitivity and understanding fully the principles that underlie the techniques, together with his or her life experience.

The study of physiognomy originally developed in the West as well as in the East and served as an integral part of everyday life and medicine in the ancient Hellenistic world and in Europe through the Renaissance. In the Zohar, a book of Jewish teachings from the Middle Ages, we read: "The character of man is revealed in the hair, the forehead, the eyes, the lips, the features of the face, the lines of the hands, and even the ears. By these seven the different types of men can be recognized." Leonardo da Vinci's notebooks contain numerous material on physiognomy. For example, he compiled a reference dictionary for his own use of heads, eyes, mouths, chins, necks, throats, shoulders, and noses upon which he drew for his famous anatomical sketches and character studies. Western literature abounds with references to physiognomy, and until the nineteenth century many great authors drew upon their knowledge of this art for development of their characters. In *Ivanhoe,* for instance, we find this description of Prince John:

> Those who remarked in the physiognomy of the Prince a dissolute audacity, mingled with extreme indifference to the feelings of others, could not yet deny to his countenance that sort of comeliness which belongs to an open set of features, well formed by nature, modelled by art to the usual rules of courtesy, yet so far frank and honest, that they seemed as if they disclaimed to conceal the natural workings of the soul.

The general principles of physiognomy can be found in a macrobiotic text—or a novel like Scott's. However, development of the art requires that the practitioner's own health and judgment be refined and involves much study and patience. My own practical study of physiognomy began in the early 1950s, shortly after I arrived in the United States and settled in New York. I used to stand on Forty-second Street and Broadway and along Fifth Avenue observing thousands of people: their body structure, their way of walking, their way of expression, their faces, their behavior, and their thinking. In cafeterias and restaurants, theaters and amusement parts, trains and subways, shops and schools, every day I observed the countless variety of human faces and forms.

Week by week, month by month, year by year, it became apparent that all physical, psychological, social, and cultural manifestations of human activity depend upon our environment and dietary habits. It became clear that hereditary factors are nothing but the result of the past environment in which our ancestors lived and the food they observed in their daily diet. The constitution we inherit at birth is largely influenced by the food our mothers ate during pregnancy. Leonardo succinctly summed up this relationship in his writings on the embryo: "The mother desires a certain food and the child bears the mark of it."

During the embryonic period, all major systems of the body gather and form the entire facial structure. These include the digestive and respiratory systems, the nervous system, and the circulatory and excretory systems. As the fetus grows, the upper and lower parts of the body develop in parallel. Following birth, each area of the face correlates with an inner organ and its functions. These major correlations are discussed below.

Correlation of Inner Organs and Facial Features

The condition of the cheeks shows the condition of the chest cavity including the lungs and breasts and their functions. The tip of the nose represents the heart and its functions, while the nostrils represent the bronchi connecting the lungs. The middle part of the nose represents the stomach, and the middle to upper part of the nose the pancreas. The eyes represent the kidneys as well as the condition of the ovaries in the case of a woman and the testicles in the case of a man. Also, the left eye represents the condition of the spleen and pancreas, and the right eye the liver and gallbladder. The irises and whites of the eyes reflect the condition of the entire body. The area on the lower forehead between the eyebrows shows the condition of the liver, and the temples on both sides the condition of the spleen. The forehead as a whole represents the small intestines, and the peripheral region of the forehead represents the large intestines. The upper part of the forehead shows the condition of the bladder. The ears represent the kidneys: the left ear the left kidney, and the right ear the right kidney. The mouth as a whole shows the condition of the entire digestive tract. More specifically, the upper lip shows the stomach; the lower lip shows the small intestines at the inner part of the lip and the large intestine at the more peripheral part of the lip. The corners of the lips show the condition of the duodenum. The area around the mouth represents the sexual organs and their functions.

Lines, spots, moles, swellings, discolorations, and other abnormalities in any of these locations indicate specific malfunctions in the corresponding inner organs as a result of improper food consumption. The markings of the hands, feet, chest, back, and all other parts of the body also offer clues to the internal physiological condition of the individual as well as mental and psychological tendencies. On the basis of these observations and other simple, safe techniques, the person's overall health can be ascertained and season-to-season, week-to-week, or day-to-day fluctuations can be monitored.

Identification of Diseased Conditions

In this way chronic ailments or precancerous conditions can be identified long before they develop and appropriate dietary adjustments taken. For example, developing obstructions, cysts, and tumors can be diagnosed through careful observation of the whites of the eyes, which represent the condition of the whole body. Precancerous conditions often correlate with the following markings:

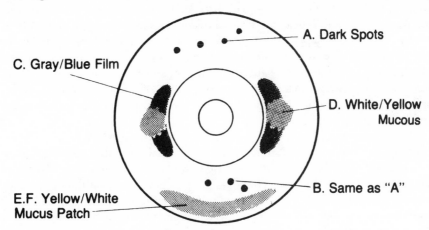

A. Calcified deposits in the sinuses are frequently indicated by dark spots in the upper portion of the white of the eye.

B. Kidney stones and ovarian cysts are often indicated by dark spots in the lower white of the eye.

C. and **D.** The accumulation of mucus and fat in the centrally located organs (liver, gallbladder, spleen, and pancreas) frequently appears in the form of a blue, green, or brownish shade, or white patches, in the white of the eye on either side of the iris, often indicating reduced functioning in these organs.

E. Accumulation of fat and mucus in and around the prostate is often indicated by a yellow or white coating on the lower part of the eyeball.

F. Fat and mucus accumulating in the female sex organs are frequently indicated by a yellow coating in the same area of the eye as E. above. Vaginal discharges, ovarian cysts, fibroid tumors, and similar disorders are also possibly shown as white/gray mucus.

Another clue to approaching cancer is a change in skin color. When cancer develops, a greenish shade will often appear in certain areas of the skin. The appearance of this color represents a process of biological degeneration. To better understand this, let us consider the order of colors in the natural world. Among the seven primary colors, red has the longest wavelength and is the warmest, brightest, and most active. Therefore, we classify red as yang. The opposite colors—purple, blue, and green—have shorter wavelengths and are cooler, darker, and more still or passive. We therefore classify them as yin. Red is the color of the more yang animal kingdom and is readily apparent in the color of the blood and general pigmentation of the skin. On the other hand, green is the color of the more yin vegetable realm and is the color of chlorophyll. Eating represents the process whereby we transform green vegetable-quality life into red animal-quality blood. It is based on the ability to change magnesium, which lies at the center of the chlorophyll molecule, into iron, the element that forms the basis of the hemoglobin in our blood.

The more yin colors—purple, blue, or gray—appear in the sky and atmosphere, both of which are more expanded or yin components of the environment, as well as often near the time of death. The more yang colors—yellow, brown, and orange—appear in the more compact world of minerals. During the transformation of vegetable life into human blood cells, waste products are eliminated through functions such as urination and bowel movements. These represent in-between stages in the transformation of vegetable into human life and therefore are yellow and brown, the colors that lie in between green and red in the color spectrum.

Cancer represents a reverse evolutionary process in which body cells decompose and change back toward more primordial vegetable life. Multiplication of these degenerating cells gives rise to tumors and manifests in a greenish shade appearing on the skin. This shading does not appear on the entire body or near the tumor itself, but in certain areas along the respective meridians of electromagnetic energy corresponding with the location of the cancer. These meridians or pathways run the length of the body and form the basis for shiatsu (Oriental massage), acupuncture, the martial arts, and some home remedies.

The light green color signifying cancer tends to show up on the hands or feet. Several examples are listed below:

Cancer Type	Region Where Greenish Shade Might Appear
Colon	Outside of either hand in the indented area between thumb and forefinger
Small intestine	Outside of the little finger
Lung/breast	Either or both cheeks and on the inside of the wrists
Stomach	Along the outside front of either leg, especially below the knee or in the extended area of the second and third toes
Bladder/uterus Ovaries/prostate	Around either ankle on the outside of the leg
Liver/gallbladder	Around the top of the foot in the outside central area, with its area extending to the fourth toe
Spleen/lymph	Inside the foot from the outer root of the big toe toward the area below the anklebone

SEASONAL APPEARANCE OF SYMPTOMS

The season of the year in which symptoms that first appear or the time of day in which discomfort is greatest can also help us determine the nature and location of the sickness. Heart and small intestine ailments arise more frequently in summer and in the late morning or noontime of the day. Spleen-, stomach-, pancreas-, and lymph-related disorders arise more during the late summer or in the afternoon. Lung and large intestine troubles often surface in the autumn and during the middle to late afternoon. Kidney, bladder, and reproductive difficulties are particularly prevalent in wintertime and during the evening or night. Gallbladder and liver disorders commonly arise in spring and are especially noticeable in early morning. In general, the incidence of cancer increases with cold weather in autumn to early winter, as excess accumulation from the summer is manifested in the formation of tumors. At this time of year, breast, skin, and other more yin type cancers appear because of the high volume of sugar, soft drinks, and dairy food that are consumed in the summertime. Conversely, in winter people tend to eat more meat, poultry, eggs, and other strong yang foods, giving rise to proportionately more yang cancers in the spring, including those of the colon, liver, ovaries, and prostate. Of course, these are not absolute, but general tendencies. Cancer may appear in any specific form at any time of the year.

Modern medicine is beginning to study the influence of some of these circadian rhythms on health and sickness. For example, medical researchers have found that heart attacks are almost twice as likely to occur in the hours after waking. Energetically, as we have seen, the circulatory system is more active in the morning and midday. Another reason is that modern people tend to eat heavy breakfasts, with an emphasis on bacon, eggs, ham, and other animal food. On top of their yang condition, these excessively yang foods can precipitate a heart attack.

Similarly, researchers report that women with breast cancer face four times the risk of recurrence and death if the have surgery near the time of their menstrual period, compared to women who have operations in midcycle. From the macrobiotic view, this is easy to understand. Prior to the menstrual period, a woman becomes more yang and should naturally make balance by taking lighter food, less animal food, and less seasoning. However, if she is eating meat, eggs, chicken, and other strong contractive foods, she becomes very yang (and often tight, irritable, angry, etc.). To offset this, in turn, she is often attracted to extreme yin in the form of sugar, sweets, light dairy food, alcohol, and other relaxing items that make her weak. Overall, extremes of meat and sugar intake make the blood acidic. In this condition, surgery—which is both extremely yangizing (shocking the system) and yinnizing (weakening it through severing the natural energy flow and through the effects of anesthesia)—can lead to increased risk of death or recurrence of the disease (especially through the impaired lymphatic system). As a rule, a woman is attracted to discharge at the full moon, not only in the form of menstruation, but also in a tendency toward more frequent shopping, spending money, cleaning out the house, and going to the doctor's or dentist's. Unless her intuition is good and she is eating well, she may endanger her health and safety by extreme behavior.

In respect to natural immunity, the number of T cells that counterbalance infections and tumors is at a high in the winter and at a yearly low in June. The reason for this, once again, is that during the winter people are usually eating stronger food, with stronger cooking, more salt, and more animal food. This creates a more yang condition in the blood and lymph system, which produces more lymphocytes. In the spring and early summer, people begin to eat proportionately more raw foods, fruits, sugars and sweets, beverages, and other stronger yin foods. Naturally, their blood and body fluids become weaker. In this way, combining our understanding of diet and environment with the unifying principle of yin and yang, we can begin to understand the cycles and rhythms of health and sickness.

There are many other factors to consider and other traditional diagnostic procedures we may use to help detect cancer before it develops or, if it has already appeared, before it spreads further. These supplementary methods include taking pulses on both wrists and touching the pressure points on the skin along the meridians of electromagnetic energy.

In contrast to modern medicine, traditional diagnosis does not require an elaborate or expensive technology and the methods employed are simple, safe, and accurate. Our own senses are the only tools employed. As our understanding of physiognomy develops, we realize that we are our own machines, and our own intuition and judgment are superior to the most advanced computer. What we see, hear, smell, taste, and touch can tell us the story of an individual's past, present, and probable future. The outer echoes the inner; the inner mirrors the outer. Learning to perceive the development of just one person can lead us to begin to understand the destiny of humanity. The person to begin with is oneself.

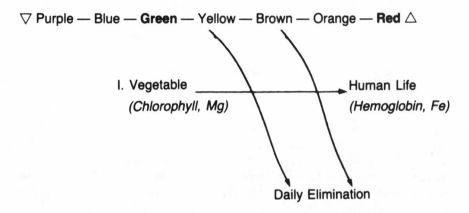

∇ Purple — Blue — **Green** — Yellow — Brown — Orange — **Red** $\triangle$

I. Vegetable _____ Human Life

(Chlorophyll, Mg)   (Hemoglobin, Fe)

Daily Elimination

The above diagram depicts the classification of basic colors from yang ($\triangle$) to yin (∇). The process of humanization (I) represents the transformation of green vegetable life into human blood and body cells. Cancer represents a reverse process (II) in which body cells decompose, often producing a greenish shade on the skin.

10

Cancer and Planetary Health

We need all realize that cancer is not solely the concern of cancer patients, their families, or the medical profession. Cancer is merely one dramatic symptom, out of many, of the deep misconceptions and ultimately self-destructive tendencies upon which we have built modern civilization. In a very real sense, we all have cancer and will be affected by the disease until a new, peaceful way of life is established in place of the old.

Cancer, as we have seen, is not a disease of certain cells or certain organs, but the means of self-protection for an entire diseased organism. If the cancer is artificially removed without changing the underlying way of eating and life that gives rise to the disease, this balance is disrupted and the whole may collapse. In modern society there are many parallels between the way we approach cancer and the way we approach relations between men and women, the breakup of the family, crime and social disorder, international conflict, and destruction of the natural environment.

"Medicine is a social science, and politics is medicine writ large," Rudolf Virchow, the German pathologist, observed more than a century ago. In medicine now, we are governed by modern concepts of cellular sovereignty—the notion that what happens in the cell or its nucleus is totally independent of the organism as a whole or its environment. Over the years modern science has convinced us that disease is the result of external invasion or an aberration in an isolated gene, hormone, or other cellular component over which we have no voluntary control or moral responsibility. Scientists assure us that if the specific factor that is causing the epidemic or abnormal cell growth can be pinpointed, a biochemical solution can be found to block its harmful effects.

Military metaphors are now used routinely to describe bodily processes and to prescribe treating. In "Closing in on Cancer," a recent article in the *New York Times,* we are informed:

These scientists want to understand how the enemy, the cancer cell, masquerades as a normal cell, slipping past the sentinels of the immune system undetected. . . . Antibodies that circulate through the bloodstream are on constant patrol. . . . The body is alerted and dispatches special killer cells and a barrage of chemical artillery to dispose of the threat. . . . It is hoped that these "poison-tagged" antibodies will act as miniature smart bombs, delivering their lethal payload to the diseased tissue—and nowhere else.

Science News, in a typical article, voiced a similar image:

What do you do with a semipowerful guided missile? Monoclonal antibodies, the proteins produced by immune system/cancer cell hybrids, have become important seek-and-bind weapons in diagnosing cancer and other illnesses. But the missiles are not as good at search-and-destroy missions— researchers have had only limited success in using monoclonal antibodies alone against cancer. Now, others are arming the antibodies with radioactivity, drugs, or toxins.

The *Boston Globe* science columnist, in an article, "The Human Body's 'Cell Wars' Defense," compared with the body's strategic defenses to the space-based Star Wars missile defense system:

We live in a sea of alien viruses and microorganisms. Many are harmful. Some are deadly. The body is protected by a stupendous array of traps, triggers, walls, moats, and chemical alarms. Some of the body's cells act as patrols, sentries, infantry, and artillery to defend the integrity of the larger society. The "cell wars" defense system never rests.

Increasingly, modern medicine is becoming nuclearized. At the present time, there are 24,000 nuclear scanners employed in hospitals around the world, producing a total of 24 million imaging studies each year. In addition, there are 18,000 radiation therapy machines in use, treating 5 million people annually. In the industrialized world, 25 percent of all patients undergo nuclear medical procedures during diagnosis or treatment.

The purely mechanical approach to science tends to trivialize traditional values and ways of life. Medically speaking, we choose to control illnesses using drugs and electronic means. Without truly understanding the causes of disease, we remove parts of the body, mechanically stimulate our organs, and gradually artificialize our bodies. On the psychological level, we understand only mechanical behavior: if we give this chemical treatment or that nuclear procedure, the patient will react this or that way. But what are the effects of such treatment? How is the treatment affecting the energy of the entire person? This we do not know.

It almost never occurs to us that we have brought disease, pain, and suffering upon ourselves because of a long-time imbalance in our way of eating, thinking, or living. In the war on cancer, heart disease, and other afflictions, as we have seen, treatments involve a variety of successively more violent means to protect healthy cells and conquer unhealthy ones. These methods are similar in design and execution to those implemented on a larger scale by the military and political leaders to protect citizens from attack in the name of national sovereignty.

Our social ills follow a development similar to our personal ills. The pattern of progressive degeneration from less to more serious conflict can be seen in disputes between families, communities, states, and nations. These conflicts generally proceed from arguments and threats to violent outbursts and aggressive behavior, from confrontation and polarization to fighting and war. Disharmony is never the fault of only one side. Yet we act as if it were and adopt an adversarial rather than a cooperative attitude. Instead of seeking a peaceful solution that reconciles and takes into account the welfare and needs of all concerned, including the environment and the next generation, we take refuge in our own short-range goals.

Terrorism, revolt, and riots occur only in proportion to society's reliance on excessive military strength and neglect of underlying social factors that create disorder in the first place. The futility of suppressing revolution with force has been demonstrated in Southeast Asia, Afghanistan, Central America, the Middle East, Los Angeles, and other American cities and other areas of recent conflict.

At the global level, this antagonistic approach has led to the doctrine of national sovereignty. In order to halt the nuclear arms race, we must transcend our allegiance to individual nation-states and begin to see ourselves as citizens of a common planet. So long as countries see themselves as separate entities, they will retain the right to build and use nuclear weapons to protect their own national security. If all states banded together and formed a world federation, limiting their sovereignty, there would no longer be competing paramount national interests to defend. Until recently, the United Nations lacked authority to intervene in the internal affairs of member states. However, with the end of the Cold War, the United Nations has begun to take a more active role in the Middle East, Southeast Asia, and other areas of conflict. Of course, unless the health and judgment of United Nations leaders and personnel are sound, another system of oppression may arise—on a world scale. Thus it is important that basic human rights, as well as diverse political, economic, social, and cultural systems, be respected.

How many times have we seen some social problem, from crime to war, from drugs to the breakdown of family values, described as a spreading cancer in the community? Like cancer in an individual, our major social problems are characterized by uncontrolled growth—excessive consumption and development—and our treatments are violent and self-destructive. In all fields of life, the use or threat of excessive force proves counterproductive. The violent means with which we produce our foods, treat our bodies, and deal with conflicts must be replaced with peaceful and harmonious methods.

OVERCOMING DUALISM

We are now at a turning point in history. One segment of modern science and medicine is moving in the direction of biotechnology, the artificial manipulation of the environment, including the creation of new life-forms in the laboratory. Between 1960 and 1990, the number of radiation-induced mutant varieties of seeds available for use in modern agriculture skyrocketed from 15 to 13,000. Sixty percent of the durum wheat in Italy, for example, is a gamma-induced mutant variety. The U.S. government recently gave approval to the genetic altering of ordinary foods without any testing of their possible effects on health and without consumer labeling. The object is to provide foods that are tastier and more varied, but the effects on human health and the environment may be catastrophic. Foods will no longer have strong ki, or natural electromagnetic energy. By blurring the boundary between species, genes from cattle, sheep, fish, and other animals may be blended into common grains, beans, vegetables, and fruits, creating even more chaotic energy and vibration. The effects on the environment—the delicate ecosystem in which everything is interrelated—cannot be gauged in the laboratory. The loss of biodiversity—the sum total of the earth's genetic variety—is inevitable, as traditional strains are replaced. Disaster—from predators, disease, altered weather patterns and climate cycles, and mutations—is inevitable.

Meanwhile, thirty-six countries have approved the use of food irradiation—an extremely dangerous and destructive technology that exposes food to highly ionized nuclear radiation—in order to prolong shelf life of spices, grain, chicken, meat, fruits, and vegetables, and other food. The potential health hazards of irradiation include reduced nutritional value of foods, creation of unique radiolytic products not found previously in foods, stimulation of carcinogenic aflatoxin-producing molds, initiation of tumors, kidney damage, and genetic abnormalities as shown in laboratory testing, production of harmful bacteria, and creation of radiation-resistant strains of mutated microorganisms.

We may decide to go further on the road to the mechanization and artificialization of the human species, or we may decide to start turning toward more natural ways of living and caring for ourselves. This is the point of decision. The further degeneration of the soil; the continuing spread of cancer, heart disease, and immune-deficiency diseases; and the outbreak of nuclear war are not inevitable. To stop or prevent such catastrophes, we must develop a new orientation toward life. Specifically, we must begin to seek out the most basic causes and to implement the most basic solutions rather than continue the present course of treating each problem separately, in terms of its symptoms alone. Issues of war and peace, and sickness and health, affect us all in one way or another and in all domains of modern life. The responsibility for finding and implementing solutions should not be left to those with the government, the military, or the medical and scientific communities alone. Global health and security will emerge only through a cooperative effort involving people at all levels of society.

Modern civilization, by orienting itself against rather than with nature, has deprived itself of the capacity to evolve with the environment. Cancer, immune-deficiency diseases, nuclear war, and environmental destruction are only the most extreme manifestations of this adversarial orientation. Instead of considering the larger ecological, social, and biological causes of the breakdown of modern life, we have focused our attention until now in the opposite direction, viewing conflict mainly as an isolated disorder, affecting certain cells within the body, criminal elements within society, and terrorist networks and dissident factions within nation-states. The remedies we employ, in our hospitals, legislatures, and world forums, involve a cessation of hostilities and containment of the disruptive forces, all the while ignoring the overall conditions that caused the disorder to develop.

The modern way of thinking that has culminated in this dead end can be described as dualistic. Dualistic thinking divides good from bad, friend from enemy, and health from sickness, seeing the one as desirable and the other as undesirable. This divisive mode of thought actually underlies all of modern society, including education and religion, politics and economics, science and industry, communication and the arts. As long as our basic point of view is one-sided, it is impossible to cure fundamentally any sickness or put an end to family disputes, criminal activity, social unrest, or conflict between nations.

From a larger perspective—such as that of the earth as a whole—we can see that no enemies really exist. On the contrary, all factors, however antagonistic to our own limited personal or national objectives, are complementary. All phenomena contain the seed of their polar opposite and are mutually influencing and changing into one another. By balancing extremes—reducing excesses, filling up empty spaces—nature makes for greater diversity and harmony as the spiral of life unfolds.

Sickness is a natural adjustment, the result of the wisdom of the body trying to keep us in natural balance. Degenerative disease is only the final stage in the sequence of events through which individuals in the modern world tend to pass because we fail to appreciate the beneficial nature of disease symptoms. In reality, disease is defending and protecting us by either eliminating or localizing undesirable factors from our body. It is a wonderful defense and adjustment mechanism that enables us to live one, two, five, or ten more years without changing our unnatural diet and artificial way of life. On the other hand, if we are willing to self-reflect, take responsibility for our sickness, and change our orientation, disease will cooperate with us and go away if it has not reached an irreversible stage.

As modern medicine is now just beginning to discover, cancer and other serious illnesses can be prevented and, in many cases, relieved naturally, without violent treatments, by adopting a balanced diet centered around whole-cereal grains and vegetables, together with other traditional basic supplemental foods, and administering safe, simple home cares. Thousands of people with cancer and heart disease, including many given up as terminal, have recovered their health and vitality by adopting natural, holistic approaches, including that presented in this book. Hundreds of thousands of others have prevented the onset of degenerative disease by changing their way of eating and living. Along with the change in diet, many persons with illness have taken the initiative to apply traditional home remedies to reduce symptoms and discharge toxic material through the skin or urine. These applications are safe, simple, and self-administered and work by helping to activate circulation and by enabling the body's own electromagnetic, healing energy to flow smoothly to the affected region.

The natural macrobiotic approach to cooking and relief of illness is peaceful and gentle. All factors are considered to be complementary, and the emphasis is on restoring balance and equilibrium. For thousands of years, humanity viewed life not as a battle in which enemies had to be violently subdued or destroyed, but as a game of limitless adventure and discovery in which opposites are gently harmonized. Health and peace will naturally follow from adopting this view.

HEALING THE EARTH

By shifting from the modern diet high in meat and sugar and processed foods toward a diet centered around whole grains and vegetables, we are benefitting not only our personal health, but also the health of the planet as a whole. "The quantity of nutritious vegetable matter consumed in fattening the carcase of an ox," Shelley, the English poet, observed, "would afford ten times the sustenance, undepraving indeed incapable of generating disease, if gathered immediately from the bosom of the earth."

In the nearly two centuries since, particularly in the last generation and the last decade, the effects of the modern way of eating—centered around beef eating and cattle production—on world health, world hunger, and the environment have become better understood.

The underlying cause of poverty and hunger in much of the world today is the modern agricultural system that utilizes the majority of arable land for livestock production and cash crops such as tomatoes, sugar, coffee, and bananas. In Third World countries, tens of millions of families growing grains and vegetables have been uprooted from their ancestral lands by large cattle ranches, sugar plantations, and other agricultural developments. Seeking food and jobs, they have crowded into cities and metropolitan areas, creating huge slums, contributing to unemployment, and becoming part of a downward spiral of hunger, disease, crime, and destitution.

About 80 percent of the world grain harvest goes to cattle and other livestock rather than to direct human consumption. There is more than enough food to feed everyone on the planet. The problem is that most of it goes to feeding cows to produce meat and dairy food. As society returns to a more plant-centered diet, world poverty and hunger will automatically decrease.

The effects of modern chemicalized agriculture on the environment are also profound. In a report on the impact of modern farming and food processing on the environment issued in the early 1980s, a panel of the American Association for the Advancement of Science concluded that adopting a diet centered on whole-grain cereals and vegetables rather than meat, poultry, and other animal foods would "have significant effects on everything from land, water, fuel, and mineral use to the cost of living, employment rates, and the balance of international trade." Based on government and industry figures, the panel summarized its findings as follows:

• **Land:** Production of animal foods uses 85 percent of all cropland and 95 percent of all agricultural land in the United States, and it is largely responsible for the extensive abuse of rangeland and forestland and for the loss of soil productivity through erosion and mineral depletion.

• **Water:** Production of animal foods uses nearly 80 percent of all piped water in the United States, and it is largely responsible for pollution of two-thirds of U.S. basins and for generating over half of the pollution burden entering the nation's lakes and streams.

• **Wildlife:** Production of animal foods is responsible for extensive destruction of wildlife through conversion and preemption of forest and rangeland habitats and through massive poisoning and trapping of predators.

• **Energy:** Production, processing, and preparation of animal food consumes approximately 14 percent of the national energy budget, which is roughly equivalent to the fuel needed to power all our automobiles, only a little less than our total oil imports, and more than twice the energy supplied by all our nuclear power plants.

• **Materials:** Processing and packaging of animal foods uses large amounts of strategically important and critically scarce raw materials, including aluminum, copper, iron and steel, tin, zinc, potassium, rubber, wood, and petroleum products.

• **Food resources:** Ninety percent of our grains and legumes and approximately one-half of the fish catch is fed to livestock, while 800 million people are going hungry.

• **Cost of Living:** Meats generally cost five to six times as much as foods containing an equivalent amount of vegetable protein, and consumption of animal foods adds approximately $4,000 (1981 figure, today $7,500) to an average household's annual budget, including the cost of increased medical care.

• **Employment:** Production and processing of animal food has led to the centralization and automation of this industry, idling thousands of farm and food workers and smaller farmers.

• **International Trade:** The value of imports of meat and other animal foods, farm machinery, fertilizers, and petroleum for production of animal foods is approximately equivalent to our national trade deficit.

In addition, over the last decade, the relation between animal food production and the world environmental crisis has become more widely recognized:

• **Rain Forest Destruction:** About 50 percent of the world's tropical rain forests have been destroyed in the last several decades. The major factor in their clearing is use of land for cattle production. Scientists have calculated that the average hamburger made from meat imported from Central or South America represents a loss of fifty-five square feet of rain forest. The rain forests contain an estimated two-thirds of all animal and plant life, and thousands, potentially millions, of species are at risk of extinction.

• **Desertification:** Modern chemical farming has depleted the topsoil, cattle ranching has resulted in loss of ground cover and barrenness in widespread regions, and cloud seeding and other artificial methods of weather modification have upset natural atmospheric patterns and weather cycles, resulting in rapid loss of arable land and spread of desert regions across Africa, Central Asia, and parts of Latin America and other areas.

• **Global Warming:** The amount of carbon dioxide and other greenhouse gases in the environment has climbed 25 percent. Scientists predict that if this rate continues, by early in the next century global warming could lead to the melting of polar ice caps, a rising of ocean levels, and the inundation of numerous islands and coastlines where hundreds of millions of people live. Already disruption of weather patterns and consequently harvest cycles has been experienced around the world. Usually we think of modern industry as the main cause of global warming. However, when we look closer, we find that modern agriculture and food processing are the largest contributors to the greenhouse effect. The production and processing of animal foods, the clearing of the rain forests (which act as the lungs of the planet, supplying oxygen and absorbing carbon dioxide), and the production of methane, a greenhouse gas, by cattle all contribute to global warming.

In human beings, cancer is a disease of chronic excess. In the planet, the environmental crisis is the result of modern civilization's chronically excessive consumption of the world's natural resources. In fact, the magnitude of the current crisis has led many people to conclude that the earth itself is terminally ill. Metaphors comparing some of these problems to cancer, heart disease, and AIDS are becoming more frequent. The buildup of toxic deposits in the land is like tumors developing in vital organs. The pollution of streams and rivers is like leukemia and lymphoma. The thinning of the ozone layer is like loss of the planet's natural immunity. In human beings, cancer thrives in oxygen-depleted cells, or an environment in which carbon dioxide, carcinogens, radioactive particles, and other toxic wastes accumulate. We need oxygen to metabolize our food properly and produce strong blood. We cannot make efficient use of caloric energy without enough oxygen. The medical profession has recently been recommending consumption of whole grains and fresh vegetables high in vitamins A, C, and E—the antioxidants—because they help regulate the availability of oxygen to the body. On a planetary scale, the buildup of carbon dioxide and other toxins indicates that the earth as a whole is developing a cancerous condition (see Table 16).

A diet based on animal foods is dangerous to the environment. In 1991 researchers at Caltech reported that cooking meat contributes to air pollution by releasing hydrocarbons, furans, steroids, and pesticide residues. In Los Angeles, long noted for its smog, the greatest source of atmospheric pollution was barbecued beef, exceeding pollution from fireplaces, gasoline- and diesel-powered vehicles, dust from roadwork, forest fires, chemical processing, metallurgy, jet aircraft, and cigarettes.

Clearly, the planet is in urgent need of healing. For many years our macrobiotic community has been saying that the outer environment reflects the inner environment and that awareness of ecology begins at the dinner table. Personal health cannot be separated from planetary health, and wholesome natural foods are the bridge between the two. If we are healthy, the environment is naturally healthy and clean. If we are sick, the environment around us begins to suffer. In turn the quality of the outside environment determines the quality of our life. If our environment is clean and wholesome, we can maintain our health and happiness. If the environment is polluted, we easily become sick and unhappy.

In the early 1990s, this view began to resonate within a wing of the environmental movement as the connection between animal food production and the global crisis became more apparent. On Earth Day 1992, several major environmental organizations launched an international coalition to reduce the number of cattle on the planet, lower beef consumption by 50 percent over the next decade, and move toward adoption of a diet centered around whole grains and vegetables as the best way to ensure personal and planetary health. Supporting the Beyond Beef Coalition are the Greenhouse Crisis Foundation, Public Citizen, Rainforest Action Network, Greenpeace U.S.A., Earth Island

TABLE 16. CORRESPONDENCE BETWEEN PERSONAL AND PLANETARY HEALTH

Personal Disorder	Planetary Disorder
Lymphoma	Water pollution, especially of rivers and streams
Leukemia	Air and water pollution, including from artificial electromagnetic radiation
Colorectal cancer	Ocean pollution, including sludge and oil spills
Ovarian/prostate cancer	Deep ocean pollution
Lung cancer	Rain forest destruction, CO_2 buildup
Breast cancer	Toxic wastes and deposits
Bone cancer	Mineral depletion
Liver cancer	Destruction of mountains, seismic and volcanic activity
Gallbladder cancer	Destruction of valleys
Kidney and bladder cancer	Poisoning of the water table, underground rivers, and lakes
Spleen cancer	Pollution of lakes
Pancreatic cancer	Destruction of grasslands, soil erosion
Stomach cancer	Destruction of forests, acid rain
Skin cancer	Desertification, drought
Brain tumors	Electromagnetic disturbances
AIDS	Ozone depletion, loss of immunity among many species of animals and plants
Heart disease	Air and water pollution, global warming

Action Group, Food First, Physicians Committee for Responsible Medicine, EarthSave, and many more.

INTO THE NEXT CENTURY

Despite continuing biological degeneration of humanity and the worsening global environmental condition, there are signs of hope and change. Modern science and medicine are clearly moving in a healthier direction, as the benefits of a grain- and vegetable-centered diet become more widely known. Red meat consumption dropped from 132 pounds per capita in 1970 to 111 pounds in 1989, and whole milk intake fell from 219 pounds to 95. As a whole, as a percentage of total calories, average fat consumption dropped from 40 percent of the modern diet to about 36 percent. Meanwhile, the intake of rice and pasta doubled between 1967 and 1988. During the last fifteen years, in the United States death from heart disease has fallen dramatically by 40 percent, largely as a result of dietary and lifestyle changes.

During the remainder of this decade and into the early twenty-first century, we can expect these trends:

• The incidence of heart attack, stroke, and other cardiovascular diseases will continue to drop sharply in the United States. In other countries, where it is currently on the rise, heart disease will also begin to fall as a result of increased nutritional awareness.

• Cancer rates will begin to decline for breast cancer, lung cancer, and colon cancer, as fat consumption drops and fiber intake rises. The overall death toll from the "War on Cancer" will begin to fall for the first time.

• Diet and nutrition will emerge as the key factors in the prevention and treatment of AIDS and other immune-deficiency diseases.

• Populations exposed to nuclear radiation, pollution, and other environmental toxins, in addition to artificial electromagnetic fields, will incorporate miso soup, sea vegetables, and other foods that are protective against contaminants in their daily diets.

• Healthier foods will be introduced into schools, hospitals, clinics, prisons, businesses, and other institutions, leading to less aggressive and antisocial behavior, increased efficiency and cooperation, and better human relations.

• Organic and natural agriculture will gradually replace chemical agriculture and become recognized as inseparable from preserving the environment and maintaining planetary health.

As Colin Campbell and Chen Junshi, the directors of the China Health Study, observed, "The occurrence of most human diseases is usually the result of exposure to many factors occurring over a long period of time." Modern medicine's analytic approach—isolating one nutrient or component and seeking a specific cause-and-effect mechanism—must be balanced by the synthetic approach in which the balance of the diet as a whole, as well as its relation to lifestyle and environmental factors, is considered.

In the future, dietary and nutritional research methods will also need to pay more attention to food quality. For example, are the foods whole or refined? Traditionally processed or artificially processed? Organically or chemically grown? Consumed seasonally or year-round? Besides scientific and medical studies, there are other avenues to knowledge and understanding, including cultural tradition, spiritual development, literary and artistic creation, and intuition and self-reflection. The medicine of the future will integrate ancient and modern, Eastern and Western, Northern and Southern, synthetic and analytic, and other complementary strands that make up the tapestry of our daily lives. As Campbell and Junshi remind us, we need always to keep in mind "the big picture"—or what has traditionally been called the macrobiotic view.

Essentially the health revolution is over. All the basic theoretical and practical information is now available to end the epidemic of degenerative disease sweeping the world and to preserve the natural environment. In medical research during the next ten years, we can expect the focus of epidemiological and case-control studies to shift to monitoring and comparing people eating the usual modern diet, the macrobiotic diet, and other more vegetarian diets. At the theoretical level, scientists will continue to develop concepts of co-carcinogenicity, synergy, oncogenes, and initiation/promotion, which are now in the formative stages, to explain conflicting results and describe complementary and antagonistic relationships. Science as a whole will move toward adopting a modern form of the traditional yin/yang principle, and a new prevention-oriented medicine, centered on diet and nutrition, will develop (see Table 17).

As the health and environmental revolution transforms modern society, the macrobiotic community will begin to shift its focus in coming decades to developing principles of a new science and developing a healthy, practical source of energy. Biological transmutation—the controlled, peaceful change of elements into one another—promises in the future to be a healthy, natural alternative to nuclear power, genetic engineering, chemicalization, irradiation, and other artificial sources of energy, products, and processes. The almost limitless natural energies streaming into our planet from the sun, moon, solar system,

TABLE 17.　THE YIN AND YANG NATURE OF THE HUMAN BODY

Yang	Yin
Blood system	Lymph system
Testosterone and male hormones	Estrogen and female hormones
DNA	RNA
Red blood cells	White blood cells
Growth-suppressing genes	Growth-enhancing genes
Inhibiting neurotransmitters	Activating transmitters
Collagen	Elastin
Sodium ions	Potassium ions
Catabolic agents such as sodium compounds	Anabolic agents such as sterols, alcohols, and amines
Interleukin, interferon, and monoclonal antibodies	Cortisone and other yin drugs
Echinacea and other yang herbs	Goldenseal and other yin herbs

galaxy, and infinite universe, as well as the turning of the Earth on its axis itself, will be harnessed to provide a simple, safe method of generating energy.

Televisions, computers, automobiles, planes, and other modern conveniences will be powered by healthy, natural forms of electromagnetic energy rather than by potentially harmful, artificial methods at present. The competition for limited resources—gas, oil, gold, and other precious metals—will become a thing of the past, further reducing a source of conflict and war. In the next century, the seeds of a new golden age may develop that will last for another ten thousand years—if we can safely pass through this time. By solving the riddle of cancer, heart disease, AIDS, and other degenerative disorders, we can heal the planet and bring health and happiness to endless generations.

PART II

A Guide to Different Cancers

Introduction to Part II

This section of *The Cancer Prevention Diet* is intended to serve as a guide to helping people recover from the more common types of cancer in modern society. The chapters may be read together as a complementary unit to the first part of the book, which emphasizes cancer prevention. Chapters may also be read individually for information on how to approach cancer in a particular site. Since many similar foods and home cares are recommended, the actual recipes and instructions have been gathered together in Part III.

It should be pointed out that guidelines suggested here are general in nature and will differ slightly for each person. After reading this book, it is recommended that anyone with cancer or their families who wish to pursue this approach see a qualified macrobiotic teacher or a medical doctor who has been trained in this way of life. Information on personal guidance sessions is available in the Resource section on page 455.

In the chapters in this section of the book, each type of cancer will be described under the following headings:

Frequency notes the extent of the disease, standard forms of medical treatment, and the current survival rates for persons undergoing treatment. Statistics are from the latest reports of the American Cancer Society, NCI, and U.S. Vital Statistics.

Structure examines in brief the physiology of the organ or body system.

Cause of Cancer discusses the progressive development of disease and the types of foods, beverages, and other substances that commonly give rise to the malignancy. Usually no one food can be said to cause cancer; rather, it is the overall way of eating that has persisted over a long period of time that needs to be changed. Yin and yang are used as tools of balance to help explain this process. A full explanation of these terms is presented in Chapter 6 of Part I.

The main categories of food are summarized as follows:

Strong Yang Foods

Refined salt	Poultry
Eggs	Fish
Meat	Seafood
Cheese	

Balanced Foods

Whole-cereal grains	Root, round, and leafy vegetables
Beans and bean products	Seeds and Nuts
Sea vegetables	Spring or well water
	Nonaromatic, nonstimulant teas
	Natural sea salt

Strong Yin Foods

Temperate Climate Fruit	Honey, sugar, and refined
White rice, white flour	sweeteners
Tropical fruits and vegetables	Alcohol
Milk, cream, yogurt	Foods containing chemicals, preser-
Oils	vatives, dyes, pesticides
Spices (pepper, curry, nutmeg, etc.)	Drugs (marijuana, cocaine, etc.)
Aromatic and stimulant beverages	Medications (tranquilizers, antide-
(coffee, black tea, mint tea, etc.)	pressants, etc.)

Medical Evidence presents data from medical studies and scientific reports linking cancer with dietary, environmental, and lifestyle factors. Sources after each item give the author or principal researcher's name, the book or professional medical journal in which the material appeared, date of publication if not included in the general discussion and volume and page numbers.

Diagnosis contrasts modern hospital techniques with simple visual methods of detection. The diagnostic methods described here are part of my observations based on the living tradition of the Far East and are explained more fully in Chapter 8 of Part I and in my book *How to See Your Health: The Book of Oriental Diagnosis* (New York and Tokyo: Japan Publications, 1980).

Dietary Recommendations explains how to help relieve a particular cancer by changing the daily way of eating. Of course, the specific guidelines for each person will differ on account of his or her condition, constitution, environment, and personal needs. Ideally, the person with cancer who wishes to begin macrobiotics will see a qualified macrobiotic teacher or schedule a personal guidance session through the Kushi Institute in Becket, Massachusetts. The guidelines in this book are offered for people living in temperate climates such as most of the United States, Europe, Russia, China, and Japan. Those living in other areas should see Appendix II, with guidelines for tropical and semitropical areas and for polar and semipolar areas, which include slight adjustments that need to be made with the environment. There are a variety of less common cancers not discussed in this book. If it cannot be clearly determined whether the condition is more yin or yang in origin, a centrally balanced diet may safely be followed, such as the one described in the chapter on lung cancer. Macrobiotic cooking instruction is essential for orientation to the new diet.

In the event a person with cancer has received or is currently undergoing medical treatment, as well as certain nutritional therapies or procedures, the dietary guidelines may need to be further modified for his or her unique situation and needs. These modifications may include proportionately increasing the volume of food consumed, especially protein, complex carbohydrate, minerals, vitamins, or saturated fat of vegetable or animal quality. For instance, chemotherapy affects protein and fat absorption. A carefully balanced macrobiotic diet would include more sources of protein and fat, such as fish and oils. More sweets, such as barley malt, may be employed in such a case, because chemotherapy also causes a craving for sweets. Cooked fruits could then supplement the usual grains, soup, legumes, and vegetables. Radiation treatment calls for increased consumption of miso soup and seaweed, which are taken along with whole grains and vegetables. Some persons with low energy or weight loss may initially need to increase the amount of fish consumed or use more unrefined vegetable oil in cooking. It is advisable for such a person to consult his or her medical doctor, nutritional consultant, or other appropriate professional. Together with proper food preparation and cooking, it may be necessary to continue periodic medical checkups to monitor the person's changing condition as these adjustments are implemented. The most important consideration is the cooperation and support of the person's family and physician. The physician must understand that the macrobiotic approach is not harmful and that it can complement whatever medical procedure is being used.

Special Drinks and Dishes presents additional beverages or side dishes that may be beneficial in some cases. The use of these special preparations, including the amount, frequency, and duration of use, will depend on each person's condition. It is advisable to see a qualified macrobiotic teacher about their use. The time frames given are averages, and the starting point begins after beginning the new way of eating. Recipes on how to prepare special drinks and dishes are given in Part III.

Home Cares lists various compresses and other applications that can be prepared in the home to reduce pain and help discharge toxic excess through the skin or urine. These remedies are inexpensive, easy to prepare, and, if used properly, safe. However, if unnecessarily applied, overused, or incorrectly administered, they may be slightly counterproductive. Their application will differ a little with the individual, and seeing an experienced macrobiotic teacher is recommended. Instructions on how to prepare home cares are given in Part III.

Other Considerations offers some way-of-life suggestions and other types of activity that may be used in conjunction with the dietary approach. Please read or reread the chapter on exercise, lifestyle, and the power of the mind in Part I. For further information on supplementary breathing, fitness, or meditative exercises, see my book *The Book of Do-in: Exercise for Physical and Spiritual Development* (New York: Japan Publications, 1979).

Personal Experience looks at actual accounts of men and women who have recovered from cancer using the approach presented in this book. Many of the these friends have sought guidance from me and after restoring their health have gone on to become wonderful macrobiotic teachers, helping many, many people. Their stories are drawn largely from case histories collected and published by the EWF and One Peaceful World, two of our nonprofit foundations. While these accounts are largely anecdotal, with varying degrees of medical documentation, we hope that they will provide a stimulus for researchers to conduct further studies of the relation between diet and cancer, including the macrobiotic approach.

11

Breast Cancer

FREQUENCY

Breast cancer is the most common form of cancer in American women (lung cancer is number one in mortality), and its incidence is on the rise (see Table 18). Between 1935 and 1965 the rate of new cases of breast cancer increased 18 percent, and between 1965 and 1975 it increased 50 percent. Since 1980, breast-cancer incidence has risen 3 percent a year, now affecting one in every nine women in the United States. Breast cancer currently accounts for about 20 percent of female cancer deaths in this country and is the leading cause of death for American women aged forty to forty-five. This year an estimated 181,000 new cases will develop and 46,300 people will die from the disease. Around the world, the death rate from breast cancer differs widely. In Britain, it is about one-third higher than in the United States, while in Japan it is four-fifths lower. A majority or more of patients with breast cancer develop metastases. Malignant tumors may spread to the lungs, bone, brain, or lymph nodes. Breast cancer may also occur in men, but it is rare.

In 1991 the General Accounting Office of the U.S. government reported to Congress that there has been no progress in preventing breast cancer or in reducing the death rate from the disease in the last twenty years.

Surgery is the most common method of treating breast cancer. The operation is called a mastectomy and includes several types of incisions, depending on the development of the tumor and the age and condition of the patient. A *lumpectomy* excises the cancerous lump and a small amount of surrounding

TABLE 18.   BREAST CANCER INCIDENCE

1940: 1 in 20 American women
1950: 1 in 15
1960: 1 in 14
1970: 1 in 13
1980: 1 in 11
1987: 1 in 10
1991: 1 in 9

Source: American Cancer Society

tissue. A *subcutaneous mastectomy* removes internal breast tissue, leaving the skin intact. A *simple mastectomy* removes the breast. A *modified mastectomy* removes the breast and lymph nodes in the armpit. A *Halsted radical mastectomy* removes the entire breast plus the lymph nodes and the pectoral muscles of the chest wall. In addition to these operations, the adrenal glands, pituitary gland, or ovaries are sometimes removed in order to regulate secretions and try to reduce tumor growth.

Radiation may be employed as an alternative or supplement to surgery. Chemotherapy is sometimes used to control metastases and to stop recurrence of the original tumor. Hormone therapy may be employed as an adjunct or alternative to chemotherapy: estrogens, antiestrogens, progestins, androgens, or adrenocortical steroids are given to control tumor growth and mestastases.

About 77 percent of women with breast cancer survive five years or more.

STRUCTURE

The female breasts or mammary glands consist chiefly of a round, compressed mass of glandular tissue known as the corpus mammae. This tissue is made up of fifteen to twenty separate lobes connected by fat. Each lobe contains a milk duct, which leads to the nipple and is further subdivided into lobules and alveoli. The breast is encased in a layer of fat tissue called the adipose capsule and is attached to the chest wall by connective tissue.

CAUSE OF CANCER

If we continue to eat poorly over a long period of time, we eventually exhaust the body's ability to discharge excess wastes and toxins. This can be serious if an underlying layer of fat has developed under the skin, which prevents discharge toward the surface of the body. Repeated overconsumption of milk, cheese, and other dairy products, eggs, meat, poultry, and other fatty, oily, or greasy foods brings about this stage. When it has been reached, internal deposits of mucus or fat begin to form, initially in areas with some direct access to the outside such as the sinuses, the inner ear, the lungs, the kidneys, the reproductive organs, and the breasts.

The accumulation of excess in the breast often results in a hardening of the breasts and the formation of cysts. Excess usually accumulates here in the form of mucus and deposits of fatty acid, both of which take the form of a sticky or heavy liquid. These deposits develop into cysts in the same way that water solidifies into ice, and the process is accelerated by the intake of ice cream, milk, soft drinks, fruit juice, and other foods that produce a cooling or freezing effect.

Women who have breast-fed are less likely to develop breast cysts or tumors. Women who do not nurse their children miss this opportunity to discharge through the breasts and therefore face a greater possibility of accumulating excess in this region of their bodies.

Many nutritionists and doctors are now aware of the relationship between the intake of saturated fats, cholesterol, and degenerative disease but often overlook the effects of sugar and dairy products, both of which contribute greatly to heart disease, cancer, and other illnesses. (See the section on pancreatic cancer for a discussion of sugar metabolism and the role of refined sugars in tumor formation, including breast cancer.)

The consumption of milk and other dairy foods in our society usually begins in infancy or early childhood. One of the major biological changes in modern times has been the progressive decline of breast-feeding. In traditional cultures, mothers usually nurse their babies for one year or more. At the beginning of the twentieth century, about 60 percent of the babies in the United States were breast-fed. By the 1970s that number had fallen sharply. A 1968 survey showed that only 11 percent of American mothers gave up in thirty to forty days. Since then, breast-feeding has experienced a rejuvenation, with 60 percent of new mothers in this country nursing their babies.

In composition, cow's milk and human milk are very different. Cow's milk contains about four times as much calcium, three times as much protein, and two-thirds as much carbohydrate as human milk. The different structure and growth rate of calves and human babies account for the varying proportion of these ingredients. For example, at birth the brain and nervous system of the calf is fully developed, and the large amount of calcium and protein is needed to increase its bone structure and muscular development. A baby calf often puts on seventy-five pounds in the first six weeks. In contrast, the body of the human infant is designed to grow slowly, gaining only two to three pounds in the first six weeks. The infant's brain, however, is only 23 percent mature at birth, and the nutrients in mother's milk are needed to complete its central nervous system.

In addition, mother's milk contains antibodies that resist the growth of undesirable bacteria and viruses, provides immunity against disease and infection (especially against rickettsia, salmonella, polio, influenza, strep, and staph), promotes strong white blood cells, which destroy harmful bacteria, and produces *B. bifidum*, a unique type of healthy bacteria found in the intestines of babies and that creates resistance to a large variety of microorganisms.

Another ingredient in milk is lactose, a simple sugar that is digested by lactase, an enzyme produced in the intestine. In most traditional societies, lactase is no longer produced after the baby is weaned from its mother's milk between ages two and four. As a result, ingestion of dairy products after that age produces indigestion, diarrhea, cramps, allergy, or other illnesses. This condition is called lactose intolerance.

In the West, however, dairy products have become a dietary staple over the course of many generations. Biologically, lactase continues to be produced in the intestine after early childhood, allowing dairy foods to be consumed into adulthood and later life. Among Caucasians, lactose intolerance is low. Only 2 percent of Danes, 7 percent of Swiss, and 8 percent of white Americans cannot digest milk and other dairy products. In contrast, about 70 percent of black Americans are lactose intolerant, as well as 90 percent of Bantus, 85 percent of Japanese, 80 percent of Eskimos, 78 percent of Arabs, and 58 percent of Israeli Jews.

Despite the body's ability to adapt to long-term dairy consumption, the excessive intake of fat and cholesterol in milk, cheese, butter, ice cream, and similar foods has taken a heavy toll as the consumption of these foods has increased. The per capita intake of dairy food in the United States now stands at 350 pounds a year, including 72 gallons of milk. In the United States there is now one cow for every two people.

In composition, milk is 28 percent fat, cheese is 50 percent, butter is 95 percent, and yogurt is 15 percent. Fatty acids and cholesterol from these foods can build up round the organs and tissues, contributing to heart disease, cancer, and other degenerative conditions. Mentally and psychologically, dairy foods affect the brain and nervous system, contributing to dullness, passivity, and dependence. Studies show that people from ethnic groups that are lactose intolerant tend to have higher IQs than those that are not. The fat from cow's milk also insulates and impedes the flow of electromagnetic energy through the body, diminishing sexual polarity and attraction between men and women.

The quality of milk and dairy food consumed today has also changed from the past. The milk itself is changed from its natural state through modern heating procedures, homogenization, sterilization, and addition of other ingredients such as vitamin D. In an effort to make them produce greater quantities of milk, modern dairy cows are fed a variety of hormones, antibodies, and other chemicals that further dilute the quality of the milk. Today 75 percent of all U.S. dairy cows are artificially inseminated and through superovulation and embryo transfer a cow can now, theoretically, give birth to a dozen calves a year instead of only one.

As a result, the dairy products available today are different from those consumed by previous generations. Until modern times, most cultures limited their dairy products to fermented foods such as yogurt, kefir, or other foods containing enzymes and bacteria, allowing them to be broken down in the digestive process in the absence of lactase. Cultured products like yogurt are superior to other dairy foods. However, they still cannot be recommended for regular consumption because they are now not traditionally and naturally processed and cannot be properly assimilated by people with sedentary lifestyles. A fermented vegetable food such as miso, tempeh, natto, or shoyu is preferable if processed naturally and is an important part of a cancer prevention diet.

In the past, animal milk (especially goat, sheep, or donkey milk) was used for infants whose mothers could not breast-feed, for certain medicinal purposes, or in small quantities with other dairy products for personal enjoyment on special occasions. The abuse of dairy food in the modern diet and its degenerating artificial quality are major factors in the rise of breast cancer, heart disease, and other serious illnesses. The quality of our food determines the quality of our blood. The quality of blood, in turn, determines the quality of mother's milk and the biological strength of the next generation.

MEDICAL EVIDENCE

• In an address before the Belgium Cancer Congress in 1923, Frederick L. Hoffman, cancer statistician for the Prudential Life Insurance Company, reported that cancer was unknown among the Indians of Bolivia and Peru. "I was unable to see a single case of malignant disease. All the physicians whom I interviewed on the subject were emphatically of the opinion that cancer of the breast among Indian women was never met with. Similar investigations of mine among the Navajo and Zuni Indians of Arizona and New Mexico have yielded identical results." Hoffman associated the rise of cancer in industrial society to overnutrition and the introduction of refined and artificial foods. Source: quoted in *Cancer* 1(1924):215–17.

• In 1942 Albert Tannenbaum, M.D., cancer researcher at Michael Reese Hospital in Chicago, reported that mice on a caloric restricted diet had substantially fewer induced breast tumors, lung tumors, and sarcoma than mice on an unrestricted diet. Source: A. Tannenbaum, "The Genesis and Growth of Tumors II: Effects of Caloric Restriction Per Se," *Cancer Research* 2:460–67.

• In another experiment in 1942, Dr. Tannenbaum reported that mice on a high-fat diet had a significantly higher incidence of spontaneous breast cancer and induced skin tumors than mice on a low-fat diet. He noted also that tumors appeared about three months earlier in the high-fat group. Source: A. Tannenbaum, "The Genesis and Growth of Tumors III: Effects of a High-Fat Diet," *Cancer Research* 2:468–75.

• In regions where total and long-term breast-feeding is practiced, breast cancer is rare. In 1969 Canadian medical researcher Otto Schaefer, M.D., reported that over a fifteen-year period only one case of breast cancer was observed in a group of Eskimo whose population grew from 9,000 to 13,000. In populations of Eskimo where breast cancer was very low but on the increase, Dr. Schaefer cited a decrease in the duration of breast-feeding or its complete elimination as a contributing factor. A 1964 study of breast cancer patients at Roswell Park Institute in New York found that breast-feeding for seventeen months decreased the risk of breast cancer. Women who had lactated for a total of thirty-six months had a much reduced risk. As for possibly transmitting some cancer-causing substance through mother's milk, two other recent studies showed no difference in the breast cancer incidence in daughters who were breast-fed by mothers who later were found to have cancer. Source: Marian Tompson, President, La Leche League International, *The People's Doctor: A Medical Newsletter* 4, no. 4 (1980):8.

• In 1973 researchers reported a high positive correlation with breast and colon cancer and total fat, animal protein, and simple sugar consumption but practically none with dietary fiber. Source: B. S. Drasar et al., "Environmental Factors and Cancer of the Colon and Breast," *British Journal of Cancer* 27:167–72.

• In a 1975 case-control study of seventy-seven breast cancer cases and seven controls, five categories of foods were associated with breast cancer: fried foods, fried potatoes, hard fat used for frying, nonmilk dairy products, and white bread. The researcher also reported that Seventh-Day Adventist women age thirty-five to fifty-four have 26 percent less breast cancer than the general population and women in the church over fifty-five have 30 percent less. The Seventh-Day Adventists, about 50 percent of whom are vegetarian, emphasize whole grains, vegetables, and fruit in their diet and avoid meat, poultry, fish, coffee, tea, alcohol, spices, and refined foods. Source: R. L. Phillips, "Role of Life-style and Dietary Habits in Risk of Cancer among Seventh-Day Adventists," *Cancer Research* 35:3513–22.

• In 1975 an epidemiologist reported that there was a five- to tenfold difference in breast cancer mortality between countries with an average per capita low-fat diet and those with a high-fat diet. Source: K. K. Carroll, "Experimental Evidence of Dietary Factors and Hormone-dependent Cancer," *Cancer Research* 35:3374–83.

• A 1976 study of the relationship of diet and breast cancer in forty-one countries found that a high intake of refined sugar was associated with increased incidence of the disease. Source: G. Hems, "The Contributions of Diet and Childbearing to Breast-Cancer Rates," *British Journal of Cancer* 37:974–82.

• Since 1949 the consumption of milk and milk products has increased 23 times in Japan, meat 13.7 times, eggs 12.9 times, and oil 7.8 times. While stomach cancer rates have declined, the incidence of breast and colon cancer has substantially increased. "Among all nutritional elements, dietary fat intake has shown the most striking increase in Japan in recent years," the epidemiological study concluded. Source: T. Hirayama, "Changing Patterns of Cancer in Japan with Special Reference to the Decrease in Stomach Cancer Mortality," in H. H. Hiatt et al. (eds.), *Origins of Human Cancer, Book A, Incidence of Cancer in Humans* (Cold Spring Harbor, NY: Cold Spring Harbor Laboratory, 1977); 55–75.

• A 1977 study reported a higher incidence of breast cancer in the unsuckled left breast of women in Hong Kong fishing villages who traditionally breastfed only with the right breast. The study of 2,372 Tanka women from 1958 to 1975 concluded that "in postmenopausal women who have breast-fed unilaterally, the risk of cancer is significantly higher in the unsuckled breast and that breastfeeding may help to protect the suckled breast against cancer." Source: R. Ing et al., "Unilateral Breastfeeding and Breast Cancer," *Lancet* 2:124–27.

• In a 1978 test, significantly more breast tumors were observed in rats fed refined sugar than in those fed rice and other starches. "These results are consistent with epidemiological data showing that age-adjusted breast cancer mortality in humans is positively correlated with sugar intake and negatively correlated with intake of complex carbohydrates," the researchers concluded. Source: S. K. Hoehn and K. K. Carroll, "Effects of Dietary Carbohydrate on the Incidence of Mammary Tumors Induced in Rats by [DMBA]," *Nutrition and Cancer* 1:27–30.

• In 1979 researchers reported that dairy products as a class increased the risk of breast cancer. Source: S. P. Gaskill et al., "Breast Cancer Mortality and Diet in the United States," *Cancer Research* 39:3628–37.

• An MIT biologist reported in 1979 that studies of women medically screened for breast cancer and women who went unscreened showed both a lower incidence of breast cancer and substantially lower mortality from breast cancer in the unscreened group. Source: M. S. Fox, "On the Diagnosis and Treatment of Breast Cancer," *Journal of the American Medical Association* 241:489–94.

• Studies of breast cancer mortality in England and Wales from 1911 to 1975 linked the rise of the disease with consumption of fat, sugar, and animal protein one decade earlier. Source: G. Hems, "Association Between Breast-Cancer Mortality Rates, Child-bearing, and Diet in the United Kingdom," *British Journal of Cancer* 41(1980):429–37.

• In 1980 scientists reported that a diet high in soybeans reduced the incidence of breast cancer in laboratory experiments. The active ingredient in the soybeans was identified as protease inhibitors, also found in certain other beans and seeds. Source: W. Troll, "Blocking of Tumor Promotion by Protease Inhibitors," in J H. Burchenal and H. F. Oettgen (eds.), *Cancer: Achievements, Challenges, and Prospects for the 1980s* (New York: Grune and Stratton), 1:549–55.

• In a case-controlled study of 577 cases and 826 controls, researchers reported in 1981 that relative risk of breast cancer increased significantly with more frequent consumption of beef and other red meat, pork, and sweet desserts. Source: J. H. Lubin et al., "Breast Cancer Following High Dietary Fat and Protein Consumption," *American Journal of Epidemiology* 114:422.

• In 1981 researchers reported a direct association between intake of serum cholesterol and breast cancer. Source: A. R. Dyer et al., "Serum Cholesterol and Risk of Death from Cancer and Other Causes in Three Chicago Epidemiological Studies," *Journal of Chronic Diseases* 34:249–60.

• In 1982 scientists at the University of Western Ontario reported that the addition of soy protein in a person's diet could reduce serum cholesterol levels irrespective of other dietary considerations. In addition to animal studies, the researchers compared human volunteers who drank either cow's milk or soy milk and reported that "both cholesterol and triglyceride values dropped substantially during the soy period." Source: *Journal of American Medical Association* 247:3045–46.

• Vegetarian women are less likely to develop breast cancer, researchers at New England Medical Center in Boston reported in 1981. The scientists found that vegetarian women process estrogen differently from other women and eliminate it more quickly from their body. The study involved forty-five pre- and postmenopausal women, about half of whom were vegetarian and half nonvegetarian. The women consumed about the same number of total calories. Although the vegetarian women took in only one-third as much animal protein and animal fat, they excreted two to three times as much estrogen. High levels of estrogen have been associated with the development of breast cancer. "The difference in estrogen metabolism may explain the lower incidence of breast cancer in vegetarian women," the study concluded. Source: B. R. Goldin et al., "Effect of Diet on Excretion of Estrogens in Pre- and Postmenopausal Incidence of Breast Cancer in Vegetarian Women," *Cancer Research* 41:3771–73.

• A fifty-year study of diet and breast cancer mortality in England and Wales between 1928 and 1977 showed that at the onset of World War II breast cancer mortality markedly fell as consumption of sugar, meat, and fat declined and consumption of grains and vegetables increased. By 1954 consumption of these foodstuffs returned to prewar levels. Breast cancer mortality did not return to prewar levels until some fifteen years later, suggesting a lag time between the ingestion and appearance of the disease. Source: D. M. Ingram, "Trends in Diet and Breast Cancer Mortality in England and Wales, 1928–1977," *Nutrition and Cancer*, no. 2 (1982); 75–80.

• In a 1984 experiment at Harvard School of Public Health, laboratory animals fed a control diet with 5 percent *Laminaria* (kombu), a brown sea vegetable, developed induced mammary cancer later than animals not fed seaweed. "Seaweed has shown consistent antitumor activity in several in vivo animal tests," the researcher concluded. "In extrapolating these results to the

Japanese population, seaweed may be an important factor in explaining the low rates of certain cancers in Japan. Breast cancer shows a threefold-lower rate among premenopausal Japanese women and a ninefold-lower rate among post-menopausal women in Japan than reported for women in the United States. Since low levels of exposure to some toxic substances have been shown to be carcinogenic, then it may be that low levels of daily intake of food with anti-tumor properties may reduce cancer incidence." Source: J. Teas, M. L. Har-bison, and R. S. Gelman, "Dietary Seaweed" [*Laminaria*] and Mammary Carcinogenesis in Rats," *Cancer Research* 44:2758–61.

• In a large case-control study in France in 1986, published in 1986, in-volving several thousand women, increased risk for breast cancer was found for consumption of dairy products. Women who ate cheese regularly had 50 per-cent more risk compared to women who didn't eat cheese, and those who drank milk regularly had 80 percent more risk. Source: M. G. Le et al., "Consump-tion of Dairy Produce and Alcohol in a Case-Control Study of Breast Cancer," *Journal of the National Cancer Institute* 77:633–36.

• In Japan, a 1987 experiment consisting of tests on six groups of female rats showed that adding sea vegetables to the diet had a significant inhibitory effect on induced mammary tumorigenesis. "Tumor incidences were 35 percent (7/20), 35 percent (7/20) and 50 percent (9/18), respectively [for groups fed nori, kombu, and another type of kombu], whereas that in the control group was 69 percent (20/29)," investigators reported. The onset of tumors was also delayed in the seaweed groups, and the weight of tumors was lower. Source: Ichiro Yamamoto et al., "The Effect of Dietary Seaweeds on 7,12-Dimethyl-Benz[a]Anthracene-induced Mammary Tumorigenesis in Rats," *Cancer Letters* 35:109–18.

• In a Chinese medical study in 1988, researchers found that the longer the mother nursed, the less at risk she was of breast cancer. Mimi Yu, associate professor of preventive medicine at the University of Southern California in Los Angeles, studied more than 500 Chinese women with breast cancer in Shanghai and 500 healthy women. The women she studied on an average nursed their various children for a cumulative total of nine years, a common pattern in China. "We believe that long periods of nursing would have the same protec-tive effect for American women," Yu reported. Source: "Breast-feeding Linked to Decreased Cancer Risk for Mother, Child," *Journal of the National Cancer Institute* 80:1362–63.

• Dairy food may be the most potent factor in the development of breast cancer. A 1989 study of 250 women with breast cancer in the northwestern province of Vercelli, Italy, found that they tended to consume considerably more milk, high-fat cheese, and butter than 499 healthy women of the same age in Italy and France. Breast cancer risk tripled among women who consumed about half their calories as fat, 13 to 23 percent of their calories as saturated fat, and 8 to 20 percent of their calories as animal protein. "These data suggest that during adult life, a reduction in dietary intake of fat and proteins of animal origin may contribute to a substantial reduction in the incidence of breast cancer in population subgroups with high intake of animal products," research-ers concluded. "[A] diet rich in fat, saturated fat, or animal proteins may be associated with a twofold to threefold increase in a woman's risk of breast cancer." Source: Paolo Toniolo et al., "Calorie-providing Nutrients and Risk of Breast Cancer," *Journal of the National Cancer Institute* 81:278–86.

• The incidence of breast cancer in first-generation Japanese migrants to Hawaii is about 60 percent of the rate in subsequent generations of Japanese born in Hawaii. In 1990 researchers at the Departments of Nutrition Sciences and Biostatistics/Biomathematics, University of Alabama at Birmingham, theorized that miso, natto, shoyu, and other traditionally fermented soybean foods may contribute to lowered disease. The consumption of these foods in Japan is about five times or more what it is among Japanese migrants to Hawaii. To test their hypothesis, the scientists initiated feeding trials with rats and found that feeding miso to the rats delayed the appearance of induced breast cancer compared with animals on the control diet. The miso- and salt-supplemented diet treatment group showed a trend toward a lower number of cancers per animal, a trend toward a higher number of benign tumors per animal, and a trend toward a lower growth rate of cancers compared with controls. "This data suggests that miso consumption may be a factor producing a lower breast cancer incidence in Japanese women," the researchers concluded. "Organic compounds found in fermented soybean-based foods may exert a chemoprotective effect." Source: J. E. Baggott et al., "Effect of Miso (Japanese Soybean Paste) and NaCl on DMBA-induced Rat Mammary Tumors," *Nutrition and Cancer* 14:103–9.

• In an extensive view of current diet and cancer research in 1990, a Scandinavian researcher concluded: "Western diet is the main factor causing the high incidence of hormone dependent cancers [breast, prostate, etc.] and CC [colon cancer] in the Western world." The researcher, chairman of the Department of Clinical Chemistry at the University of Helsinki, particularly cited studies of macrobiotic women in the United States who ate more whole grains and fiber than controls and enjoyed greater freedom from chronic illness. Source: Herman Adlercreutz, "Western Diet and Western Diseases: Some Hormonal and Biochemical Mechanisms and Associations," *Scandinavian Journal of Clinical Laboratory Investigations* 50: Suppl. 201:3–23.

• Whole grains, cereals, and other foods high in fiber may help protect against breast cancer. In laboratory tests, scientists at the American Health Foundation found in 1991 that a high-fiber diet reduced induced cancer in rats by about 50 percent. "We found that by doubling the amount of fiber in a diet that is similar to our Western diet, you can significantly reduce the amount of mammary cancer," concluded researcher Leonard Cohen. Sources: L. A. Cohen et al., "Modulation of N-Nitrosomethylurea-induced Mammary Tumor Promotion by Dietary Fiber and Fat," *Journal of the National Cancer Institute* 83:496–500, and "Fiber Is Linked to Reduced Breast Cancer Risk," *Boston Globe*, April 3, 1991.

• In laboratory experiments, animals fed soybeans or soy products experienced a reduction in the number of induced mammary tumors compared to controls. Source: S. Barnes et al., "Soybeans Inhibit Mammary Tumors in Models of Breast Cancer," in Pariza (ed.), *Mutagens and Carcinogens in the Diet* (New York: Wiley-Liss, 1990), 239–53.

• In a presentation before the American Cancer Society, a researcher from the University of Alabama at Birmingham reported that rats supplied a soybean-rich diet developed significantly fewer breast tumors than the control group.

Dr. Stephen Barnes reported that scientists are presently involved in collecting and analyzing different varieties of soybeans, as well as various soybean products, including tofu, tempeh, and miso, to identify how they inhibit tumor growth. Source: "Tofu Chic: The Role of Soybeans in Breast Cancer Prevention, *Oncology Times,* July 1990.

• At a workshop sponsored by the NCI in 1991 on the role of soy products in cancer prevention, medical researchers presented evidence that soybeans and soy products such as tofu, miso, and tempeh can help prevent the onset of induced cancer in laboratory animals. "The consensus of the meeting was that there are sufficient data to justify studying the impact of soybean intake on cancer risk in humans." Source: Mark Messina and Stephen Barnes, "The Role of Soy Products in Reducing Risk of Cancer," *Journal of the National Cancer Institute* 83:541–46.

• Moderately strong X ray tests, including upper gastrointestinal series and barium enemas, significantly raise the risk of breast cancer in women who carry a particular gene that occurs in more than 1 million American women. Source: M. Swift et al., "Incidence of Cancer in 161 Families Affected by Ataxia-Telangiectasia," *New England Journal of Medicine* 325(1991):1831–36.

• In 1993 scientists reported that diets rich in soyfoods, especially miso soup, produced genistein, a natural substance that blocked the growth of new blood vessels that feed a tumor. Researchers from Children's University Hospital in Heidelberg, Germany, reported that genistein also deterred cancer cells from multiplying and could have significant implications for the prevention and treatment of solid malignancies, including those of the brain, breast, and prostate. Source: "Chemists Learn Why Vegetables Are Good for You," *New York Times*, April 13, 1993.

DIAGNOSIS

A majority of breast lumps are discovered by palpitation by the woman or her partner. Although 80 percent of lumps are classified as benign, doctors like to take a soft-tissue X ray of the entire breast called a mammogram. If a malignancy is suspected, a biopsy will be taken to determine whether the growth is a cyst or a tumor. Hormone tests, X rays of the chest and skeleton, bone-marrow aspiration, and scans of gallium, liver, and bone will generally follow. Until the mid-1970s mammography was widely offered as a preventive measure to detect cancer in the early stages. However, in 1976 Dr. John Bailar III, editor of *Journal of the National Cancer Institute,* reported that breast X rays could cause as many deaths through radiation as they could save through early detection. Since then, the radiation dosage for mammography has sharply declined in many cases. The American Cancer Society currently recommends monthly breast self-examination by women 20 years or older; a screening mammogram by age 40; an annual or biennial mammogram from age 40 to 49; and an annual mammogram after age 50. In addition, a physical examination by a doctor is recommended every three years for women age 20 to 40 and annually over age 40. The mammography controversy flared up again in 1993 when the National Cancer Institute reported that a comprehensive review of data showed that there was no benefit from the procedure for women under fifty and that mammograms failed to detect up to 40 percent of tumors.

In addition to self-examination of the breasts, Oriental medicine looks for signs of developing mammary disorders in the condition and complexion of the cheeks. As a result of parallel embryonic development, the cheeks reflect underlying changes in the chest region, including the lungs and breasts, and in the reproductive region.

Cheeks with well-developed, firm flesh and a clean, clear skin color show sound respiratory and digestive functions, especially if there are no wrinkles or pimples in the area. Red or pink cheeks, except during vigorous exercise or when out in cold weather, show abnormal expansion of the blood capillaries, caused by heart and circulatory disorders due to the overconsumption of yin foods and drinks, including fruits, juices, sugar, and drugs. Milky white cheeks are caused by the overconsumption of dairy products such as milk, cheese, cream, and yogurt. A pinkish shade mixed with the white indicates excessive intake of flour products and fruits. Both these colors indicate accumulation of fat and mucus in various regions of the body, including the breasts, lungs, intestines, and reproductive organs.

Fatty spots that are dark, red, or white in color on the cheeks are a sign of fat accumulation in either the lungs or breast and often accompany the beginning of cyst or tumor formation. Coffee and other stimulant, aromatic beverages may contribute to the appearance of this color on the cheeks. Pimples on the cheeks show the elimination of excessive fat and mucus caused by the intake of animal food, dairy products, and oils and fats. If these pimples are whitish in color, the main cause is milk and sugar. If yellowish, the cause is cheese, poultry, and eggs. A green shade on the cheeks shows that cancer is developing in the breasts, lungs, or large intestine.

Certain colors and marks appearing on the white of the eye also indicate abnormal conditions in the corresponding areas of the body. In the case of the breasts, a transparent or pale white color in the upper outer region of the eye shows the presence of stagnated fat and mucus, which may be growing into a cyst or tumor. Cataracts also may indicate cyst formation. If these colorings or swellings occur in the right eye, the right breast is affected; if in the left eye, the left breast.

Green vessels appearing along the Heart Governor meridian or Lung meridian from the wrist toward the elbow on the inside, softer side of the arm also show the development of cancerous conditions in the breast or lung region. A similar condition is indicated by the appearance of green and dark colors, together with irregular swelling on the inside of the wrist.

DIETARY RECOMMENDATIONS

The primary cause of most cases of breast cancer is long-time consumption of dairy food, including milk, cheese, cottage cheese, yogurt, butter, and ice cream, along with excessive consumption of chicken, eggs, meat, and other fatty animal foods, as well as sweets, sugar, chocolate, honey, and other sweeteners and sugar-treated foods and beverages. All these foods are to be strictly

avoided. Tropical fruits, temperate-climate fruit juices, and vegetables of tropical origin such as potatoes, yams, sweet potatoes, asparagus, tomatoes, and
eggplant also should not be consumed. Because they are excessively mucus-
producing, all flour products are to be avoided except for occasional consumption of nonyeasted unleavened whole wheat or rye bread if craved.
Chemicalized and artificially produced and treated foods and beverages are to
be completely eliminated. Even unsaturated vegetable oil is to be completely
avoided or minimized in cooking for a one- or two-month period. All ice-cold
foods and drinks should be avoided. Although they are not the cause of breast
cancer, all stimulants, spices, coffee, wine and other alcoholic drinks, and
aromatic, fragrant beverages and drugs should be avoided because they enhance tumor development.

There is a type of breast cancer called inflammatory breast cancer that
appears as a red inflammation on the surface of the breast and spreads quickly.
This form of breast tumor is caused predominantly by extreme yin foods,
including excessive oil (both in cooking and salads), sugar, chocolate, and other
sweets, dairy food, fruit, stimulants, etc. The following general dietary guidelines are recommended for breast cancer.

• **Whole Grains:** 50 to 60 percent of daily consumption, by volume, should
be whole-cereal grains. The first day prepare plain pressure-cooked short-grain
brown rice. Then the next day prepare brown rice pressure-cooked with 20 to
30 percent millet, then rice with 20 to 30 percent barley, then rice with 20 to
30 percent aduki beans or lentils, and then plain brown rice again. A delicious
morning porridge can be made by taking leftover rice, adding a little more
water to soften, and seasoning with a little miso at the end and simmering for
two to three minutes more. Except for morning porridge, which may be soft,
the grain should be on the firm side, rather than creamy. In pressure cooking,
the ratio of grain to water should be about 1:2. For seasoning, cook with a small
postage stamp–sized piece of kombu instead of salt, though in some cases sea
salt may be used depending on the person's condition. Other grains can be used
occasionally, including whole wheat berries, rye, corn, and whole oats, though
oats should be avoided for the first month. Buckwheat and seitan should be
minimized. Good-quality sourdough bread (preferably steamed) may be enjoyed two to three times a week if craved, and noodles, both udon and soba,
may also be taken two to three times a week. Avoid all hard baked products
until the condition improves, including cookies, cake, pie, crackers, muffins,
and the like.

• **Soup:** 5 to 10 percent soup, consisting of one or two cups or bowls per day
of soup cooked with wakame sea vegetable and various land vegetables such as
onions and carrots and seasoned with miso or shoyu. Occasionally a small
volume of shiitake mushroom may be added to the soup. The miso may be
barley miso, brown rice miso, or soybean (hatcho) miso and should be naturally
aged two to three years. For breast cancer, millet soup with sweet vegetables
such as squash, cabbage, onions, and carrots may be prepared often. Grain
soups, bean soups, and other soups may be taken from time to time, but avoid
puréeing soups with oats. For breast cancer, the consistency of soups, and food

in general, should be neither too creamy nor too salty. If the soup is too salty, a breast lump can remain tight and not heal.

• **Vegetables:** 20 to 30 percent vegetables, cooked in a variety of forms. Root vegetables such as burdock, carrots, and daikon should be used regularly. Round vegetables such as cabbage, onions, and fall-season squash and pumpkin and hard or leafy vegetables such as watercress, broccoli, and dandelion are also recommended and can be prepared separately or together. As a rule of thumb, the following dishes may be prepared, though the frequency may differ from person to person: nishime-style vegetables, three times a week; squash-aduki-kombu dish three times a week; dried daikon, one cup, three times a week; carrots and carrot tops or daikon and daikon tops, three times a week; blanched vegetables, five to seven times a week; pressed salad, five to seven times a week; raw salad and salad dressing, avoid; steamed greens, five to seven times a week; sautéed vegetables, two to three times a week, using water the first month instead of oil, then occasionally a small volume of sesame oil may be brushed on the skillet; kinpira, sautéed in water, two-thirds of a cup, two times a week, then oil may be used after three weeks; dried tofu, tofu, tempeh, or seitan with vegetables, two times a week.

• **Beans:** Five percent small beans, such as aduki beans, lentils, chickpeas, or black soybeans, may be used daily, cooked together with sea vegetables such as kombu or with onions and carrots. Other beans may be used altogether two to three times a month. For seasoning, a small volume of unrefined sea salt or shoyu or miso can be used. Bean products, such as tempeh, natto, and dried or cooked tofu may be used occasionally, but in moderate volume. Avoid making the tofu too creamy and use firm rather than soft tofu.

• **Sea Vegetables:** Five percent or less sea vegetable dishes, including wakame and kombu, daily when cooking grain, in soup, etc. A sheet of toasted nori may also be taken daily. A small dish of hijiki or arame should be prepared two times a week. All other sea vegetables are optional.

• **Condiments:** Condiments to be available on the table are gomashio (sesame salt), on the average made with 1 part salt to 18 parts sesame seeds (reduced to 1:16 after two months); kelp or wakame powder; umeboshi plum; and tekka, though all other regular macrobiotic condiments may be used if desired. These condiments may be used daily on grains and vegetables, but the volume should be moderate to suit individual appetite and taste.

• **Pickles:** Pickles, made at home in a variety of ways, are to be eaten daily, 1 tablespoon in all, though salty pickles are to be minimized.

• **Animal Food:** Fish and other animal food is to be avoided. However, in the event that animal food is craved, a small amount of white-meat fish may be eaten once every two weeks. The fish should be prepared steamed, boiled, or poached and garnished with grated daikon or ginger. After two months, fish may be eaten once a week. Strictly avoid blue-meat and red-meat fish (especially tuna) and all shellfish.

• **Fruit:** Avoid all tropical fruits. The less temperate-climate fruit the better until the condition improves. If cravings develop, a small volume of cooked fruit with a pinch of sea salt or dried fruit (also preferably cooked) may be taken. Avoid all fruit juices and cider.

• **Sweets and Snacks:** Avoid all sweets and desserts, including good-quality macrobiotic desserts, until the condition improves. To satisfy a sweet tooth, use sweet vegetables every day in cooking, drink sweet vegetable drinks (see special drinks below), sweet vegetable jam, and amasake (up to eight ounces a week). Mochi, rice balls, vegetable sushi, and other grain-based snacks may be eaten frequently. Limit rice cakes, popcorn, and other dry or baked snacks, as they may harden the tumor. In the event of cravings, a small volume of barley malt or rice syrup may be taken.

• **Nuts and Seeds:** Nuts and nut butters are to be avoided due to their high amount of fat and protein, except for chestnuts. Unsalted, roasted seeds such as sunflower seeds and pumpkin seeds may be consumed as a snack, up to one cup altogether per week.

• **Seasonings:** Seasonings, such as unrefined sea salt, shoyu, and miso, are to be used moderately in order to avoid unnecessary thirst. Avoid mirin and garlic. If you become particularly thirsty after a meal or between meals, you should cut back on these seasonings until the normal level of thirst returns.

• **Beverages.** Beverage consumption and other dietary practices can follow the general recommendations in Part I, including bancha twig tea as the main drink with the meal. Strictly avoid the beverages on the "infrequent" and "avoid" list and don't take grain coffee for the first two to three months after starting this new way of eating.

In the event of hunger pains, which women sometimes get with this condition, one or two balls of brown rice with half an umeboshi plum put inside and wrapped with toasted nori may be eaten. However, less overall eating may be beneficial. In some cases, skipping breakfast for a day or on the weekend is very beneficial for breast cancer and many other conditions.

The most important thing in connection with dietary practice is chewing very well, until all food becomes liquid in the mouth and well mixed with saliva. Chew very, very well, at least 50 times, preferably 100 times, per mouthful. It is also important to avoid overeating and eating within three hours of sleeping.

As noted in the introduction to Part II, persons who have received or who are currently undergoing medical treatment may need to make further dietary modifications.

SPECIAL DRINKS AND DISHES

Several special drinks or side dishes may need to be taken, depending on the individual case. Please see a qualified macrobiotic teacher for guidance. Amounts and frequencies given here are averages; these will differ from person to person.

• **Sweet Vegetable Drink:** Take one small cup every day for the first month, then every other day the second month, and then several times a week after that as desired.

• **Carrot-Daikon Drink:** Take one small cup every day, every other day, or every third day for the first ten to fourteen days depending on the case. Then reduce the amount by about half for the next two weeks and then stop.

• **Ume-Sho-Kudzu Drink:** Take one small cup two times a week for four to six weeks and then stop.

• **Lotus Root–Kombu Drink:** Grate fresh lotus root, cook with a small amount of kombu, and add water and a little shoyu at the end. Take one cup every three days for one to two weeks.

• **Grated Daikon:** Grate about one half a small cup of fresh daikon, add a few drops of shoyu, and take two to three times a week.

HOME CARES

• **Body Scrub:** Scrubbing the whole body, including the abdominal region and the spinal region, with a towel that has been immersed in hot water and squeezed out is very helpful for better circulation of blood, lymph, and other body fluids, as well as for activating physical and mental energies.

• **Compress Guidelines:** For a small number of breast tumors, a compress may be needed to gradually help draw the excess mucus and fat from the inner parts of the mammary tissues toward the surface of the skin. Eventually, the fatty mucus, sticky substances, and unclean blood that make up the tumor will dissolve and discharge through the skin or urine and bowel. Please see a qualified macrobiotic teacher for guidance on the proper use and frequency of a compress or plaster. Several types are used depending on the person's condition. Precede the compress or plaster with application over the affected area of a towel that has been soaked in hot water and squeezed out for about three to five minutes to stimulate circulation.

• **Green Vegetable Compress:** Mix about 50 percent green clay and 50 percent finely chopped and ground up cabbage leaves or other natural plant leaves and apply over the area to help facilitate the discharge of accumulated toxic matter. A little water may be added to the mixture if it is too dry. (Good-quality clay can usually be obtained in the cosmetic section of a natural foods store.) The clay-cabbage compress may be left in place about four hours or overnight, and it may be applied daily for up to one month and then as needed.

• **Miso–Brown Rice Plaster:** Mash cooked brown rice; mix with 50 percent miso paste and 5 percent grated ginger. Mix in a mortar if necessary. Place a two-centimeter–thick layer of this mixture on a cotton cloth and then place the cloth directly on the affected area of the breast. Leave for three hours or longer, or keep on overnight until waking up in the morning. Can also be applied to swollen lymph nodes in the neck and shoulder region if necessary.

• **Kombu Plaster:** Soak kombu in water ten to twenty minutes, until soft, and then mash. Mix together with one-third vegetable greens and one-third grated ginger. Add a little flour and water. Put this paste directly on the breast, cover with cotton and a cloth bandage, and keep on for three hours. Reduce the ginger if burning is felt. Apply every day for two weeks and then as needed.

• **Buckwheat Plaster:** In cases where a breast has already been surgically removed and the surrounding lymph nodes, neck, and in some cases arm have become swollen, a buckwheat plaster can be applied separately following a brief (two- to three-minute) application of a ginger compress.

• **Medical Attention:** In the event the lymph glands under the armpit and along the arm become swollen due to the cancer spreading from the breast through the lymph system, medical attention is often necessary. Again, a qualified macrobiotic teacher, nutritionist, or medical associate or professional should be consulted. Massage is often helpful in reducing such swelling.

OTHER CONSIDERATIONS

• Breast cancer patients are subject to depression and should do everything possible to maintain a cheerful and calm attitude. Smile, be optimistic, dance, sing, and enjoy each day for itself.

• In addition to the daily body scrub, soaking the feet at night in hot water, or occasionally in hot gingerroot water, will help bring down the energy of the body and help eliminate excess through the skin.

• Avoid wearing wool and synthetic fibers. At the minimum wear cotton underwear and use cotton sheets and pillowcases.

• Avoid wearing metallic jewelry, including rings, bracelets, and necklaces. These pick up excess charges from the atmosphere and transmit them to the internal organs via the meridians running along the fingers and hands. It is fine, though, to wear a wedding ring.

• Avoid watching television for long stretches. Radiation weakens the chest area. Similarly, avoid other artificial sources of electromagnetic energy such as video terminals, smoke detectors, and hand-held electrical appliances.

• If possible, avoid birth-control pills and estrogen additive therapy. These are extremely weakening and can accelerate breast cancer. Doctors will sometimes recommend estrogen drugs because in medical tests it has been shown that older women taking estrogen get less heart disease and more women in old age die from heart disease than breast cancer. From an energetic view, most heart disease results from intake of overly yang foods like meat, poultry, and eggs, so estrogen, which is classified as extremely yin, will help reduce risk of heart attack and stroke. However, it contributes to increased risk of breast cancer, which is caused by too much yin. Women who adopt a macrobiotic way of eating commonly experience a rapid improvement in blood values, including reduced cholesterol levels. There is therefore no need to take estrogen to protect against heart ailments if you are eating predominantly grains and vegetables.

• Breast-feed your baby if you are able. There is no danger of transmitting breast cancer to your child, and breast-feeding will have a protective effect on both mother and baby.

PERSONAL EXPERIENCE

Metatastic Breast Cancer

In October 1972, Phyllis W. Crabtree, a fifty-year-old homemaker, nursery school teacher, and grandmother from Philadelphia, had an operation for cancer in which her uterus, ovaries, and Fallopian tubes were removed. By January 1973, the tumor metastasized, and she had a modified radical mastectomy of the right breast.

In the hospital, her son Philip, who had studied macrobiotic cooking, brought her miso soup, brown rice, and bancha tea. The first food offered Phyllis by the hospital had been a bowl of Froot Loops.

Breast surgery was a very frightening experience for her. "One of the most terrifying is the signing of that paper which gives a doctor the right to cut out or off any part that he deems necessary," she observed afterward. "By the time I was admitted for the mastectomy, it was my fourth admission in ten weeks, my fourth signing, and this time I knew what they were going to take. For each operation, there was an initial trip for biopsy, an okay from the frozen section, and then a return trip for surgery when more lab work had been completed. Another very simple hospital procedure that was sheer horror for me was the presurgical shave and shower. Watching the surgical nurse shave my chest from armpit to armpit and washing my breasts for what might have been the last time was a very emotional procedure. Before the biopsy, as I washed (and the tears flowed almost as fast as the shower) I wondered if I would have none, one, or two the next day." Mrs. Crabtree was so distraught from the experience that she had to see a psychiatrist afterward to help her deal with her loss.

Over the next three years, she gradually began to implement macrobiotics with the support of her son, daughter, and husband. She cut out sugar from her diet, increased vegetables, and reduced her intake of red meat, dairy food, and martinis. In the summer of 1976, however, the newspapers and television were filled with stories about a connection between cancer and contraceptives and hormone medication. Mrs. Crabtree, who had taken these drugs, became depressed again and suspected that cancer was spreading to her liver.

Once again her son impressed upon her the need to follow the diet closely and to take full responsibility for her condition and recovery. In March 1977, she attended the EWF cancer and diet conference in Boston and came to see me. "I listened and had an appointment with Michio Kushi," she recalled later. "One phrase from the classroom kept haunting me: 'There are no cancer victims, only cancer producers.' Michio recommended a healing diet and sent me off to eat far more strictly than ever before."

The next summer Mrs. Crabtree returned, and I told her that she was 60 percent healed and to continue eating carefully. By autumn of 1978, Phyllis had completed the five-year "cure" period for her original illness and outlived 85 percent of women who had had similar operations on uterus and breast.

"I'm grateful to macrobiotics for more than a cancer 'cure,' " she stated. "For myself, there had been an improvement in my aching back (caused by osteoporosis) and a urinary infection (both ailments of thirty years' duration). The migraine headaches are fewer in number and less in intensity and duration. Even my motion sickness has lessened.

"My husband has benefited from the diet through weight control. Michio's lectures in Los Angeles many years ago were instrumental in returning Phil to us from his 'hippy' world. My daughter adopted a baby girl because she had been unable to conceive. She now has three daughters, two of them 'macrobiotically brewed.' "

Source: Phyllis W. Crabtree, "A Grandmother Heals Herself," *East West Journal*, November 1978, 74–81.

Breast Cancer

In February 1986, Anne Kramer was diagnosed with breast cancer and underwent a modified radical mastectomy of her left breast. Doctors found metastatic carcinoma in four lymph nodes, plus microscopic tumor emboli in small auxiliary blood vessels. "My oncologist recommended chemotherapy for a year, possibly longer," Anne recalls. "A second opinion from another oncologist was the same—a year or more of chemotherapy. He suggested that I probably had several thousand cancer cells floating around in my bloodstream. It wasn't a happy picture." Meanwhile, a routine hospital blood test revealed her cholesterol level to be 243.

While recovering from the mastectomy, Anne started to read about scientific research relating diets high in fat content to breast cancer. One study reported that Japanese women eating traditionally had a much lower incidence of breast cancer and a lower recurrence rate compared to Western women eating standard American high-fat foods. Anne decided she wanted to try a low-fat dietary approach, but was too weak from chemotherapy to begin. After three months of treatment, including Tamoxifen, she learned about macrobiotics from a friend and began to read *The Cancer Prevention Diet*. "I read the book and immediately started cooking meals recommended for my illness," Anne explains. "I knew this macrobiotic diet was what I was looking for. I believed it would help me heal myself of breast cancer. My feelings of helplessness went away. I became more optimistic about the outcome of my disease."

At first, it was not easy to shop and prepare the new foods, especially since Anne had almost no energy and felt sick and nauseated most of the time. She attributed this to the chemotherapy treatments. "At least I didn't have to worry about getting hair in the food," she looks back. "I didn't have any left on my head! I believed in this new diet and followed the directions strictly. Aveline Kushi's peaceful recipes made me feel calm and in charge of my getting well." Anne also performed visualization exercises three times a day.

After two months on the diet, Anne went in for another mammogram on her right breast. She was anxious because her doctor had warned her of the possibility of new tumors where calcification spots had been found. "The mammograms revealed that the calcification spots were gone! I was elated."

In September 1986, Anne decided to stop chemotherapy despite the opposition of her oncologist. "My mind rebelled at the thought of another six months of that poison," she observes. "On several occasions the doctor couldn't perform chemotherapy treatments on me because my white blood cell count was dangerously low. I promised my body I would not undergo any further chemotherapy treatments."

Later that fall Anne met Bonnie Breidenbach, a macrobiotic teacher in the Detroit area who helped her fine-tune her diet. Bonnie also told her about a doctor who had a therapy group for cancer patients. She attended the group sessions for awhile and found sharing her feelings and experiences on the diet very encouraging and supportive.

It is now almost seven years later and Anne is healthy. Repeated mammograms, bone scans, chest x-rays, and blood tests have shown no trace of cancer. Anne is in her early sixties, her cholesterol reading is 170, and she has enrolled in the Kushi Institute Extension Program in Cleveland to learn more about macrobiotics. "I enjoy the program and I'm enjoying life. I am grateful that my husband is supportive and went on the diet with me from the start. I am also grateful that my child, grandchildren, and eighty-nine-year-old mother are benefiting from this diet as well. I am also thankful to God for giving me illness and health to help me appreciate life."

Source: Ann Fawcett and the East West Foundation, *Cancer-Free: 30 Who Triumphed Over Cancer Naturally* (Japan Publications, 1992).

12

Lung Cancer

FREQUENCY

In the last several decades, the incidence of lung cancer has risen more sharply in the United States than that of any other form of cancer. Today it is the leading cause of cancer deaths in both men and women, accounting for 28 percent of all cancer deaths in 1991. In men, incidence fell slightly for the first time in 1984, reflecting several decades of reduced smoking and reduced fat consumption. From 1950 to 1977 incidence in American women more than tripled, from 4 per 100,000 to 15 and has been increasing 4 to 5 percent a year since then (44 percent between 1979 and 1986). In the late 1980s, lung cancer surpassed breast cancer as the most lethal malignancy among women (as women's rates of smoking and fat consumption continued to rise). Three out of five lung cancer patients are men, usually between the ages of forty and seventy. Altogether lung cancer will kill an estimated 146,000 Americans this year and 168,000 new cases will develop. In other parts of the world, incidence differs widely. In Scotland, for instance, it is about twice as high as in the United States. In Portugal, lung cancer occurs only one-eighth as frequently.

Lung cancers commonly spread to or from the liver, brain, or bone. Ninety percent of cases consist of four types: 1) *epidermoid carcinomas*, which are located centrally and spread by invasion to nearby tissues; 2) *adenocarcinomas*, which usually affect only one lobe of the lung but spread to other sites; 3) *large-cell carcinomas*, which are similar to adenocarinomas; and 4) *oat-cell carcinomas*, which are fast-growing. Early detection of lung cancer is not common, and 50 percent of tumors are considered inoperable. Surgery followed by radiation treatment is favored by the medical profession for the first three types. This may take the form of a lobectomy, involving removal of a lobe, or a pneumonectomy, removal of the entire lung. Oat-cell carcinoma is treated with chemotherapy. Drugs may also be given to those with the other forms of tumors to control pain. Overall 13 percent of men and women with lung cancer currently survive five years or more. Chemotherapy for oat-cell carcinoma may produce regression lasting one to two years.

STRUCTURE

The lungs are twin respiratory organs situated along with the heart in the thoracic cavity. They are conical in shape and divided into five lobes. There are three on the right side and two on the left. The lobes are further subdivided into bronchi and alveoli. The alveoli consist of thousands of tiny air sacs. During breathing, oxygen enters the lungs and is picked up by the blood. The surface of the alveoli contains an array of blood vessels that total about 100 square yards. Oxygenated blood goes to the heart, from which it is pumped through the arteries to the cells. In the body's cells, oxygen combines with metabolized sugar or fat to produce energy, leaving behind carbon dioxide and water as by-products. The carbon dioxide is picked up by the blood and carried to the lungs, where it is breathed out. The lungs are also a major site for receiving electromagnetic energy from the surrounding environment and for stimulating certain digestive processes, especially the eliminatory function of the large intestine.

CAUSE OF CANCER

Modern medicine has focused considerable attention on lung cancer because of its steady increase. Cigarette smoking has been cited as the major cause, and epidemiologists say up to 80 or 90 percent of lung tumors could be prevented by eliminating tobacco. Other researchers have noted an association between lung cancer and increased pollution in the environment or workplace. In Houston, for example, lung cancer deaths increased by 53 percent during the 1970s. This seemed to correspond with a boom of petrochemical plants and refineries in the area. Lung cancer is also higher among asbestos workers, copper miners, and those who work with lead and zinc. In the last several years, the role of diet in protecting against lung cancer has received increased attention. Several medical studies show that people who regularly consume carrots and dark green or yellow vegetables containing beta-carotene, a precursor to vitamin A, have lower lung cancer rates than other people.

Each of these hypotheses is related to understanding the spread of lung cancer. However, the underlying cause of the disease is not smoking, pollution, or a temporary vitamin deficiency, but rather a long-time imbalance in the entire daily way of eating. Situated in the middle region of the body, the lungs are relatively balanced in structure, combining both expanded (yin) and contracted (yang) features. Respiratory disorders, including lung tumors, result from excessive intake of extreme foods from both the yin and yang categories, including meat, eggs, poultry, dairy products, refined flour, sugar, fats and oils, fruits and juices, alcohol, stimulants, chemicals, and drugs.

As we have seen in the progressive development of disease, excess intake of acid, mucous-forming, and fatty foods eventually results in accumulations in various parts of the body, including the sinuses, inner ear, breasts, lungs, and kidney and reproductive organs. In the case of the lungs, aside from the obvious symptoms of coughing and chest congestion, mucus often fills the air sacs, and breathing becomes more difficult. Occasionally, a coat of mucus in the bronchi can be loosened and discharged by coughing, but once the sacs are surrounded it becomes more firmly lodged and can remain there for a long period. Then, if air pollutants or cigarette smoke enters the lungs, their heavy components, especially various carbon compounds, are attracted to and remain in this sticky environment. In severe cases, these deposits can give rise to tumors. However, the underlying cause of this condition is the accumulation of sticky fat and mucus in the alveoli and in the blood and capillaries surrounding them.

The subject of tobacco and its role in cancer is best understood in relation to daily diet. For centuries North American Indians have smoked tobacco without developing cancer and have utilized the plant for many medicinal purposes. One of the main differences between the Indian's use of tobacco and our own is that they ate a balanced diet high in corn and other cereal grains, wild grasses, locally grown or foraged vegetables, fresh seasonal fruit, seeds, and a small to moderate amount of fresh game. Current studies suggest that in societies where a traditional way of eating is still followed and where smoking is widespread there is no clear correlation between smoking and lung cancer.

The quality of modern tobacco is also a contributing factor in the increase of respiratory illnesses. The original Indian tobacco was grown naturally without phosphate fertilizers or artificial pesticides and was air-dried. Modern flue-cured tobacco is subjected to heavy amounts of chemicals during cultivation, and the drying process is sped up from about three months to six days. Commercial cigarettes also often contain 5 to 20 percent sugar by weight, as well as humectants to retain moisture and other synthetic additives to enhance flavor and taste. In countries where tobacco is not flue-cured or mixed with sugar, such as Russia, China, and Taiwan, medical studies generally indicate no significant correlation between smoking and lung cancer. Laboratory studies also show that mice on a low-fat diet will not get lung cancer from smoking but when put on a high-fat diet will develop tumors. Thus chemically refined tobacco and a diet high in fat, sugar, oil, and other sticky foods will combine synergistically and increase the risk of lung cancer.

Similarly, a healthy pair of lungs can withstand and neutralize a great deal of air pollution, metallic dust, or chemical irritants in the environment. This is why nonsmokers who eat a balanced diet are usually not bothered physically by cigarette smoke in their vicinity. Their lungs are working properly and naturally filter airborne particulates with no perceived discomfort. However, nonsmokers whose lungs are coated with fat, mucus, and acid from eating a meat and sugar diet or a vegetarian diet high in dairy foods and sweets will often feel irritated as these particles from the smoke enter and are trapped in their lungs. Of course, cigarette pollution should be avoided, and insofar as possible, it is not advisable to work in or live near chemical industries or hazardous waste sites. However, some people are relatively more immune than others to toxic substances owing to their daily diet and physical constitution or inherited characteristics formed primarily by their mother's diet during pregnancy.

In Far Eastern medicine, tobacco is classified as a yang substance due to its contracting and drying effects. Smokers are generally thinner (more yang) than nonsmokers, and most smokers put on weight (become more yin) when they stop. Thus smoking contracts the body and has an alkalizing effect on the blood. As the Indians found, pure tobacco used in moderation can have a soothing effect and can increase immunity to colds, infections, and chronic ailments brought about by an overly acidic condition.

The principles of contraction (yang) and expansion (yin) can also be used to understand why many people in modern society are attracted to smoking and why they abuse tobacco by consuming it in far greater quantities than the Indians. Nicotine, the major ingredient in tobacco, is very yang. Farmers in the South have often sprayed tobacco juice on crops to ward off parasites and prevent blights. In the body, a similar process occurs. Disease-promoting bacteria cannot thrive in an alkaline environment. The human blood is normally slightly alkaline in pH. A daily diet of whole grains, cooked vegetables, and seasonal fruit produces this slightly yang condition. However, the modern diet containing a large percentage of meat and sugar has a net effect of making the blood acid. Acid-forming foods also include eggs, poultry, dairy products, refined flour and flour products, and stimulants. In order to restore proper pH and balance acidic (yin) blood, the body is physiologically attracted to nicotine (yang). Biochemically, nicotine raises sugar levels in the blood. Chain smokers are often hypoglycemic and suffer from low blood sugar and their daily diet also lacks complex carbohydrates. This condition is brought about by intake of excessive fat, protein, sugar, or alcohol and can result in pancreatic and liver malfunction, weak adrenals, and erratic emotional behavior. The weaker the blood, the greater the desire to smoke. The more one smokes, the more carbon monoxide is produced in the blood and the harder the heart has to work.

In addition to excessive yang effects, smoking can produce excessive yin effects. Recent studies reported that smoking can increase a person's risk of leukemia by 30 percent. New studies have also found that smokers experience greater memory loss and ability to concentrate than nonsmokers. Both leukemia and memory loss are classified as strong yin characteristics, evidently arising from the sugar and chemicals added to modern cigarettes.

The Indians smoked at most only a handful of cigarettes a day and often went for long periods without smoking at all. And, of course, their tobacco did not contain sugar or chemicals. Throughout history, almost all traditional societies around the world existed happily without tobacco, and there is no biological necessity to smoke. Perhaps the North American Indians alone were attracted to this extreme yang pastime because their own staple food, corn, is the most expanded, yin form of grain and this was the way they had found to achieve a balance with their natural environment.

The unifying principle of yin and yang helps us to understand the physiology of smoking and the synergistic role chemicalized tobacco plays in overworking the circulatory and respiratory systems and promoting lung cancer. Though aggravated by tobacco, the epidemic of lung cancer in the West is primarily a disease of overnutrition and corresponds with the rise of chemical agriculture and changing patterns of food consumption, especially following World War II. Return to a daily way of eating centered on whole grains, vegetables, locally grown fruit, and a minimum of animal products will make lung cancer as rare an occurrence as it was in the early part of the century. The vitamin A and beta-carotene contained in certain foods are protective, though they are some examples of several nutritional elements beneficial to the lungs. Establishment of a regionally based natural system of agriculture will result in a substantial reduction of pollution in the environment as well as improved health. Less chemicals will be needed for crops, less petroleum for transcontinental shipment of produce and livestock, and less mining of metals for heavy farm equipment.

In exploring the roots of lung cancer, we find that many social problems are also related to the way we eat, and these problems cannot be resolved apart from changing our daily way of eating.

MEDICAL EVIDENCE

• In 1773 Bernard Payrilhe, professor of chemistry at Ecole Santé and professor-royal of the College of Surgery in Paris, urged that cancer be treated by drinking carrot juice. His proposal won first prize from the Academy of Lyon on the subject of "what is cancer?" In a treatise on cancer four years later, he wrote that "with respect to medicinal ailments, barley, rice, etc. will be of great use." Sources: B. Peyrilhe, M.D., *A Dissertation on Cancerous Diseases* (London, 1777), and Michael Shimkin, *Contrary to Nature* (Washington, DC: National Institutes of Health, 1977), 183.

• In the early twentieth century, cancer began to appear among North American Indians as they began to adopt the diet of modern society. In the 1920s, J. L. Bulkley, M.D., a physician who lived among native Alaskans for twelve years, reported that he did not see a trace of cancer and attributed their lack of degenerative disease to a balanced diet. "The common cereals, which they raised, were ground and baked in the ashes of their fires, unleavened, and with little if any seasoning other than salt." A U.S. government official who helped compile health statistics among tribes in the continental United States noted: "Originally the Indians lived mostly on wild game and fish, with corn and dried berries, but, of course, as their conditions have changed, their diet has changed with them. . . . Like the white man, they now live very largely from tin cans and paper bags. . . . During the first years of my service, the scarcity of cancer among the Indians was a subject of comment. Now cases frequently come to my notice." Source: J. L. Bulkley, M.D., "Cancer among Primitive Tribes," *Cancer* 4(1927):289–95.

• In 1958 Hugh Sinclair, a researcher at Oxford University in England, reported that rats will not develop lung cancer by smoking alone, controlling for other factors. "Just let someone feed a rat a high-meat diet, rich in peroxide fat, and see how quickly it gets lung cancer when it smokes cigarettes." Source: Wayne Martin, *Medical Heroes and Heretics* (Old Greenwich, CT.: Devin-Adair, 1977), 84.

• A 1967 study indicated that vitamin A protected against cancer in laboratory animals. Of 113 hamsters dosed with a tumor-inducing chemical, one of sixty animals treated with vitamin A developed lung cancer, while sixteen of fifty-three controls got cancer. Source: U. Saffiotti et al., "Experimental Cancer of the Lung," *Cancer* 20: 857–64.

• After twenty years of tobacco research, Dr. Richard Passey of London's Chester Beatty Research Institute reported an association between flue-dried tobacco, especially that to which sugar had been added, and lung cancer. However, he found no significant link between traditional sugar-free, air-dried tobacco and cancer. In one experiment, he gave twenty flue-cured high-sugar cigarettes a day to a group of twelve rats and twenty air-dried low-sugar cigarettes to another dozen rats. On the sixty-second day, three rats in the flue-cured group had died. The other high-sugar rats were too weak to continue the experiment and four more died shortly thereafter. The dead rats had lung lesions and cancerous changes. At this point, the daily quota of the air-dried low-sugar group was increased to forty cigarettes day. After 251 days, six healthy survivors remained. Three died of heatstroke, two died of undetermined causes, and one had an abscess near the kidney but not the lungs. Epidemiological studies show that England and Wales, which have the highest male lung cancer rate in the world, also have the highest sugar content in cigarettes, about 17 percent. France, where tobacco is air-dried and contains only 2 percent sugar, has one-third less lung cancer. The United States, where sugar in tobacco averages 10 percent, has one-half the male lung cancer mortality rate of Great Britain. Still, the U.S. tobacco industry reportedly is the nation's second largest consumer of sugar, after the canning industry. "Investigators from some other countries where cigarettes are made of air-dried tobacco—the Soviet Union, China, and Taiwan, among them—are unable to find any correlation between smoking and cancer." Source: "Tobacco: Is There a 'Cure' for Cancer?", *Medical World News*, March 16, 1973, 17–19.

• In 1977 a case-control study in Singapore among Chinese women found that those who consumed green, leafy vegetables rich in vitamin A were about one-half as likely to contact lung cancer as other women. Source: R. MacLennan et al., "Risk Factors for Lung Cancer in Singapore Chinese, a Population with High Female Incidence Rates," *International Journal of Cancer* 20:854–60.

• In 1978 epidemiologists reported that cancer of the lung, breast, and colon increased two to three times among Japanese women between 1950 and 1975. During that period, milk consumption increased 15 times, meat, eggs, and poultry consumption climbed 7.5 times, and rice consumption dropped 70 percent. In Okinawa, with the highest proportion of centenarians, longevity was associated with lowered sugar and salt intake and higher intake of protein and green-yellow vegetables. Source: Y. Kagawa, "Impact of Westernization on the Nutrition of Japan," *Preventive Medicine* 7:205–17.

• In 1979 an epidemiologist visiting Shanghai reported that "Chinese scientists are not convinced that cigarette smoking is the major cause of lung cancer." According to medical statistics, smokers in China are only slightly more susceptible to lung cancer than nonsmokers and "the effect of cigarette smoking disappeared after controlling for chronic bronchitis." Source: B. Henderson, "Observations in Cancer Etiology in China," *National Cancer Institute Monograph* 53:59–65.

• In 1981 a case-control study of 375 women in Hawaii indicated that "cigarette smoking is clearly not the only cause, nor even the major cause, of lung cancer in all populations of women." The researchers found that native Hawaiians who smoked had a 10.5 relative risk of lung cancer, women of Japanese origin 4.9, and those of Chinese origin 1.8. The researchers speculated that dietary factors were possibly the primary cause of lung cancer and that smoking was a contributing factor. Source: M. W. Hinds et al., "Differences in Lung Cancer Risk from Smoking among Japanese, Chinese, and Hawaiian Women in Hawaii," *International Journal of Cancer* 27:297–302.

• A 1981 Chicago study found that regular consumption of foods containing carotene, a precursor to vitamin A, protected against lung cancer. Over a period of nineteen years, a group of 1,954 men at a Western Electric plant were monitored, and those who regularly consumed carrots, dark green lettuce, spinach, broccoli, kale, Chinese cabbage, peaches, apricots, and other carotene-rich foods had significantly lower lung cancer rates than controls. Source: R. B. Shekelle et al., "Dietary Vitamin A and Risk of Cancer in the Western Electric Study," *Lancet* 2:1185–90.

• In 1982 a British medical researcher reviewed epidemiological studies in Wales, England, the United States, Sweden, Japan, Singapore, and Thailand and concluded that tobacco was not the major cause of lung cancer. "Recorded increases in lung cancer in both sexes during this century are enormously larger than those expected from the changes in tobacco consumption . . . factors other than smoking must have been the dominant causes. . . ." Source: P. R. J. Burch, "Cigarette Smoking and Lung Cancer: A Continuing Controversy," *Medical Hypotheses* 9:293–306.

• In 1986, the U.S. Surgeon-General reported that the passive inhalation of cigarette smoke by nonsmokers was associated with lung cancer. Earlier, a British study found that nonsmokers exposed to smoke contracted lung cancer twice as often as those not exposed. Source: *Health Consequences of Involuntary Smoking: A Report of the Surgeon General,* Washington, D.C., 1986, and J. L. Repace, "Consistency of Research Data on Passive Smoking and Lung Cancer," *Lancet* 1(1984):506.

• In a review of the relation of diet, lifestyle, and lung cancer in 1987, researchers found that calories from dietary fat were highly significantly associated with lung cancer mortality. For example, male lung cancer deaths are highest in Western European countries, where a high-fat diet is consumed, and lowest in Thailand, the Philippines, Honduras, Guatemala, and Japan, all countries where a low-fat diet is eaten. While noting that smoking is still the major causative factor of lung cancer, the scientists theorized that a high-fat diet might also trigger the process by which cigarette smoke is harmful to the lungs. It is conceivable that "tobacco smoke is readily oxidized to the ultimate carcinogen as a consequence of a high-fat diet." Source: Ernst L. Wynder, James R. Hebert, and Geoffrey Kabat, "Association of Dietary Fat and Lung Cancer," *Journal of the National Cancer Institute* 79:631–37.

• In a 1991 study of several thousand Finnish men, researchers reported a 60 percent lower rate of lung cancer among men who ate diets high in grains, vegetables, and fruits containing carotenoids, vitamin C, and vitamin E. Source: P. Knekt et al., "Dietary Antioxidants and the Risk of Lung Cancer," *American Journal of Epidemiology* 134:471–79.

• In a 1991 case-control study, men with lung cancer, bladder cancer, prostate cancer, larynx cancer, colorectum cancer, and esophagael cancer had from 10 to 24 percent lower intake of vegetables and fruits high in carotene than controls. Source: W. C. Ruth et al., "A Case-Control Study of Dietary Carotene in Men with Lung Cancer and in Men with Other Epithelial Cancers," *Nutrition and Cancer* 15, no.1:63–68.

• In a 1991 Italian study, researchers reported that diet may modify the carcinogenic effect of tobacco in lung cancer. An ecological analysis carried out by the American Health Foundation showed a positive association between lung cancer mortality rates in forty-three countries and dietary fats. In southern Italy people tend to consume more vegetable-quality foods, including cereals, pulses, fruit, vegetables, and vegetable oil, while those in northern Italy tend to consume more animal foods, including beef, eggs, butter, milk, and cheese. The lung cancer rate in southern Italy, however, was almost half that of northern Italy, though the proportion of smokers was slightly higher in the south. The researchers concluded: "Our data suggest that the effect of smoking alone on the development of lung cancer might be modified by dietary habits, in particular the total amount of saturated and polyunsaturated fats and fruit and vegetables consumed." Source: Emanuela Taioli et al., "Possible Role of Diet as Host Factors in the Aetiology of Tobacco-induced Lung Cancer," *International Journal of Epidemiology* 20, no. 3:611–14.

• In further studies of the twenty-four-year cohort study of 1,878 men employed by the Western Electric Company in Chicago, researchers reported in 1991 that men who ingested 500 milligrams or more of dietary cholesterol a day faced almost twice the risk of lung cancer as those who ate less than 500 milligrams. Eggs were singled out as the chief cause. Source: R. B. Shekelle et al., "Dietary Cholesterol and Incidence of Lung Cancer," *American Journal of Epidemiology* 134:480–84.

• A nonsmoking woman faces a 30 percent higher risk of lung cancer if her husband smokes, according to a three-year study of the effects of passive smoking. Source: *Cancer Epidemiology, Biomarkers & Prevention*, January 1992 and Jane E. Brody, "New Study Strongly Links Passive Smoking and Cancer," *New York Times*, January 8, 1992.

DIAGNOSIS

Doctors employ a variety of means to test for lung cancer, including chest X rays, chest tomogram, bone, liver, and gallium scans, fluoroscopy, bronchoscopy, and sputum examination. If tumors are indicated, their location will be sought by various types of biopsies as well as thoracoscopy, a surgical procedure in which the lung is deflated and examined, or a mediastinoscopy, a small incision in the front of the neck by which lymph nodes are removed for examination.

Oriental medicine diagnoses the condition of the lungs by observing their corresponding region of the face: the cheeks. Weak and underactive lungs, as well as tuberculosis, are indicated by a sallow, pale, or slightly puffy appearance on the cheeks. The person often experiences poor circulation, labored breathing, weak chest muscles accompanied by rounding and tensing of the shoulders, a drooping posture, and an inclination toward anemia or overweight. Over time, this condition of the lungs can lead to pleurisy, emphysema, asthma, and possible lung or breast cancer. This form of lung condition results from excessive consumption of hard fats, particularly eggs and cheese as well as dry, baked, and salty foods, which lead to excessive fluid consumption, the lack of fresh or lightly cooked crisp green vegetables, excessive smoking, and a lack of exercise.

An excessive and hyperactive functioning of the lungs is reflected by a variety of other signs. These include pimples on the cheeks, showing excesive storage of fatty acid and mucus as a result primarily of dairy food and sugar. White cheeks indicate excessive animal fats from dairy foods. Red cheeks show overactive blood capillaries in the lungs caused by too much fruit and juices, spices, sugar, and coffee or tea. A drawn, overly tight appearance on the cheeks is produced by overconsumption of salt, fish, or poultry as well as dry or baked goods. This drawn appearance sometimes includes vertical lines on the cheeks indicating restricted blood flow, contracted alveoli, and tightened chest muscles and may lead to pneumonia. Brown blotches on the cheeks represent acidosis resulting from sugar consumption, and this is a serious precancerous condition. Green colorations on the cheeks or a light green shadow on the outer vertical edges of the cheeks is a sign of breast or lung cancer. Beauty marks show a past fever in the lungs and moles on the cheeks indicate excess protein and sugar intake. The various signs of excess mucus and fat storage in the lungs can indicate developing allergies, nasal congestion, bronchitis, whooping cough, tuberculosis, or cancer. Overactive lungs are often accompanied by constipation or other difficulties in the large intestine, the lung's complementary opposite organ.

A skilled Oriental diagnostician will also examine the person's lung meridian, which runs along the arms and the seam between the thumb and first finger, for colors and blemishes. One common sign of lung problems is a weakness or tension in the thumb, the ending of the lung meridian. The practitioner of Far Eastern medicine will also take pulses on the wrist and press the abdominal, chest, and back regions to substantiate the visual diagnosis and diagnose the exact type of lung ailment.

DIETARY RECOMMENDATIONS

Lung tumors are one of the deeper forms of cancer, and usually the lungs are filled in part or in whole with mucus and fatty substances. The primary cause of lung cancer is dairy food, especially cheese. To prevent and relieve lung cancer, first, all extreme foods from the yang category are to be avoided or minimized, including meat, poultry, eggs, dairy products, and seafood, as well as baked flour products. It is also necessary to avoid extreme foods and beverages from the yin category, including sugar and all other sweets, fruits and juices, spices and stimulants, and alcohol and other drugs, as well as all artificial, chemicalized, and refined food. In preparing food, beware of using an excessive volume of oil. However, after the first month of starting the macrobiotic approach, during which no oil should be used, a reasonable amount of unrefined vegetable oil may frequently be used in sautéing vegetables. No raw, uncooked foods should be eaten. Dietary recommendations for daily consumption, by volume, should be as follows.

• **Whole Grains:** Fifty to 60 percent of daily consumption, by volume, should be whole-cereal grains. The first dry prepare plain pressure-cooked short-grain brown rice. On subsequent days, brown rice pressure-cooked with 20 to 30 percent millet, then rice with 20 to 30 percent barley, then rice with 20 to 30 percent aduki beans or lentils, and then plain rice again. A delicious morning porridge can be made by taking leftover rice, adding a little more water to soften, and seasoning with a little miso at the end and simmering for two to three minutes more. In ordinary pressure cooking, the ratio of grain to water should be about 1:2. For seasoning, cook with a small postage stamp–sized piece of kombu instead of salt, though in some cases sea salt may be used depending on the person's condition. Other grains can be used occasionally, including whole wheat berries, rye, corn, and whole oats, though oats should be avoided for the first month. However, buckwheat and seitan should be limited in use because they are very contracted relative to other grains and grain products. Flour products, even unrefined whole wheat bread, chapatis, pancakes, or cookies, should be totally avoided or limited in volume for a period of a few months. Whole-grain pasta and noodles may be eaten a couple times a week.

• **Soup:** Five to 10 percent soup, consisting of one or two cups or bowls per day of soup cooked with wakame sea vegetable and various hard green leafy or root vegetables and seasoned lightly with miso or shoyu. Occasionally a small volume of shiitake mushroom may be added to the soup. The miso may be barley miso, brown rice miso, or soybean (hatcho) miso and should be naturally aged two to three years. Grain soups, bean soups, and other soups may be taken from time to time.

• **Vegetables:** Twenty to 30 percent vegetables, cooked in a variety of forms, mainly steamed, boiled, and after one month without oil occasionally sautéed. Among vegetables, broccoli, leafy green tops of carrots, turnips, and daikon, and watercress are especially recommended. Root vegetables such as carrots, daikon, and burdock are also very beneficial, and cabbages, onions, pumpkin, and acorn and butternut squash may also be eaten regularly. Lotus root is especially good for all sorts of lung disorders and helps to ease breathing. Lotus root can be used frequently as a part of other vegetable dishes.

As a rule of thumb, the following dishes may be prepared, though the frequency may differ from person to person: nishime-style vegetables, three times a week; squash-aduki-kombi dish, three times a week; dried daikon, one cup, three times a week; carrots and carrot tops or daikon and daikon tops, three times a week; blanched vegetables, five to seven times a week; pressed salad, five to seven times a week; raw salad, avoid the first month, then once in ten to fourteen days; steamed greens, five to seven times a week; sautéed vegetables, two times a week, prepared with water the first month, then with sesame or corn oil once or twice a week after that; kinpira, two-thirds cup, two times a week; dried tofu, tofu, tempeh, or seitan with vegetables, two times a week.

• **Beans:** Five percent small beans, such as aduki beans, lentils, chickpeas, or black soybeans, may be used daily, cooked together with sea vegetables such as *kombu* or with onions and carrots. Other beans may be used altogether two to three times a month. For seasoning, a small volume of unrefined sea salt or shoyu or miso can be used. Bean products, such as tempeh, natto, and dried or cooked tofu may be used occasionally, but in moderate volume.

• **Sea Vegetables:** Five percent or less sea vegetable dishes, including wakame and kombu, daily when cooking grain, in soup, etc. A sheet of toasted nori may also be taken daily. A small dish of hijiki or arame should be prepared two times a week. All other sea vegetables are optional.

• **Condiments:** Condiments to be available on the table are gomashio (sesame salt), on the average made with 1 part salt to 18 parts sesame seeds; kelp or wakame powder; umeboshi plum; and tekka, though all other regular macrobiotic condiments may be used if desired. These condiments may be used daily on grains and vegetables, but the volume should be moderate to suit individual appetite and taste.

• **Pickles:** Pickles, made at home in a variety of ways, are to be eaten daily, one tablespoon in all, though salty pickles are to be minimized. Rice bran (nuka) pickles are the most suitable.

• **Animal Foods:** Fish and other animal food is to be avoided. However, in the event that animal food is craved, a small volume of white-meat fish may be eaten once every ten days to two weeks. The fish should be prepared steamed, boiled, or poached and garnished with grated daikon or ginger. Strictly avoid blue-meat and red-meat fish and all shellfish.

• **Fruit:** The less the better until the condition improves. If cravings develop, a small volume of cooked fruit with a pinch of sea salt or dried fruit (also preferably cooked) may be taken. Avoid all fruit juices and cider.

• **Sweets and Snacks:** Avoid all sweets and desserts, including good-quality macrobiotic desserts, until the condition improves. To satisfy a sweet tooth, use sweet vegetables every day in cooking, drink sweet vegetable drink (see special drinks below), and use sweet vegetable jam. Mochi, rice balls, vegetable sushi, and other grain-based snacks may be eaten frequently. Limit rice cakes, popcorn, and other dry or baked snacks, as they harden the tumor. In the event of cravings, a small volume of amasake, barley malt, or rice syrup may be taken.

• **Nuts and Seeds:** Nut and nut butters are to be avoided due to their high amount of fat and protein, except for chestnuts. Unsalted, roasted seeds such as sunflower seeds and pumpkin seeds may be consumed as a snack, up to one cup altogether per week.

• **Seasonings:** Seasonings, such as unrefined sea salt, shoyu, and miso, are to be used moderately in order to avoid unnecessary thirst. Avoid mirin and garlic. If you become particularly thirsty after a meal or between meals, you should cut back on these seasonings until the normal level of thirst returns.

• **Beverages:** Beverages and other dietary practices can follow the general recommendations in Part I including bancha twig tea as the main beverage. Strictly avoid the beverages on the "infrequent" and "avoid" list and don't take grain coffee for the first two to three months after starting this new way of eating.

The most important thing in connection with dietary practice is chewing very well, until all food becomes liquid in the mouth and well mixed with saliva. Chew very, very well, at least 50 times, preferably 100 times, per mouthful. It is also important to avoid overeating and eating within three hours of sleeping.

As noted in the introduction to Part II, persons who have received or who are currently undergoing medical treatment may need to make further dietary modifications.

SPECIAL DRINKS AND DISHES

Several special drinks may need to be taken, depending on the individual case. Please see a qualified macrobiotic teacher for guidance. Amounts and frequencies given here are averages; these will differ from person to person.

• **Sweet Vegetable Drink:** Take one small cup every day for the first month, then every other day the second month, and then several times a week after that as desired.

• **Carrot-Daikon Drink:** Take one small cup every day or every other day for one month, then two times a week for the second month.

• **Carrot-Lotus Drink:** Grate one half a small cup of carrots and one half a small cup of fresh lotus root. Add twice the volume of water, simmer three or four minutes, and drink and eat daily or every other day for one to one-and-a-half months.

• **Lotus Tea.** In the event of coughing, drink one half-cup of liquid squeezed from grated fresh lotus root. Warmed up and taken like a tea, this is particularly effective in easing throat or chest congestion. The remaining lotus root may also be cooked in soup or eaten with a little shoyu. Lotus root prepared in various forms with other vegetables is helpful in general for lung cancer and other lung and breathing disorders, including asthma and bronchitis. Raw slices of lotus root, seasoned with umeboshi juice or rice vinegar, may also be taken frequently as a side dish.

• **Lotus Seeds:** Lotus seeds cooked with kombu or wakame sea vegetable seasoned with a moderate amount of shoyu or miso are also helpful for the lungs. One cup of this mixture may be eaten daily.

• **Grated Daikon:** Grate about one half a cup of fresh daikon, add a few drops of shoyu, and take two to three times a week.

HOME CARES

• **Body Scrub:** Scrubbing the whole body, including the abdominal region and the spinal region, with a towel that has been immersed in hot water and squeezed out is very helpful for better circulation of blood, lymph, and other body fluids, as well as for activating physical and mental energies.

• **Compress Guidelines:** For a small number of lung tumors, a compress may be needed to help gradually draw out excess mucus and fat. Please see a qualified macrobiotic teacher for guidance on the proper use and frequency of a compress or plaster. Several types are used depending on the person's condition. Precede the compress or plaster with application of a towel that has been soaked in hot water and squeezed out over the affected area for about three to five minutes to stimulate circulation.

Mustard Plaster: A mustard plaster applied on the chest, preferably both front and back, can also help alleviate severe coughing.

Lotus Plaster: A lotus-root plaster, consisting of grated lotus root, mixed with white flour to hold consistency, and well mixed with 5 to 10 percent grated ginger, may be applied to loosen up the congested lung. This plaster may be kept on for a few hours.

OTHER CONSIDERATIONS

• Smoking should be strictly avoided by people with lung disorders, especially cancer. Nicotine, tars, and other carbon compounds in tobacco become lodged in the air sacs of the lungs. This causes further accumulation of fat, mucus, and other dietary substances that cause the tumor to form.

• Lung conditions are closely related to the proper functioning of the large intestine. Smooth, regular bowel movements daily can help the smooth functioning of the lungs and improve breathing. If the intestines are constipated or stagnated, it is especially necessary to chew all food very, very well, up to 100 times, and not to overeat. This will help restore proper elimination.

• Those who suffer with lung cancer tend to be depressed, sad, and melancholy. It is important to keep a positive, optimistic, happy mood. Good breathing exercises are very helpful.

• Avoid wearing wool and synthetic fibers. At the minimum wear cotton underwear and use cotton sheets and pillowcases.

• Avoid wearing metallic jewelry, including rings, bracelets, and necklaces. These pick up excess charges from the atmosphere and transmit them to the internal organs via the meridians running along the fingers and hands. It is fine, though, to wear a wedding ring.

• Avoid watching television for long stretches. Radiation weakens the chest area. Similarly, avoid other artificial sources of electromagnetic energy such as video terminals, smoke detectors, and hand-held electrical appliances that can weaken the lungs and respiratory system.

• Avoid smoggy and dusty air as well as atmospheres contaminated with industrial gases of chemical fumes. Visit the countryside or seashore or take long walks in the woods. At home, maintain a clean, orderly environment. Carbon dioxide in the house may accelerate tumor growth, so place green plants in the living room and other spaces to secure a fresh supply of oxygen.

• Avoid inhaling asbestos fibers. Many household products contain asbestos, including some types of aprons, potholders, and other cooking fabrics, and some floor tiles and other building and construction materials. Use natural materials and furnishings whenever possible.

PERSONAL EXPERIENCE

Cancer of the Lung, Female Organs, and Intestines

Kim Bright, the cook at Mother Nature's Restaurant in Fairfield, Connecticut, took one look at the curly-haired woman behind the counter and knew she was ill. Offering to help, Kim suggested she come back for a macrobiotic consultation the next day. Elizabeth Masters was so sick that she could no longer work or walk. During the last six months, she had undergone many X rays, blood tests, and other medical procedures. She was diagnosed with hypoglycemia, kidney failure, congestive heart failure, and allergies. The doctors gave her drugs, but she did not get better. She found that red meat made her feel sick, so she quit eating it and started going to a local vegetarian restaurant.

Elizabeth had an appointment with her doctor at noon, but she decided to see Kim earlier in the day, at 9:00 A.M. She had been praying for a miracle. As she later looked back, perhaps it was no coincidence that a macrobiotic chef happened to be cooking that night.

Kim told Elizabeth that she appeared to have a large tumor in her right lung and cancer of the female organs. She outlined a healing diet emphasizing whole grains and vegetables. "I felt relieved to know that I had been properly diagnosed," Elizabeth recalls. "I intuitively knew from my green color that I had cancer. The diet made sense to me, so I was anxious to start."

Later that day, however, at the doctor's office she received another shock. When further tests and probings showed nothing, Elizabeth and her husband got upset and mentioned that they had seen another "doctor" who suspected cancer. "They scurried around, looked at the tests and X rays again, and discovered their error," Elizabeth recounts. "Their diagnosis was cancer of the female organs, intestines, and a large tumor in the lower lobe of the right lung. They told me I had only two weeks to live."

But rather than staying in New Haven and having radical surgery and medical treatment at Yale University Hospital, Elizabeth decided to return home to Maine. "Over their objections, I decided to give the diet a try. I could see food had created my illness, so I wanted to give my body a chance to heal itself with the proper way of eating. I went home to live or die."

Over the years, Elizabeth had experienced many difficulties. Born in Missouri to parents who were unable to care for her because of alcohol problems and violence, she grew up at her grandmother's. As a child, she suffered from swollen adenoids and tonsils, and a local physician removed them by holding a rusty tin can filled with cotton over her nose and giving her ether. When she awoke, she was offered ice cream but chose hot dogs and sauerkraut instead. She had come to like the fresh meats, eggs, and dairy food of the countryside.

After years of neglect and abuse as a child, Elizabeth left home at fifteen and found a friend to live with. Working hard, going to school, and continuing to eat the modern American diet, she continued to have problems with her menstrual cycle and her abdomen was always distended. In high school an appendix ruptured and ovarian cysts were removed surgically. Elizabeth married at age twenty and gave birth to her first child at age twenty-one. The marriage lasted five years. Elizabeth didn't really know what was wrong, just felt she had to get out, and went to work and began fitting in with the coffee and doughnut for breakfast, hamburger for lunch, and ice cream for supper crowd.

At age twenty-five, Elizabeth married again and had her second child. She worked at a very stressful job in the aircraft industry, ran a cattle ranch, and continued to eat a diet high in animal food. This marriage lasted fifteen years, though her health problems continued—losing weight, gaining weight, distended stomach, emotional outbursts, an enlarged pancreas—for which she took various medical drugs, including Librium, Valium, antibodies, and allergy shots. When this marriage failed, she took a job that required a lot of traveling.

Elizabeth noticed changes in herself that she didn't like—low self-esteem (which showed itself in poor personal grooming, excessive weight, compulsive overeating, and excessive alcohol consumption). She lived life in the fast lane. She would eat excessively, then miss three days of work—sleeping all the time—to let her body recover. Again, excessive menstruation, along with diarrhea, low energy, and extreme pain, caught up with her. This was when she sought medical help and became more vegetarian.

After two weeks eating macrobiotically, Elizabeth was still alive. Able to get out of bed and walk for the first time in months, she returned to work. But after a few months, it became apparent that she was not really getting better, and she came to see me in Brookline, Massachusetts. I asked if she could quit work and cook for herself. She wasn't sure she'd have the courage to quit, but when she returned to work her boss came in and told her the company had lost the contract it was working on and could no longer keep her as an employee. With the decision made for her, she began to take macrobiotic cooking classes and concentrate solely on her recovery.

That was nine years ago. Today Elizabeth is in good health and lives with her husband in Maine. She has graduated from the Kushi Institute in Becket, speaks and teaches at centers in New England, and spreads macrobiotics wherever she goes. She is a living testament to the power of food, faith in the universe, and the body's amazing healing abilities.

Source: Gale Jack, "Given Two Weeks to Live—Seven Years Ago: Elizabeth Masters's Story," *One Peaceful World Newsletter*, Autumn/Winter 1991.

13

Colon and Rectal Cancer

FREQUENCY

Cancer of the large intestine, including the colon and rectum, is the second most deadly cancer in the United States (lung cancer being number one). It is also known as colorectal cancer, bowel cancer, and cancer of the gut. This year an estimated 58,300 people in the United States will die of this disease, and about 156,000 new cases will develop. Rectal cancer is slightly more prevalent in men, colon cancer more frequent in women, and each type is on the increase in both sexes. About 54 percent of tumors appear in the rectum, 23 percent in the sigmoid colon, 13 percent in the ascending or right colon, 8 percent in the transverse colon, 3 percent in the descending colon, and 1 percent in the anus. Bowel cancer is much less common in the Far East. In Japan, the rate is about one-fourth the American incidence.

Current medical treatment calls for surgical removal of part or all of the large intestine. After the tumor and some healthy adjacent tissue are taken out, the ends of the remaining part of the colon are sewn together. If this is not possible, a colostomy is performed, in which an opening is made in the skin and a disposable plastic bag is worn to collect feces. Radiation and chemotherapy may be administered after surgery in an attempt to control metastases, though a major study in 1985 published in the *New England Journal of Medicine* reported that these follow-up treatments—for nine of the ten most common cancers, including large-intestinal cancer—were no more effective than no treatment and, in some cases, could lead to death or further disability.

Cancer of the large intestine often spreads to the lungs or liver and, in women, the ovaries. Fifty-six percent of patients who have surgery for colon or rectal cancer can expect to live five years or more. This is one of the higher survival rates achieved by modern cancer therapy. However, unless the way of life, including way of eating, is changed, tumors tend to recur in the intestinal tract or elsewhere, occasioning further surgery.

STRUCTURE

The large intestine meets the small intestine at the cecum, turns upward (ascending colon), crosses the abdomen (transverse colon), winds down (descending colon), makes an S-shaped turn (sigmoid colon), and extends straight (rectum) to the anus. Altogether, the entire bowel tract is about five feet long. Like other organs, the large intestine can be classified according to its relative degree of expansion and contraction, or yin and yang. In structure, the large intestine is yin—long, soft, expanded, smooth. In contrast, its complementary opposite, the lungs, are more yang—small, firm, compact, textured.

The major functions of the large intestine are 1) to absorb water, vitamins, and minerals through its mucus-lined tissue to be sent to the liver for distribution through the body, and 2) to eliminate waste and excessive nutrients from the body, including iron, magnesium, calcium, and phosphates. The large intestine's functions are complementary to the lungs, which 1) regulate delivery of oxygen to the heart for distribution in the bloodstream, and 2) regulate elimination of carbon dioxide and other gaseous wastes from the body. Interestingly, the total number of cases of cancer of the large intestine and cancer of the lung are almost the same: 120,000 and 122,000, respectively. Without drawing too much from this correlation, this close incidence may suggest an underlying relationship between the origin and development of these two forms of cancer. Oriental medicine has traditionally treated them as a pair of organs that are antagonistic and complementary to each other.

CAUSE OF CANCER

People living in modern society suffer from a multitude of intestinal disorders. These include diarrhea, constipation, gas, enteritis, colitis, hernia, appendicitis, obesity, hemorrhoids, diverticular disease, and spastic or irritable colon. In general, these conditions arise from overeating, inadequate chewing of poor-quality food, overworking, and not enough exercise. The colon becomes further abused because of irregular patterns of eating, especially snacking between meals and eating before bedtime, which puts an increased burden on the inner organs.

A sedentary lifestyle, including long hours watching television or the habit of riding in cars for short distances instead of walking, is another major factor contributing to intestinal ailments. In traditional societies, where intestinal disorders and cancer of the colon are rare, people are much more orderly and active. They eat only two or three times a day, rarely eat between meals or before going to sleep, and approach their daily activity as creative participants rather than as passive spectators.

The traditional diet, which has protected hundreds of human generations from cancer and other degenerative diseases is high in what today we call fiber or roughage. Fiber includes the insoluble cellulose found in the cell walls of cereal grains, vegetables, and fruit; the endosperm of seeds; and the lignins or substances that constitute the woody pulp of growing plants. Whole grains are the best source of fiber, containing about four to five times as much as fruit. In the large intestine, fiber works like a sponge to absorb water, bile acids, and other waste products, giving bulk to the feces and propelling them quickly through the system. Fiber also serves to modify cholesterol metabolism, bind trace metals, and neutralize various irritants, residues, and toxins that accumulate in the intestinal lining. In addition, there are several hundred different kinds of bacteria in the colon that synthesize enzymes and vitamins, especially the B-complexes. A regular diet of fibrous whole grains and vegetables is necessary for the proper functioning of these bacteria.

The consumption of meat, dairy products, and other animal foods, on the other hand, weakens the digestive tract and can lead to various colonic disorders. Unlike grains and vegetables, which do not usually putrefy before they are eaten, animal protein starts to decompose as soon as the animal is killed. This process is offset by refrigeration or the addition of preservatives in the form of spices or chemicals. But putrefaction resumes as soon as the animal protein is cooked and eaten, and by the time it reaches the colon, decay has set in. The harmful bacteria from this decay tend to accumulate in the large intestine.

In addition to the synthesizing yang group of bacteria in the colon, there is a yin group of bacteria, which decomposes the remaining food particles into elementary compounds. These bacteria can break down a small amount of animal fat and protein in the colon, but the volume of these foods ingested by many people today cannot be properly metabolized. As a result, excess ammonia and bile acids begin to accumulate in the bowel tract. Along with the harmful bacteria produced by the putrefaction of animal food, these substances give rise to mutations in the lining of the large intestine, injure and kill cells, and lower the body's natural immunity to infection.

The shape, size, color, texture, and frequency of the bowel movement indicate the specific condition of the large intestine and overall health of the individual. People consuming a traditional or macrobiotic diet high in whole grains usually pass from thirteen to seventeen ounces of solid waste a day. Those consuming a high-fat, high-protein diet discharge only three to four ounces a day. On the whole-grain diet, food takes about thirty hours to travel from the mouth through the gastrointestinal tract. On the modern diet, transit time averages two to three days and in elderly people can take up to two weeks. Nearly 100 percent of the foods in humanity's traditional diet contain fiber, and this way of eating produces a bowel movement that is large and long, light in color, and soft in consistency and floats in water. Only 11 percent of the calories from the modern diet come from foods with fiber, and the bowel movement tends to be small, compact, dark in color, and hard in consistency and sink in water. Lack of fiber in the diet slows down the movement of feces and allows the buildup of harmful bacteria. Furthermore, the muscles of the large intestine must work harder to propel small, compact wastes. As pressure builds, small sacs erupt in the lining of the colon called diverticula. These pockets, in turn, can become inflamed as harmful bacteria and waste material become trapped.

Cancer of the large intestine is generally preceded by spastic colon, colitis, or diverticulosis and the growth of polyps. Though usually classified as benign nodules by modern medicine, polyps should be viewed as a precancerous condition. Polyps, or abnormal growths in the mucosa of the colon, represent a defensive measure on the part of the large intestine to limit the passage of harmful material. When the colon can no longer protect itself with benign resistance, full-fledged obstructions in the form of cancerous tumors result. Of course, these blockages may be cut out by surgery. But unless daily diet, the source of the disease, is changed, cancer will spread to other organs and eventually the patient will die.

Nearly 75 percent of intestinal cancer in the United States occurs in the rectum and sigmoid or lower colon—the compact yang end of the gut. This suggests overconsumption of meat, eggs, salty cheeses, poultry, and other extreme yang foods as major causative factors. However, the intestines can also become loose and sluggish from excessive intake of sugar, alcohol, refined flour, and other extreme yin substances, resulting in cancer of the ascending colon. Tumors in the transverse or descending colon result from a combination of extreme yin and yang foods and beverages.

Over the last decade there has been increased scientific interest in the relationship between diet and colon cancer. Among the major forms of cancer, colon and breast cancer are now generally associated with a high-fat, high-protein diet by epidemiologists and clinical researchers. Still, the progressive development of intestinal sickness is not widely understood. Modern medicine continues to employ a variety of laxatives, enemas, and colonics to speed up elimination, relieve constipation, and reduce pain. In the long run, these medications only further expand and weaken an already overactive bowel tract. Additional complications then develop requiring a still stronger application of temporary, chemical antidotes. We must begin to look at the other end of the digestive system for a permanent solution to intestinal disease. A balanced diet centered around whole grains offers lasting relief from colonic ills and the promise of improved health and vitality in the future.

MEDICAL EVIDENCE

• In 1809 Dr. William Lambe published a book associating cancer with a diet high in meat and other animal products. He reported that tumors in the digestive system could be progressively reduced and eliminated by a diet centered on plant foods. "We may conclude that it is the property of this regimen, and, in particular, of the vegetable diet, to transfer diseased action from the *viscera* to the exterior parts of the body—from the central parts of the system to the periphery. . . ." Source: Dr. William Lambe, *Effects of a Peculiar Regimen in Scirrhous Tumors and Cancerous Ulcers* (London: J. Mawman, 1809).

• In the midnineteenth century Ellen White, prophet and leader of the Adventist movement, encouraged her followers to give up meat, rich casseroles, and pastries and eat plain food, prepared in the simplest manner, according to climate and season. "Those who eat flesh are but eating grains and vegetables second-hand, for the animal receives from these things the nutrition that produces growth. The life that was in the grains and vegetables passes into the eater. We receive it by eating the flesh of the animal. How much better to get it direct, by eating the food that God provided for our use. . . . People are continually eating flesh that is filled with tuberculous and cancerous [substances]." Source: Ellen White, *Ministry of Healing* (Mount View, Ca.: Pacific Press Publishing Association, 1905), 313.

• At the beginning of the twentieth century, British cancer specialist and

Fellow of the Royal College of Surgeons W. Roger Williams linked the rise of cancer in Western society to excess protein, especially animal protein, and asserted that cancer was a disease of the whole body, not just separate organs. In his 519-page book, *The Natural History of Cancer*, he asserted:

> Tumour formation has too commonly been regarded as an isolated patho-logical entity, having no connection with other biological processes. Yet between tumour formation and morphological variation in general there is, I believe, real affinity; and in ultimate analysis both may be regarded as the outcome of the cumulative effects of changed conditions of existence. Of these conditions the most important seems to me to be changed environ-ment and excess of food. . . . Malignant tumours in mankind and animals consist mainly of albuminous or protein substances; and it seems not un-reasonable to suppose that they may be the outcome of excess of these substances in the body, and especially of such of them as serve for nuclear pabulum. When excessive quantities of such highly stimulating forms of nutriment are ingested, by beings whose cellular metabolism is defective, I believe there may thus be excited in those parts of the body where vital processes are most active, such excessive and disorderly proliferation as may eventuate in cancer. . . . It has been clearly established, that cancer is of most frequent occurrence among the well-to-do, highly nourished com-munities of occidental Europe; and, within the limits of these communities, as I have proved, the disease is commonest among the well-to-do groups. Source: W. Roger Williams, M.D., *The Natural History of Cancer* (New York: William Wood 1908), 12–13.

• During World War I, Mikkel Hindhede, M.D., superintendent of the State Institute of Food Research, persuaded the Danish government to shift its agricultural priorities from raising grain for livestock to grain for direct human consumption. Accordingly, in the face of a foreign blockage, the Danes ate primarily barley, whole-rye bread, green vegetables, potatoes, milk, and some butter. In the nation's capital, the death rate from all causes, including cancer, fell 34 percent during 1917 to 1918. "It was a low protein experiment on a large scale, about 3 million subjects being available," Hindhede reported to his medical colleagues: ". . . People entered no complaints; there were no diges-tive troubles, but we are accustomed to the use of whole bread and we knew how to make such bread of good quality." Sources: M. Hindhede, "The Effects of Food Restriction during War on Mortality in Copenhagen," *Journal of the American Medical Association* 74 (1920):381–82.
• In 1932 an English medical writer linked cancer with diet and an artificial way of life, recommending brown rice and other whole foods for relieving gastrointestinal tumors. "Brown breads, standard bread or whole-meal bread or unpolished rice are also helpful by furnishing coarse particles for that stimula-tion of the bowels, so desireable for their movement." Source: John Cope, *Cancer: Civilization: Degeneration* (London, 1932).
• After serving as a surgeon for the British in Africa from 1941 to 1964, Denis P. Burkitt, M.D., concluded that cancer and other degenerative diseases were rare and in some cases virtually unknown among traditional societies.

Over the course of thirteen years, the internationally renowned cancer specialist (after whom Burkitt's lymphoma is named) reported that in one South African hospital with 2,000 beds only six patients were observed with polyps, a condition of the colon that sometimes precedes cancer. He attributed the "replacement of carbohydrate foods such as bread and other cereals by fat (and animal fat in particular)" with the rise of cancer and other degenerative diseases during the last century. Burkitt also cited studies showing that forty to fifty years ago the incidence of colon cancer among African-Americans was less than among whites but higher than among rural Africans today. In recent years, as American blacks began to eat less grains, especially cornmeal, and more fat and protein, their rate of intestinal cancer rose to that of whites. Source: Denis P. Burkitt, M.D., *Eat Right—to Stay Healthy and Enjoy Life More* (New York: Arco, 1979), 11, 66–71.

• In the early 1960s, Dr. Maud Tresillian Fere, a physician living in New Zealand, reported curing herself of colon cancer by adopting a whole-grain diet that excluded meat, fish, cheese, sugar, stimulants, spices, and refined salt. She theorized that cancer and other degenerative diseases resulted from excess acidity or alkalinity. "In good health our blood and lymph are slightly alkaline, as also are our bodies. . . . It is no good having a bit of one's body cut out, as in a cancer operation, if the irritant poison is in one's whole body. One must eat the right food in the right proportion and so purify the bloodstream, thus rendering the operation unnecessary." Source: Dr. Maud Tresillian Fere, *Does Diet Cure Cancer?* (Northamptonshire, England: Thorsons, 1971), 18–21.

• In 1961 surgeon Donald Collins reported that five of his long-time patients had cured themselves of rectal cancer by eating an organically grown diet. He noted that each of the five patients lived for a further twenty-one to thirty-two years, and medical tests showed they died from causes other than cancer. "The only constant factor in the lives of these five persons was the fact that they all ate home-raised organically grown foods that were free from chemical preservatives and insect repellant sprays." Source: D. C. Collins, M.D., "Anti-Malignancy Factors Apparently Present in Organically Grown Foods," *American Journal of Proctology* 12:36–37.

• In 1968 a major epidemiological study indicated that dietary habits and environmental influences are the chief determinants of the world's varying cancer rates and not genetic factors as some scientists had believed. Data showed that in the course of three generations Japanese migrants in the United States contracted colon cancer at the same rates as the general American population. In contrast, the regular colon cancer rate in Japan remained about one-fourth the American incidence. Source: W. Haenszel and M. Kurihara, "Studies of Japanese Migrants," *Journal of the National Cancer Institute* 40:43–68.

• In 1969 scientists reported a high correlation between animal protein consumption and colon cancer incidence. Source: O. Gregor et al., "Gastrointestinal Cancer and Nutrition," *Gut* 10:1031–34.

• In 1973 British researchers found a high positive correlation between colon and breast cancer and total fat and protein consumption. Source: B. S. Drasar and D. Irving, "Environmental Factors and Cancer of the Colon and Breast," *British Journal of Cancer* 27:167–72.

• In 1973 British scientists reported that bran and fiber in the diet inhibited the production of bile salts by intestinal bacteria in the colon. The researchers contrasted this with white flour and sugar and hypothesized that the refining of foods might be a cause of cancer of the large intestine. Source: E. W. Pomare and K. W. Heaton, "Alteration of Bile Salt Metabolism by Dietary Fibre," *British Medical Journal* 4:262–64.

• In 1974 researchers for the NCI linked colon cancer with high beef consumption. "The evidence suggests that meat, particularly beef, is a food associated with malignancy of the large bowel." Source: J. W. Berg and M. A. Howell, "The Geographic Pathology of Bowel Cancer," *Cancer* 34:807–14.

• A 1975 study found that laboratory animals fed a diet consisting of 35 percent beef fat experienced a significant increase in intestinal tumors. Source: N. D. Nigro et al., "Effect of Dietary Beef Fat on Intestinal Tumor Formation by Azoxymethane in Rats," *Journal of the National Cancer Institute* 54:439–42.

• In 1975 Harvard Medical School researchers reported that Boston-area macrobiotic people eating a diet of whole grains, beans, fresh vegetables, sea vegetables, and fermented soy products had significantly lower cholesterol and triglyceride levels and lower blood pressure than a control group from the Framingham Heart Study eating the standard American diet. The average serum cholesterol in the macrobiotic group was 126 milligrams per deciliter, versus 184 for controls. Analysis further showed that consumption of dairy foods and eggs significantly raised cholesterol and fat levels in those eating macrobiotically, although fish was consumed as much as dairy and eggs combined. "The low plasma lipid levels of the vegetarians," the researchers concluded, "resemble those reported for populations in nonindustrialized societies," where heart disease, cancer, and other degenerative illnesses are uncommon. Source: F. M. Sacks et al., "Plasma Lipids and Lipoproteins in Vegetarians and Controls," *New England Journal of Medicine* 292:1148–51.

• In 1975 an epidemiological study associated cancer of the large intestine among women in twenty-three countries with either increased meat consumption or lowered consumption of cereal grains. Source: J. Cairns, "The Cancer Problem," *Scientific American* 233, no. 11:64.

• Epidemiological studies in 1977 reported the strongest correlation between cancer of the large intestine and per capita consumption of eggs, followed by beef, sugar, beer, and pork. Source: E. G. Knox, "Foods and Diseases," *British Journal of Preventive Social Medicine* 31:71–80.

• In 1977 an Indian cancer researcher asserted that the virtual absence of colon cancer among Punjabis in northern India appeared to be due to their high-fiber diet. The Punjabis' diet consists primarily of whole-grain chapatis, thick dal made with lentils, vegetable curry, and a small amount of fermented milk products. In South India, where colon cancer is prevalent, the staple is polished white rice and considerably more fat, oil, and spices are used in cooking. The researcher further concluded that thorough chewing seemed to lower the risk of cancer. "The proper chewing of meals ensuring that mucous-rich saliva mixed with the food seemed to be protective factors. Source: S. L. Malhotra, "Dietary Factors in a Study of Cancer Colon from Cancer Registry, with Special Reference to the Role of Saliva, Milk and Fermented Milk Products, and Vegetable Fibre," *Medical Hypotheses* 3:122–26.

• In 1977 researchers associated consumption of dietary fat and age-adjusted mortality from cancer of the colon in forty-one countries. Source: E. L. Wynder and B. S. Reddy, "Diet and Cancer of the Colon," in Myron Winick (ed.), *Nutrition and Cancer* (New York: John Wiley, 1977), 57.

• A 1978 case-control study in New York reported that a decreased risk of colon cancer was associated with frequent ingestion of vegetables, especially cabbage, Brussels sprouts, and broccoli. Source: S. Graham et al., "Diet in the Epidemiology of Cancer of the Colon and Rectum," *Journal of the National Cancer Institute* 61:709–14.

• In 1980 scientists reported an increased risk of both colon and rectal cancer from elevated consumption of calories, total fat, total protein, saturated fat, oleic acid, and cholesterol. The highest risk was found for saturated fat consumption and there was evidence of a dose-response relationship. Source: M. Jain et al., "A Case-Control Study of Diet and Colo-Rectal Cancer," *International Journal of Cancer* 26:757–68.

• In a 1981 study of twenty-one macrobiotic individuals, Harvard medical researchers reported that the addition of 250 grams of beef per day for four weeks to their regular diet of whole grains and vegetables raised serum cholesterol levels 19 percent. Systolic blood pressure also rose significantly. After the macrobiotic individuals returned to a low-fat diet, cholesterol and blood pressure values returned to previous levels. Source: F. M. Sacks et al., "Effects of Ingestion of Meat on Plasma Cholesterol of Vegetarians," *Journal of the American Medical Association*, 246:640–44.

• A preliminary 1981 report implicated refined sugar in the development of induced colon tumors in rats. Test animals given a 1.6 percent glucose solution developed approximately twice the number of tumors as controls. Source: D. M. Ingram and W. M. Castleden, "Glucose Increases Experimentally Induced Colorectal Cancer," *Nutrition and Cancer* 2:150–52.

• Men in Finland consume a lot of fat and have the highest heart disease rate in the industrialized world. Yet they have one of the lowest colon cancer rates (one-third that of the United States). Researchers around the world have found that whole-cereal grains protect against colon cancer by reducing bile acid concentrates in the large intestine and giving bulk to the feces. In 1982 investigators found that Finnish men consume large amounts of whole rye bread and had bowel movements three times bulkier than men in other Western countries, as well as reduced amounts of bile acid buildup. Source: H. N. Englyst et al., "Nonstarch Polysaccharide Concentrations in Four Scandinavian Populations," *Nutrition and Cancer* 4:50–60.

• In a 1984 study, beans lowered bile acid production by 30 percent in men with a tendency toward elevated bile acid. Bile acids are necessary for proper fat digestion but in excess have been associated with causing cancer, especially in the large intestine. Case-control studies showed that pinto and navy beans were effective in lowering bile acid production in men at high risk for this condition. Source: J. W. Anderson, "Hypocholesterolemic Effects of Oat-Bran or Bean Intake for Hypercholesterolemic Men," *American Journal of Clinical Nutrition* 40:1146–55.

• A 1984 study on health and exercise found that men with sedentary jobs have a 60 percent higher risk of developing colon cancer than those who are more active. The sedentary group included accountants, lawyers, musicians, and bookkeepers. The active group included carpenters, gardeners, plumbers, and mail carriers. Source: D. H. Garabrant et al., "Job Activity and Colon Cancer Risk," *American Journal of Epidemiology* 119, no. 6:1005–14.

• In 1986 Norwegian scientists examined the colons of 155 people in their fifties who had no signs of colon cancer. Half had polyps growing in the colon; the half with no polyps ate more cruciferous vegetables. The less cruciferous vegetables consumed, the greater the risk for polyps and the larger and more abnormal the polyps. Source: G. Hoff et al., *Scandinavian Journal of Gastroenterology* 21:199.

• In a 1987 case-control study in Belgium, researchers found that consumption of simple sugars, including monosaccharides and disaccharides, was related to increased risk of colon and rectal cancer. The relative risks for the highest compared to the lowest consumption level was 1.7 times for colon cancer, 2.4 for rectal cancer. Source: A. J. Tuyns et al., "Colorectal Cancer and the Intake of Nutrients," *Nutrition and Cancer* 10:181–96.

• Eating more whole grains, vegetables, and fruit may lower a person's risk for colorectal cancer by up to 40 percent, according to a 1990 study. Researchers at the Fox Chase Cancer Center in Philadelphia looked at thirty-seven studies involving 10,000 people in fifteen countries and reported that those who ate a diet high in whole grains and other plant-quality foods had about 40 percent less risk of this disease. Source: Bruce Tock, Elaine Lanza, and Peter Greenwald, "Dietary Fiber, Vegetables, and Colon Cancer: Critical Review and Meta-analyses of the Epidemiologic Evidence," *Journal of the National Cancer Institute* 82:650–61.

• Women who eat beef, lamb, or pork as a daily main dish are at two and a half times the risk for developing colon cancer as women who eat meat less than once a month. The conclusion, drawn from a study published in 1990 of 88,751 nurses over a ten-year period, found that the more fish and poultry in the diet, the less chances of getting colon cancer. "The substitution of other protein sources, such as beans or lentils, for red meat might also be associated with a reduced risk of colon cancer in populations that consume more legumes," researchers concluded. Investigators also found that eating the fiber from fruit appeared to reduce the risk of colon cancer. The fruits mentioned as possibly protective included apples and pears.

"The less red meat the better," recommended Dr. Walter Willett, professor of epidemiology and nutrition at the Harvard School of Public Health, who directed the study. "At most, it should be eaten only occasionally. And it may be maximally effective not to eat red meat at all." Sources: Walter C. Willett et al., "Relation of Meat, Fat, and Fiber Intake to the Risk of Colon Cancer in a Prospective Study among Women," *New England Journal of Medicine* 323:1664–72, and Anastasia Toufexis, "Red Alert on Red Meat," *Time*, December 24, 1990.

• Researchers at the Harvard School of Public Health reported that men with the lowest fat intake, averaging 24 percent of calories, had only half the rate of colon polyps, a common precursor of colon cancer, as men eating the usual amount of fat. "A modest reduction [of fat such as proposed by current medical guidelines] will not appreciably reduce the risk," said Dr. Tim Byers of the Centers for Disease Control in Atlanta. He described an effective cancer prevention diet as one that included six servings a day of whole grains and legumes and five or six servings of vegetables and fruits. Source: "Very Low Rate of Fat in Diet Is Advised to Fight Cancer," *Boston Globe*, April 23, 1991.

DIAGNOSIS

In a doctor's office or hospital, cancer of the large intestine is usually diagnosed through a rectal examination; blood, urine, and stool tests; X rays; a proctosigmoidoscopy, in which a rigid tube is inserted through the rectum to provide a view of the lower colon; or a colonoscopy, in which the tube is inserted and air is forced in to expand the complete colon for viewing.

Traditional Oriental medicine analyzes the condition of the bowel tract with simple external means rather than complex internal ones. In facial diagnosis, the lower lip corresponds to the large intestine, and by observing its condition we can take preventive or remedial dietary action to counter intestinal disorders, including bowel cancer. A swollen lower lip signifies a swollen, yin condition of the large intestine. In modern society, up to 75 percent of the population have swollen lower lips, indicating irregular bowel movements and enteritis or inflammation of the intestinal tract. Usually a swollen lower lip indicates constipation from a combination of excessive yin and yang foods. However, if the lip is wet, diarrhea is indicated. An extremely contracted, yang lower lip shows overconsumption of meat and other protein. The virtual absence or receding of the lower lip shows a tendency toward cancer of the sigmoid colon or rectum.

The different colorations of the lower lip further show specific disorders: white indicates fatty mucous deposits in the colon; pale shows weak metabolism of nutrients and anemia; bright red indicates expansion and hyperactivity of the blood capillaries and tissue; yellow around the edges of the lips shows hardening of fatty deposits in the large intestine and blockages in the liver and gallbladder; blue or purple shows stagnation of feces and blood in the colon; and a green shade around the mouth probably indicates colon cancer.

These discolorations may also occur around areas along the meridian of the large intestine, especially on the area around the base of the thumb on the inside of the hand. A blue or green color in this region may indicate developing intestinal cancer. Also, the fleshy part of the outside of the hand between the thumb and index finger often takes on a green or bluish hue in the case of colon cancer. If this coloring appears on the left hand, the descending colon is affected. If on the right hand, the ascending colon is diseased.

The condition of the color is also revealed in the forehead. The right part of the forehead shows the ascending colon, the upper forehead the transverse colon, and the left part the descending colon. Swellings, colorations, patches, pimples, or spots indicate where fat deposits, ulcers or cancerous growths are developing in the colon.

General skin color also offers clues to intestinal disorders. A purplish shading, from the consumption of extremely yin foods and beverages; a brown shade, from excessive yang animal food and yin tropical vegetables and fruits; and yellow, white, hard fatty skin, from the consumption of excessive eggs, poultry, cheese, and other dairy foods, are early warning signs of overactive intestines and general digestive troubles.

DIETARY RECOMMENDATIONS

For cancers of the large intestine—the ascending, transverse, and descending colon and the rectum—it is advisable to eliminate all animal food, including beef, pork, and other kinds of meat, chicken and eggs, and cheese and other dairy food, which are the primary cause of this type of cancer. Even fish and seafood, which may be high in fat and cholesterol, should be avoided for an initial period. Furthermore, any greasy, oily, or fatty foods and beverages are to be stopped. Sugar, sugar-treated food and beverages, refined flour, soft drinks, tropical fruits and vegetables, various nuts and nut butters, spices, stimulants, and aromatic food and drinks are also to be discontinued. Flour products, though not a main cause of this malignancy, may contribute to stagnation and blockages and make recovery more difficult and therefore should be strictly avoided, even good-quality sourdough bread, for an initial period. Dietary guidelines for daily consumption, by volume, are generally as follows.

• **Whole Grains:** 50 to 60 percent of daily consumption, by volume, should be whole-cereal grains. The first day prepare plain pressure-cooked short-grain brown rice. On subsequent days, alternate brown rice pressure-cooked with 20 to 30 percent millet, then rice with 20 to 30 percent barley, then rice with 20 to 30 percent aduki beans or lentils, and then plain rice again. A delicious morning porridge can be made by taking leftover rice, adding a little more water to soften, and seasoning with a little miso at the end and simmering for two to three minutes more. In ordinary pressure cooking, the ratio of grain to water should be about 1:2. For seasoning, cook with a postage stamp–sized piece of kombu instead of salt, though in some cases sea salt may be used, depending on the person's condition. Other grains can be used occasionally, including whole wheat berries, rye, corn, and whole oats, though oats should be avoided for the first month. However, for a contracted condition such as colorectal cancer, buckwheat and seitan should be limited in use because they are very contracted relative to other grains and grain products. Flour products, even unrefined whole wheat bread, chapatis, pancakes, or cookies, should be totally avoided or limited by volume for a period of a few months. Whole-grain pasta and noodles also should not be used more than a couple times a week in small volume.

• **Soup:** 5 to 10 percent soup, consisting of one or two cups or bowls per day of soup cooked with wakame sea vegetable and various hard green leafy vegetables such as kale or collards and seasoned lightly with miso or shoyu. Occasionally a small volume of shiitake mushroom may be added to the soup. The miso may be barley miso, brown rice miso, or soybean (hatcho) miso and should be naturally aged two to three years. Grain soups, bean soups, and other soups may be taken from time to time.

• **Vegetables:** 20 to 30 percent vegetables, cooked in a variety of forms, mainly steamed, boiled, and after one month without oil occasionally sautéed. For cancer of the ascending colon, lighter and quicker cooking, which preserves freshness and crispness, is preferred over longer cooking with a strong, salty taste. Leafy vegetables are preferable to root vegetables for this cancer, though root vegetables should also be used occasionally. For cancer of the transverse colon, leafy vegetables and round vegetables such as cabbage, onions, and pumpkin and squash may be used almost equally. The cooking style should be medium, neither too short nor too long. For cancer of the descending colon and rectum, round and root vegetables should receive more emphasis than leafy vegetables, though the latter are also necessary. For any of these conditions, seasoning with unrefined sea salt, shoyu, and miso or condiments is to be moderate. After one month with limited oil, sautéed vegetables made with unrefined sesame or corn oil can also be consumed frequently.

As a rule of thumb, the following dishes may be prepared, though the frequency may differ from person to person: nishime-style vegetables, three times a week; squash-aduki-kombu dish, three times a week; dried daikon, one cup, three times a week; carrots and carrot tops or daikon and daikon tops, three times a week; blanched vegetables, five to seven times a week; pressed salad, five to seven times a week; raw salad, avoid the first month, then once in ten to fourteen days; steamed greens, five to seven times a week; sautéed vegetables, once a week, then after the first month more often; kinpira, two-thirds of a cup, two times a week; dried tofu, tofu, tempeh, or seitan with vegetables, two times a week.

• **Beans:** Five percent small beans, such as aduki beans, lentils, chickpeas, or black soybeans, may be used daily, cooked together with sea vegetables such as kombu or with onions and carrots. Other beans may be used altogether two to three times a month. For seasoning, a small volume of unrefined sea salt or shoyu or miso can be used. Bean products, such as tempeh, natto, and dried or cooked tofu, may be used occasionally, but in moderate volume.

• **Sea Vegetables:** Five percent or less sea vegetable dishes, including wakame and kombu, daily when cooking grain, in soup, etc. A sheet of toasted nori may also be taken daily. A small dish of hijiki or arame should be prepared two times a week. All other sea vegetables are optional.

• **Condiments:** Condiments to be available on the table are gomashio (sesame salt), on the average made with 1 part salt to 18 parts sesame seeds; kelp or wakame powder; umeboshi plum, and tekka, though all other regular macrobiotic condiments may be used if desired. These condiments may be used daily on grains and vegetables, but the volume should be moderate, to suit individual appetite and taste. As a condiment, a small amount of miso sautéed in sesame oil with the same volume of chopped scallions can be used daily on grains. One teaspoon of sautéed whole dandelions is also helpful for cancer of the large intestine.

• **Pickles:** Pickles, made at home in a variety of ways, are to be eaten daily, one tablespoon in all, though salty pickles are to be minimized. Rice bran (nuka) pickles are the most suitable.

• **Animal Food:** Fish and other animal food is to be avoided. However, in the event that animal food is craved, a small volume of white-meat fish may be eaten once every ten days for the first three months, then once a week. The fish should be prepared steamed, boiled, or poached and garnished with grated daikon or ginger. After two months, fish may be eaten once a week. Strictly avoid blue-meat and red-meat fish and all shellfish.

• **Fruit:** The less the better until the condition improves. If cravings develop, a small volume of cooked fruit with a pinch of sea salt or dried fruit (also preferably cooked) may be taken. Avoid all fruit juices and cider.

• **Sweets and Snacks:** Avoid all sweets and desserts, including good-quality macrobiotic desserts, until the condition improves. To satisfy a sweet tooth, use sweet vegetables every day in cooking, drink sweet vegetable drink (see special drinks below), and eat sweet vegetable jam and amasake. Mochi, rice balls, vegetable sushi, and other grain-based snacks may be eaten frequently. Limit rice cakes, popcorn, and other dry or baked snacks, as they may harden the tumor. In the event of cravings, a small volume of barley malt or rice syrup may be taken.

• **Nuts and Seeds:** Nuts and nut butters are to be avoided due to their high amount of fat and protein, except for chestnuts. Unsalted, roasted seeds such as sunflower seeds and pumpkin seeds may be consumed as a snack, up to one cup altogether per week.

• **Seasonings:** Seasonings, such as unrefined sea salt, shoyu, and miso, are to be used moderately in order to avoid unnecessary thirst. Avoid mirin and garlic. If you become particularly thirsty after a meal or between meals, you should cut back on these seasonings until the normal level of thirst returns.

• **Beverages:** Beverages and other dietary practices can follow the general recommendations in Part I, including bancha twig tea as the main beverage. Strictly avoid the beverages on the "infrequent" and "avoid" list and don't take grain coffee for the first two to three months after starting this new way of eating.

The most important thing in connection with dietary practice is chewing very well, until all food becomes liquid in the mouth and well mixed with saliva. Chew very, very well, at least 50 times, preferably 100 times, per mouthful. It is also important to avoid overeating and eating with three hours of sleeping.

As noted in the introduction to Part II, persons who have received or who are currently undergoing medical treatment may need to make further dietary modifications.

SPECIAL DRINKS AND DISHES

Several special drinks or side dishes may need to be taken, depending on the individual case. Please see a qualified macrobiotic teacher for guidance. Amounts and frequencies given here are averages; these will differ from person to person.

• **Sweet Vegetable Drink:** Take one small cup every day for the first month, then every other day the second month.

• **Carrot-Daikon Drink:** Take one small cup every day or every other day for one month, then two times a week for the second month.

• **Shiitake-Kombu Dish:** For relieving tumors, a small dish of shiitake mushrooms cooked with kombu, seasoned with miso while cooking, is helpful. One tablespoon may be consumed daily.

• **Daikon-Kombu Dish:** A dish of dried, shredded daikon soaked in water and cooked with kombu and seasoned with either miso or shoyu is also helpful for colon cancers if consumed daily or several times a week.

• **Brown Rice Cream:** In the event of appetite loss, genuine brown rice cream can be consumed with a piece of umeboshi plum and a small amount of gomashio or tekka.

• **Other Special Drinks:** In the event that part of the descending colon or rectum has become narrowed or blocked by tumorous growth, the bowel channel may be widened or opened by one of the following special measures:

1. Drink two to three cups per day of liquid made from boiling spring water with dried shiitake mushrooms, grated daikon, and a small portion of grated ginger, with a slight taste of shoyu. (Grated lotus root may be used instead of either shiitake mushrooms or grated daikon.)

2. Drink two or three cups per day of boiled water in which dried tangerine or orange peel has cooked. The same liquid can be used for an enema if needed.

3. Drink miso soup, two to three cups daily, cooked with sliced daikon or radish, garlic or ginger, and onion or scallion.

4. Eat a dish of cooked agar-agar (kanten) seasoned with apple juice or barley malt together with grated ginger a couple of times per day.

• **Grated Daikon:** Grate about one half a small cup of fresh daikon, add a few drops of shoyu, and take two to three times a week.

HOME CARES

• **Body Scrub:** Scrubbing the whole body, including the abdominal region and the spinal region, with a towel that has been immersed in hot water and squeezed out is very helpful for better circulation of blood, lymph, and other body fluids, as well as for activating physical and mental energies.

• **Compress Guidelines:** For a small number of colon tumors, a compress may be needed to help gradually draw out excess mucus and fat. Please see a qualified macrobiotic teacher for guidance on the proper use and frequency of a compress or plaster. Several types are used, depending on the person's condition. Precede the compress or plaster with application of a towel that has been soaked in hot water and squeezed out over the affected area for about three to five minutes to stimulate circulation.

• **Taro Plaster:** For intestinal and rectal tumors, a taro potato plaster may be applied for three to four hours following administration of a ginger compress for three to five minutes. This plaster may be repeated daily.

• **Buckwheat Plaster:** In the event of swelling in the abdominal region, repeated application of a buckwheat plaster can help absorb excessive liquid. The buckwheat plaster should be kept warm while being applied.

• **Green Vegetable Plaster:** In the event of pain, a ginger compress applied for about three to five minutes and a plaster of mashed green leafy vegetables mixed with 20 to 30 percent white flour in order to make a paste is helpful. The vegetable plaster should be preceded by a ginger compress. Gentle massage and acupuncture treatment may also help relieve pain and bowel-tract stagnation.

• **Gas Formation:** To eliminate intestinal gas, all food should be chewed very well. It is also helpful to eat less, even skipping breakfast for a period of a few weeks.

• **Intestinal Warmth:** Avoid exposing the abdominal region to cold air or consuming cold beverages, which have a paralyzing effect on the intestines. Keeping the abdominal region warm is essential for restoring smooth digestive functions. For that purpose, a small volume of scallions or garlic cooked in miso soup or in *bancha* tea, consumed daily or several times a week, is helpful.

• **Weight Loss:** People with cancer and their physicians are concerned that weight loss is not beneficial, and thus a tendency arises to overconsume, especially food rich in protein and fat. Actually, this practice serves to enhance the cancerous condition, especially in the case of the large intestine. Having an energetic and tireless condition is more of a barometer to health than maintaining previous weight.

• **Rice Fasting:** For a short period—seven to fourteen days—persons with large-intestinal cancer may eat only pressure-cooked brown rice served with either umeboshi plum or gomashio (sesame salt) and with toasted nori. The rice and condiments should be chewed very, very well. In making gomashio, the proportion of roasted sea salt to crushed sesame seeds should be from 1 to 16 to 1 to 18. Along with the brown rice, one to two cups of miso soup and one or two dishes of cooked vegetables may be consumed every day. This limited rice diet is very beneficial to cleansing and revitalizing the intestinal tract. However, it should not be continued longer than two weeks without proper supervision of a qualified macrobiotic teacher, nutritionist, or medical associate or professional.

OTHER CONSIDERATIONS

• Those who suffer with intestinal cancer tend to be depressed, sad, and melancholy. It is important to keep a positive, optimistic, happy mood. Good breathing exercises are very helpful not only for lung metabolism, but also for the smooth functioning of the large intestine.

• Avoid wearing wool and synthetic fibers. At the minimum wear cotton underwear and use cotton sheets and pillowcases.

• Avoid watching television for long stretches. Radiation weakens the intestinal area. Similarly, avoid other artificial sources of electromagnetic energy such as video terminals, smoke detectors, and hand-held electrical appliances.

PERSONAL EXPERIENCE

Colon Cancer

Osbon Woodford was born in Macon, Georgia, in the mid-1940s, and nearly all the food that he ate during his first twenty years growing up was homemade.

However, it was laced with lard, cooked in lard, and seasoned with grease left over from bacon or fatback. Sugar, in various forms, was also plentiful. Over the next twenty years, he lived primarily on fast food and highly processed foods from the supermarkets.

In April 1987 Osbon was diagnosed with colon cancer and several days later underwent surgery at Riverside Methodist Hospital in Columbus, Ohio. Doctors found metastases to eleven lymph nodes, and their prognosis was poor. His wife was told there was nothing that could be done. And he would probably live six months to a year.

Seeking alternatives, Osbon began macrobiotics, eating whole grains, vegetables, legumes, and sea vegetables daily. Along with the change in way of eating, he reduced his stress level through meditation and self-reflection.

In February 1990 Osbon's oncologist pronounced him cured after his CEA tests repeatedly registered normal low-level and no signs of recurrence or metastasis appeared. Today Osbon is completing studies at the Kushi Institute Extension Program in Cleveland, Ohio, and planning to help others as a result of his experience.

Source: Ann Fawcett and the East West Foundation, *Cancer-free: 30 Who Triumphed over Cancer Naturally* (New York and Tokyo: Japan Publications, 1991).

Colon Cancer

In 1982 Cecil Dudley experienced pain in his abdomen and his doctor prescribed a tranquilizer for "gas." About this same time, Dudley took a course at Ohio State University titled Avoid Dying of Cancer—Now or Later. While the course was attended primarily by medical and nursing students, it was offered without charge to senior citizens. During the course, Dudley, who was then seventy-five years old, learned that everyone over fifty should be tested for blood in the feces with a simple test called the hemoccult II slide method.

Dudley conducted the test at home. It proved positive, and a barium enema later revealed that he had a tumor in the colon. Following surgery, Dudley learned about macrobiotics and attended a seminar on diet and degenerative disease at the Kushi Institute, where he learned about cooking, home care, and macrobiotic principles. With the support of his wife, Margaret, he has experienced constant improvement. "I increased my amount of exercise. As a result, I experienced weight control from a lowered fat intake. My cholesterol went from 219 to 137, and I feel physically and mentally more alert and good enough to take several trips a year. My CEA levels are well within the normal range and there is no sign of a recurrence of the cancer."

Source: Ann Fawcett and the East West Foundation, *Cancer-free: 30 Who Triumphed over Cancer Naturally* (New York and Tokyo: Japan Publications, 1991).

14

Oral and Upper Digestive Cancers: Mouth, Larynx, Pharynx, and Esophagus

FREQUENCY

Cancers of the upper digestive system, including the mouth, throat, and esophagus, will account for 21,600 estimated deaths in the United States this year and some 53,900 new cases. Men are about twice as likely to contract these forms of cancer as women. Esophagael cancer is one of the fastest-growing malignancies in the United States, and the death rate has increased 20 to 25 percent in the last thirty years. Among sufferers of Barrett's esophagus, a precancerous condition characterized by persistent heartburn or stomach regurgitations, the incidence of esophagael cancer has soared 100 percent and the age of onset is steadily falling. Death from cancer of the larynx has increased 114 percent among women over the last generation, though it remained steady for men. During the same time frame, oral cancer mortality fell 23 percent among men and rose 13 percent among women. The incidence of upper digestive cancer is also particularly high in the Far East.

Cancers in the head and neck do not usually metastasize, but spread by local invasion. About 90 percent of these tumors are classified as squamous-cell carcinomas. They grow slowly and tend to recur within several years of treatment. Cancer of the esophagus often spreads to the liver, the lungs, or the membrane surrounding the lungs.

Surgery and radiation are widely used by modern medicine to treat these forms of cancer. In the case of esophageal cancer, partial removal of the diseased section will be rectified by taking a portion of the large intestine and surgically linking it with the remaining part of the esophagus and the stomach. This procedure is called an esophagogastric anastomosis. If the whole esophagus is taken out, the spleen and end of the pancreas are usually removed as well. Again, part of the intestinal wall or plastic tubing will be inserted to connect the severed ends of the digestive tract.

For head and neck tumors, surgery is usually employed to remove the tumor and part of the healthy tissue surrounding it. Plastic surgery will follow if this results in the disfiguration of the face. The voice is often lost as a consequence of surgery to the throat area. Radiation therapy may also be used as a primary treatment, depending on the type and size of the tumor. Chemotherapy may be used in conjunction with radiation if the tumor is advanced or has spread to the bone. The survival rate for esophageal cancer is 3 percent. The five-year cure rate is higher for head and neck cancers: lips, 84 percent; tongue, 32 percent; mouth, 45 percent; larynx, 63 percent; and pharynx, 21 percent.

STRUCTURE

The upper digestive tract extends from the lips to the stomach and consists of the mouth, the larynx, the pharynx, and the esophagus. The larynx is also known as the voice box, the pharynx as the throat, and the esophagus as the gullet. Food enters the body through the mouth and moves spirally up and down in the process of chewing. Digestion alternates between alkaline (yang) and acidic (yin) secretions at various stages along the alimentary canal. From the mouth, where alkaline substances are released, food travels to the stomach, where acids are secreted. From there it moves to the duodenum, where alkaline enzymes from the small intestine and pancreas are activated. Finally, remaining foodstuffs are absorbed by the acidic substances in the villi of the small intestine.

In the mouth the digestive process begins with the secretion of saliva, a clear, watery fluid that has a pH of 7.2, making it slightly salty or alkaline. The main function of saliva is to begin gradually breaking down carbohydrates for further absorption in the stomach and complete digestion in the small intestine. Ptyalin, an enzyme in saliva, is released during chewing and initiates this process.

The pharynx is a mucous-lined tube situated at the back of the mouth, nasal cavity, and larynx. Its muscles push food to the esophagus, a flat canal about ten to twelve inches long extending from the lower neck through the chest to the stomach.

CAUSE OF CANCER

Tumors of the upper digestive system, except for the tongue, are a more yin form of cancer. They are caused primarily by long-term consumption of expansive yin substances, including milk and dairy products, oily and greasy foods, sugar and other sweeteners, tropical fruits and vegetables, coffee and black tea, spices, vitamin pills and protein supplements, alcohol, drugs, and medications. In the Far East, a diet centered around refined white rice, the use of sugar and refined oil, the increasing use of chemical seasonings and flavors, and the popular practice of chewing betel-nut leaves, a gumlike wad of spices, are the main factors contributing to the high rise of mouth, throat, and esophageal cancers in that part of the world.

As we have seen, digestion begins in the mouth, and the primary function of saliva is to alkalinize (make more yang) entering foodstuffs. A meal consisting primarily of whole grains and other balanced foods will begin to be broken down in the mouth as the enzyme in saliva slowly metabolizes starch into maltose, a disaccharide. Thorough chewing is essential for this process, and it is especially necessary to balance the acidity of extreme yin foods, drinks, and medications. If chewing is minimal or light, not enough saliva will be secreted to neutralize the excess volume or strong quality of incoming yin. As a result, these expansive substances will be prematurely absorbed into the blood system in the mouth, throat, esophagus, or stomach. This makes for a thinner condition of the blood and other bodily fluids, ultimately giving rise to illness, loss of vitality, and degeneration of the organism.

The progressive development of disease in the upper digestive system, as in other systems of the body, takes the form of localized inflammations, ulcers, cysts, and, finally, tumors. Mouth cancer is often preceded by leukoplakia, a disease characterized by the growth of thick white patches on the inside of the cheeks, gums, or tongue. Cancer of the esophagus is commonly accompanied by difficulty in swallowing as the gullet moves to restrict the the passage of harmful and irritating substances by creating a natural obstruction.

Cancer of the tongue, a small, compact organ, is a more yang form of mouth cancer and is caused by the excessive intake of yin accompanied by overly yang food. Cancer of the tongue could result from long-term consumption of sardines and cream cheese, smoked white fish cooked with spices, overconsumption of salt and fatty, greasy, and oily foods, or other extreme combinations.

Cancer of the throat is caused by consumption of both extreme yin and yang foods and beverages, including overconsumption of greasy and oily foods, dairy foods, flour products, and sugar, and other sweeteners.

MEDICAL EVIDENCE

• A 1961 study found that consumption of green and yellow vegetables was lower for esophageal cancer patients than controls. Source: E. L. Wynder and I. J. Bross, "A Study of Etiological Factors in Cancer of the Esophagus," *Cancer* 14:389–413.

• A 1975 study in the Caspian littoral region of Iran, an area of high esophageal cancer, indicated lower intake of lentils and other pulses, cooked green vegetables, and other whole foods. Source: H. Hormozdiari et al., "Dietary Factors and Esophageal Cancer in the Caspian Littoral of Iran," *Cancer Research* 35:3493–98.

• Heavy consumption of alcohol increases the risk of cancer of the mouth, throat, larynx, esophagus, and liver. These forms of cancer appear about fifteen times more frequently in heavy drinkers and smokers than in those who neither smoke nor drink. Source: Samuel S. Epstein, M.D., *The Politics of Cancer* (New York: Doubleday, 1979), 474–75.

• Mormon males in California have 55 percent less esophageal cancer and females 39 percent less than other Californians. A 1980 epidemiological study associated lowered cancer risk with the Mormons' diet, high in whole grains, vegetables, and fruit, moderate in meat, and low in stimulants, alcohol, tobacco, and drugs. Source: J. E. Engstrom, "Health and Dietary Practice and Cancer Mortality among California Mormons," in J. Cairns et al. (eds.), *Cancer Incidence in Defined Populations, Banbury Report 4* (Cold Spring Harbor, NY: Cold Spring Harbor Laboratory), 69–90.

• A 1981 epidemiological study found that populations with a low risk of esophageal cancer in Africa and Asia consume more millet, cassava, yams, and peanuts than high-risk groups. Source: S. J. van Rensburg, "Epidemiologic and Dietary Evidence for a Specific Nutritional Predisposition to Esophageal Cancer," *Journal of the National Cancer Institute* 67:243–51.

• Research studies in Colombia, Chile, Japan, Iran, China, England, and the United States have indicated an association between increased cancer of the esophagus and stomach and exposure to high levels of nitrate or nitrite in the diet and drinking water. Foods generally containing or producing these substances include hams, sausages, bacon, and other cured meats, baked goods and breakfast cereals, and fruit juices. Source: *Diet, Nutrition, and Cancer* (Washington, DC: National Academy of Sciences, 1982), 12:19–21.

• "Diets high in plant foods—i.e., fruits, vegetables, legumes, and whole-grain cereals—are associated with a lower occurrence of coronary heart disease and cancer of the lung, colon, esophagus, and stomach." Source: National Research Council, *Diet and Health* (Washington, DC: National Academy Press, 1989).

• Preliminary studies indicate that precancerous lesions of the mouth can be neutralized by foods high in beta-carotene. Source: "3 Promising Weapons against Disease," *New York Times*, September 25, 1991.

• In a 1991 case-control study, men with lung cancer, bladder cancer, prostate cancer, larynx cancer, colorectum cancer, and esophagael cancer had from 10 to 24 percent lower intake of vegetables and fruits high in carotene than controls. Source: W. C. Ruth et al., "A Case-Control Study of Dietary Carotene in Men with Lung Cancer and in Men with Other Epithelial Cancers," *Nutrition and Cancer* 15, no. 1:63–68.

• In a case-control study in Italy, researchers reported in 1991 a positive association between cancer of the oral cavity and pharynx and frequent consumption of refined pasta or rice, cheese, eggs, and alcohol. Source: S. Franceschi et al., "Nutrition and Cancer of the Oral Cavity and Pharynx in Northeast Italy," *International Journal of Cancer* 47:20–25.

• In 1992 Gladys Block, formerly of the NCI and now a researcher at the University of California at Berkeley, reviewed fifteen epidemiological studies and found that people who were in the top quarter for eating foods high in vitamin C, such as green leafy vegetables, had only one-half to one-third the rate of esophagael and stomach cancer of those in the lowest quarter. Source: "Vitamins Win Support as Potent Agents of Health," *New York Times*, March 10, 1992.

DIAGNOSIS

Cancers of the mouth and throat are commonly detected by X rays to the chest, skull, and jaw; an upper GI series; various endoscopies; and a biopsy. Esophageal tumors will be diagnosed with these methods as well as liver and bone scans to check for metastases and a bronchoscopy to see whether the tumor has spread to the bronchial tubes.

Cancers of the upper digestive organs can be pinpointed, however, without the intervention of high technology, including potentially harmful X ray radiation. In visual diagnosis, the upper lip corresponds with the condition of the upper digestive system. Specifically, the top part of the upper lip reflects the condition of the esophagus and the lower part of the upper lip reveals the state of the stomach. Swellings, discolorations, or patches in this region indicate corresponding troubles in the respective digestive organs. For example, a pinkish-white hue on the lips shows overconsumption of sugar, fruits, fats, and dairy products. White patches show excessive intake of dairy foods and fat.

The condition of the gums and mouth cavity offers other clues to general health. Swallow gums, often accompanied by pain and inflammation, are caused by overconsumption of liquid, oil, sugar, fruits, and juices. Receding gums are caused by either the overconsumption of yang foods—including animal food, salts, and dried food—or overconsumption of yin foods, including sugar, honey, chocolate, soft drinks, and fruit juices. Abnormally red or purple gums that are not swollen are caused by a combination of yang animal food or salts and yin sugar, fruits, juices, soft drinks, and chemicals. Similar colors accompanied by swelling are caused by the overconsumption of yin foods and drinks. Pale, whitish gums indicate poor circulation as well as a lack of hemoglobin in the bloodstream, due to anemia caused by nutritional imbalance.

Pimples appearing on the inner wall of the mouth cavity are eliminations of excessive protein, fat, oil (from either animal or plant sources), sugar, or sugar products. Bleeding gums, in most cases, are caused by broken blood capillaries, which have been weakened by a lack of salt and other minerals in the bloodstream. In rare cases, they can also be caused by an overconsumption of animal food, dry flour products, salts, and minerals and a lack of fresh fruits and vegetables, as in the case of scurvy. Inflammation deep in the throat, with or without swollen tonsils, is caused by the overconsumption of such yin foods as fruits, juices, sugar, soda, ice-cold drinks, and milk.

The back region of the tongue, the root area below the uvula, also corresponds to the esophagus. Discolorations, inflammation, pimples, or patches here indicate disorders in the gullet.

DIETARY RECOMMENDATIONS

For all cancers in the upper digestive tract, including the mouth, gums, lips, tongue, larynx, pharynx, and esophagus, it is of primary importance that fatty and oily foods, including animal foods such as meat, poultry, eggs, and dairy food of any kind, as well as vegetable oil, be avoided. Sugar, chocolate, fruits, juices, soda, and all food and beverages treated by sweeteners, as well as heavily chemicalized and artificialized food and beverages, are to be avoided. All stimulants including alcohol, coffee, black tea, aromatic herb drinks, curry, mustard, and peppers should be discontinued. Avoid refined flour products and limit even unrefined flour products. Dietary guidelines are as follows.

• **Whole Grains:** Fifty to 60 percent of daily consumption, by volume, should be whole-cereal grains. The first day prepare plain pressure-cooked short-grain brown rice. On subsequent days, alternate brown rice pressure-cooked with 20 to 30 percent millet, then rice with 20 to 30 percent barley, then rice with 20 to 30 percent aduki beans or lentils, and then plain rice again. A delicious morning porridge can be made by taking leftover rice, adding a little more water to soften, and seasoning with a little miso at the end and simmering for two to three minutes more. In ordinary pressure cooking, the ratio of grain to water should be about 1:2. For seasoning, cook with a postage stamped–sized piece of kombu or a pinch of sea salt, depending on the person's condition. Other grains can be used occasionally, including whole wheat berries, rye, corn, buckwheat, and whole oats, though oats should be avoided for the first month. Good-quality sourdough bread may be enjoyed two to three times a week, and noodles, both udon and soba, may also be taken two to three times a week. Avoid all hard baked products until the condition improves, including cookies, cake, pie, crackers, muffins, and the like.

• **Soup:** Five to 10 percent soup, consisting of one or two cups or bowls per day of soup cooked with wakame sea vegetable and various land vegetables such as onions and carrots and seasoned with miso or shoyu. Occasionally a small volume of shiitake mushroom may be added to the soup. Millet soup made with sweet vegetables is especially beneficial for this condition. The miso used in seasoning soups may be barley miso, brown rice miso, or soybean (hatcho) miso and should be naturally aged two to three years.

• **Vegetables:** Twenty to 30 percent vegetables, cooked in a variety of forms. Hard, leafy vegetables are to be emphasized, supplemented with root vegetables and round vegetables such as onions, pumpkin, autumn squash, and cabbage. As a general rule, the following dishes may be prepared, though the frequency may differ from person to person: nishime-style vegetables, four times a week; squash-aduki-kombu dish, three times a week; dried daikon, one cup, three times a week; carrots and carrot tops or daikon and daikon tops, three times a week; blanched vegetables, five to seven times a week; pressed salad, five to seven times a week; raw salad and salad dressing, avoid; steamed greens, five to seven times a week; sautéed vegetables, two to three times a week, using water the first month and then a small volume of sesame oil thereafter; kinipira, two-thirds of a cup, two times a week; tofu, dried tofu, tempeh, or seitan with vegetables, two times a week.

• **Beans:** Five percent small beans, such as aduki beans, lentils, chickpeas, or black soybeans, may be used daily, cooked together with sea vegetables such as kombu or with onions and carrots. Other beans may be used altogether two or three times a month. For seasoning, a small volume of unrefined sea salt or shoyu or miso can be used. Bean products, such as tempeh, natto, and dried or cooked tofu, may be used occasionally, but in moderate volume.

• **Sea Vegetables:** Five percent or less sea vegetable dishes, including wakame and kombu, daily when cooking grain, in soup, etc. A sheet of toasted nori may also be taken daily. A small dish of hijiki or arame should be prepared two times a week. All other sea vegetables are optional.

• **Condiments:** Condiments to be available on the table are gomashio (sesame salt), on the average made with 1 part salt to 18 parts sesame seeds (reduced to 1:16 after two months); kelp or wakame powder; umeboshi plum; and tekka, though all other regular macrobiotic condiments may be used if desired. These condiments may be used daily on grains and vegetables, but the volume should be moderate to suit individual appetite and taste.

• **Pickles:** Pickles, made at home in a variety of ways, are to be eaten daily, one tablespoon in all, though salty pickles are to be minimized.

• **Animal Food:** Meat, poultry, eggs, and other strong animal food are to be avoided. A small volume of white-meat fish may be eaten once a week. The fish should be prepared steamed, boiled, or poached and garnished with grated daikon or ginger. After two months, fish may be eaten twice a week if desired. Strictly avoid blue-meat and red-meat fish and all shellfish.

• **Fruit:** None the best, the less the better, including both tropical and temperate-climate fruit, until the condition improves. If cravings develop, a small volume of cooked fruit with a pinch of sea salt or dried fruit (also preferably cooked) may be taken. Avoid all fruit juices and cider.

• **Sweets and Snacks:** Avoid all sweets and desserts, including good-quality macrobiotic desserts, until the condition improves. To satisfy a sweet tooth, use sweet vegetables every day in cooking, drink sweet vegetable drink (see special drinks below), and eat sweet vegetable jam. Mochi, rice balls, vegetable sushi, and other grain-based snacks may be eaten frequently. Limit rice cakes, popcorn, and other dry or baked snacks, as they may harden the tumor. In the event of cravings, a small volume of amasake, barley malt, or rice syrup may be taken.

• **Nuts and Seeds:** Nuts and nut butters are to be avoided due to their high amount of fat and protein, except for chestnuts. Unsalted, roasted seeds such as squash seeds and pumpkin seeds may be consumed as a snack, up to one cup altogether per week.

• **Seasonings:** Seasonings, such as unrefined sea salt, shoyu, and miso, are to be used moderately in order to avoid unnecessary thirst. Avoid mirin and garlic. If you become particularly thirsty after a meal or between meals, you should cut back on these seasonings until the normal level of thirst returns.

• **Beverages:** Beverages and other dietary practices can follow the general recommendations in Part I, with bancha twig tea as the main beverage. Strictly avoid the beverages on the "infrequent" and "avoid" list and don't take grain coffee for the first two to three months after starting this new way of eating.

Chewing thoroughly is essential for all types of cancer, but especially for cancers in the mouth and upper alimentary tract. Chew each mouthful 50 times, or preferably 100 times. Liquefying and mixing food well with saliva contributes to the prevention and improvement of this condition. Also, it is important to avoid overconsumption of liquid, though bancha tea or water should be consumed if thirst arises. It is also important to avoid overeating and eating within three hours of sleeping.

As noted in the introduction to Part II, persons who have received or who are currently undergoing medical treatment may need to make further dietary modifications.

SPECIAL DRINKS AND PREPARATIONS

Persons with upper digestive cancer may also consume some special drinks and dishes, which, taken in small volume, can strengthen blood quality. These dishes include:

• **Sweet Vegetable Drink:** Take one small cup every day for the first month, then two to three times a week the second month.

• **Carrot-Daikon Drink:** Take one small cup two to three times a week for two to four weeks, and then once every three days for one month.

• **Buckwheat Noodles or Paste:** Buckwheat noodles or buckwheat paste, made with buckwheat flour cooked with chopped scallions, is helpful for upper digestive cancers if consumed two to three times per week.

• **Ume-Sho-Kuzu Drink:** A cup of kuzu drink can be helpful if drunk daily for a one- to two-week period and occasionally thereafter.

• **Grated Daikon:** Grate about half a small cup of fresh daikon, add a few drops of shoyu, and take two to three times a week.

• **Miso-Scallion Condiment:** One teaspoon of miso sautéed with sesame oil together with the same volume of scallions and a small volume of grated ginger or garlic added while cooking may be used as a condiment for the meal.

• **Brown Rice Cream:** In the event that the esophagus is blocked by a tumorous obstruction and the person is unable to eat, or if the tumor has been removed and a tube has been inserted from the nose, the diet should be liquefied by cooking with more water and by mashing food substances. Rice cream is also helpful and may be consumed with miso soup as well as other mashed and liquefied vegetables, beans, and sea vegetables.

HOME CARES

• **Body Scrub:** Scrubbing the whole body, including the throat and neck, with a towel that has been immersed in hot water and squeezed out is very helpful for better circulation of blood, lumph, and other body fluids, as well as for activating physical and mental energies.

• **Compress Guidelines:** For a small number of tumors in the upper digestive system, a compress may be needed to gradually help draw out excess mucus and fat. Please see a qualified macrobiotic teacher for guidance on the proper use and frequency of a compress or plaster. Several types are used depending on the person's condition. Precede the compress or plaster with application of a towel that has been soaked in hot water and squeezed out over the affected area for about three to five minutes to stimulate circulation.

• **Taro Plaster:** For throat and esophageal cancers, a taro potato plaster can be applied to the area daily for three to four hours, immediately following application of a ginger compress for about three to five minutes. In some cases, a taro plaster causes mucus and fat to gather too rapidly for comfort, in which event a lotus-root plaster can be applied to slow the discharge. This is made by mixing an equal volume of grated fresh lotus root and grated taro potato with a small amount of white flour to hold them together, and mixing with 5 to 10 percent grated fresh ginger. The lotus plaster may be applied for a few hours daily over a few weeks' period.

• **After Surgery:** In the event that the esophagus is blocked by a tumorous obstruction and the person is unable to eat, or if the tumor has been removed and a tube has been inserted from the nose, the diet should be liquefied by cooking with more water and by mashing food substances. Rice cream is also helpful and may be consumed with miso soup as well as other mashed and liquefied vegetables, beans, and sea vegetables. Carrot and lotus-root drink is also helpful in this case.

OTHER CONSIDERATIONS

• Avoid synthetic clothing, especially around the area of the throat, neck, head, and chest, and use cotton underwear, clothing, and sleepwear if possible.

• Maintaining clean, fresh air inside the home is important, and for this purpose green plants can be placed in each room. Indoor air circulation can also be maintained by frequently opening the windows.

• Avoid frequent exposure to artificial radiation, including medical and dental X rays, smoke detectors, television, video terminals, and hand-held appliances, which are weakening to the lymph and blood and to the upper digestive and digestive system.

• Try to be happy, positive, and outgoing. Singing, dancing, and playing are particularly beneficial in improving overall health and mentality and harmonizing with the rhythms of nature.

• Light exercise, including breathing fresh air outdoors and ten to fifteen minutes a day practicing long exhalations through the nostrils, will promote harmonious mental and physical metabolism and contribute to overall relaxation.

PERSONAL EXPERIENCE

Granular Myoblastoma on the Vocal Cord

In the spring of 1979, Laura Anne Fitzpatrick discovered that her voice became raspy when she tried out for cheerleader at her high school in Sherborn, Massachusetts. Doctors told her that she had a benign tumor on the vocal cords known as a granular myoblastoma, and in August she had it surgically removed. By January 1980, however, the tumor had reappeared, and Laura underwent a second operation, this time with advanced laser-beam surgery, at University Hospital in Boston. A month later the swelling returned, and doctors feared yet another recurrence of the obstruction.

During this period, Laura and her family saw a television program on macrobiotics. After attending a seminar on cancer and diet at the EWF, Laura came to see me for a consultation, and I recommended the Cancer Prevention Diet. I warned her to completely avoid oil in cooking and advised her to go to bed with a taro plaster wrapped around her neck. Laura's family, including her parents and two sisters and three brothers still living at home, was very supportive and started the macrobiotic way of eating as well. "John and I both wanted to support Laura, and we also began to eat in this new way as much as we could," her mother later noted. "We changed our stove from electric to gas, and the adventures continued as we truly tried to understand the principles behind the diet."

Laura experienced many changes in her body as the toxins from many previous years of imbalanced eating were rapidly released. She began to feel more energy and her voice started improving. In the spring of 1980, she returned for a medical checkup, and her doctor was surprised to find that the operation was unnecessary. Laura continued to improve through the fall. However, in November she began to deviate from the diet and use oil in cooking.

On Thanksgiving she had turkey. By Christmas her symptoms started to return and her voice grew weak. The doctors told her the tumor had returned and would have to be removed.

Laura and her family asked the hospital for a two-month reprieve from surgery and returned to see me. "[Michio] scolded me humorously," Laura recalled of that visit, "and I decided I was ready to get back to basics and resume the diet he had recommended. . . . I again began to discharge a lot of mucus and felt a tremendous cleansing coming very rapidly. I resumed the taro potato compresses each night. One humorous sidelight of this was that my father's T-shirts were disappearing, and he would find them with mysterious brown spots from the remains of the taro potato. I found that whenever I missed the ginger and taro potato plaster compress for a few days, the mucus would not discharge as freely. I prepared all the compresses by myself and the routine became normal."

At the college she was now attending, Laura found it difficult to get the proper food and care she needed. But with the help of her family she succeeded. In March 1981 she returned for a medical checkup, and her doctor told her the condition had improved and stabilized and there was no need for surgery. "I learned from this experience that the diet makes sense," Laura concluded. "I feel I am well on my way to a full and complete recovery." Today, twelve years later, Laura is happily married and in excellent health. Source: "Granular Myoblastoma on the Vocal Cord," *The Cancer Prevention Diet* (Brookline, MA: East West Foundation, 1981), 87–89.

15

Stomach Cancer

FREQUENCY

In the United States, an estimated 13,300 persons will die from stomach cancer this year, and 24,400 new cases will develop. Overall, deaths from stomach cancer have sharply declined by about two-thirds in the United States during the last thirty years. This is attributed largely to the decreased consumption of sausage, luncheon meats, and other meats preserved in large amounts of salt or containing nitrosamines. Men suffer the illness about one and a half times as often as women, blacks slightly more than whites. It is more prevalent in older than in middle-aged or younger persons. Stomach or gastric cancer, as it is also known, accounts for about 5 percent of all cancers in the United States. In Japan, however, it is the leading type of cancer, with an incidence six times higher than in the United States.

Surgery is the standard medical treatment, though many cases are considered inoperable because stomach cancer is usually detected only in the late stages of development. The operation is called a gastrectomy, and the stomach may be partly or totally removed. In total gastrectomies, regional lymph nodes, the spleen, and part of the small intestine are also removed. Chemotherapy or radiation may follow. From 12 to 14 percent of patients who undergo this treatment survive five years or more.

STRUCTURE

The stomach is a relatively hollow gourd-shaped organ located in the upper left of the abdominal cavity between the esophagus and the small intestine. The layers of the stomach include 1) the mucosa, or interior lining of the stomach, which secretes digestive enzymes; 2) the connective tissue between the submucosa and the muscles of the stomach; 3) the muscular coat, which enables the stomach to contract and expand and move decomposing food toward the intestines, and 4) the serosa, or outer coating.

The mucosa contains millions of tubular glands, which secrete hydrochloric acid or pepsin as well as small amounts of mucin, antianemia materials, and inorganic salts. The upper, expanded region of the stomach, known as the fundus and the body, secretes hydrochloric acid, the stronger of the two acids. The lower, more compact section of the stomach, called the pylorus, secretes pepsin. These acids decompose protein into its various amino acids. Together with muscular peristalsis, enzymatic actions convert solid food into semiliquid chyme, an acid substance that relaxes the lower pyloric valve, allowing the chyme to pass from the stomach into the duodenal section of the small intestine.

CAUSE OF CANCER

In order for the digestive juices in the stomach to be secreted properly, food must first be alkalized by saliva in the mouth. Hence the necessity for thorough chewing of each mouthful of food. Whole grains, especially those cooked with a pinch of sea salt, pass through the stomach to the small intestine, where they are absorbed in the villi and converted into red blood cells and other healthy circulatory fluids. In contrast, morsels of food from refined grains such as white flour and white rice, as well as refined sugar, start to be absorbed directly in the stomach and enter the body fluids prematurely, producing a thinner quality of blood and lymph. Stomach cancer results from long-term consumption of extreme yin foods and beverages such as refined grain, flour, sugar and other sweets, soda and ice-cold drinks, alcohol, aromatic and stimulant beverages, chemicals and drugs. Strong yang foods, which overtax the stomach, can also cause cancer, including foods high in animal protein and salts, as well as high-fat, oily, and greasy foods. Repeated oversecretion of stomach acids to neutralize and process an excess of these foods results in irritating the stomach lining, ulcerations, and eventually the formation of tumors. Depending on the location and type, stomach cancer can metastasize to nearby lymph nodes, the pancreas, liver, or ovaries (Krukenberg tumor). It can also spread to the lungs, bones, and occasionally the skin through the lymphatic system.

The yin form of stomach cancer, affecting the upper expanded region of the stomach, is caused by overconsumption of extremely expansive substances, especially refined grains, sugar, foods containing chemical additives or preservatives such as MSG, and food grown with chemical fertilizers or pesticides. Cancer in the more compact pylorus in the lower stomach results from overconsumption of meat, eggs, fish, or other overly yang products. Over the last twenty years, the rate of stomach cancer in the United States has fallen about 75 percent. In a recent issue of *Life* magazine, in the article, "The Endless Quest for a Cure," medical writer Jeff Wheelwright concludes: "The trend towards more vegetables, fruit, and fiber in the American diet . . . may be the main reason for the decline."

MEDICAL EVIDENCE

• In 1887 Ephraim Cutter, M.D., a physician from Albany, New York, wrote a book in which he postulated that "cancer is a disease of nutrition." Cutter presented nine case histories of cancer relieved by putting the patient on a balanced diet and concluded that the question was not vegetable versus animal food, but the "proper proportion of animal to vegetable food." He listed mental depression and stress as contributing factors and reported one case of stomach cancer "evidently caused by living in the suburbs and having business in the city, taking a light lunch there, and returning late in the day, all tired out, and having a hearty supper with much condiments." Cutter speculated that "cancer may be cured in times to come by food." Source: Ephraim Cutter, M.D., *Diet in Cancer* (New York: Kellogg, 1887), 19–26.

• From 1904 to 1911 British surgeon Robert McCarrison traveled in the Hunza, a remote Himalayan kingdom in the then Northwest Territory of India. There he was astonished to discover a completely healthy culture in which the infectious and degenerative diseases of modern civilization, including colonial India, were unknown. "I never saw a case of asthenic dyspepsia, of gastric or duodenal ulcer, of appendicitis, of mucous colitis, or of cancer," he informed his medical colleagues. McCarrison hypothesized that the unusual health and longevity of the Hunza people was due primarily to their daily diet consisting of whole wheat chapatis, barley, and maize, supplemented by leafy green vegetables, beans and legumes, apricots, and a small amount of dairy products and goat's milk only on feast days. The Hunzas did not eat refined white rice, sugar, black tea, or spices as did most of the Indian population. In 1927 Sir Robert McCarrison assumed the post of director of nutritional research in India and to test his theory began a series of laboratory experiments. Feeding the Hunza diet and the regular Indian diet to rats over a period of four years, he discovered that animals fed the modern, refined diet of Bengal and Madras contracted cysts, abscesses, heart disease, and cancer of the stomach. Rats fed the Hunza whole-grain diet remained healthy and free of all disease. Sources: Robert McCarrison, M.D., "Faulty Food in Relation to Gastro-intestinal Disorder," *Journal of the American Medical Association* 78 (1922) 1–8, and G. T. Wrench, M.D., *The Wheel of Health* (London: O. W. Daniel, 1938).

• A 1966 case-control study found that stomach cancer cases had consumed fried foods more frequently than controls, especially bacon drippings and animal fats used for cooking. Source: J. Higginson, "Etiological Factors in Gastrointestinal Cancer in Man," *Journal of the National Cancer Institute* 37:527–45.

• In 1971 a Japanese cancer researcher reported a significant negative association between per capita tofu intake and stomach cancer. Source: T. Hirayama, "Epidemiology of Stomach Cancer," in T. Murakami (ed.), *Early Gastric Cancer, Gann Monograph on Cancer Research* (Tokyo: University of Tokyo Press) 1:3–19.

• A 1974 case-control study observed that high-starch foods such as refined white bread and sugar were consumed more frequently by gastric cancer cases than controls. Source: B. Modan et al., "The Role of Starches in the Etiology of Gastric Cancer," *Cancer* 34:2087–92.

• In 1978 medical researchers reported that Brussels sprouts, cabbage, turnips, cauliflower, broccoli, and other vegetables high in a substance identified as indoles lessened the incidence of stomach and breast cancer in laboratory animals by 77 percent. Source: L. W. Wattenberg and W. D. Loub, "Inhibition of Polycyclic Hydrocarbon-induced Neoplasia by Naturally Occurring Indoles," *Cancer Research* 38:1410–13.

• In 1981 Japan's National Cancer Center reported that people who eat miso soup daily are 33 percent less likely to contract stomach cancer than those who never eat miso soup. The thirteen-year study, involving about 265,000 men and women over forty, also found that miso soup is effective in reducing the risk of "hypertensive diseases, ischemic heart disease and all other causes of death." Source: T. Hirayama, "Relationship of Soybean Paste Soup Intake to Gastric Cancer Risk," *Nutrition and Cancer* 3:223–33.

• A 1981 case-control study of 100 gastric cancer patients and controls in Shanghai showed significantly lower cancer risk among those who regularly consumed soy milk. Source: S. K. Xing, "Personal Communication," *Chinese Journal of Preventive Medicine*, 15:2.

• In 1979 researchers at Tokyo Medical and Dental University reported that traditional Oriental diagnostic techniques for stomach cancer compared favorably with Western detection methods. Using a Meridian Imbalance Diagram based on twenty-three different ratios of measurements along the yin and yang meridians of the upper and lower limbs, the scientists compared Oriental and Western diagnosis in twenty-two patients complaining of stomach problems and nineteen healthy controls. These findings were then evaluated against postoperative reports. For example, ten of the patients were later confirmed to have stomach cancer. "This shows the existence of a pattern of Oriental diagnosis corresponding to a specific Western diagnosis," the researchers concluded. Source: Jean Pierre Garnery, M.D., et al., "Oriental Diagnosis in Stomach Cancer Patients," *American Journal of Chinese Medicine* 7, no. 1:91–99.

• Epidemiology studies indicate that vitamin C–containing foods such as green leafy vegetables and citrus fruits may offer protection against stomach cancer, and animal experiments show that vitamin C can protect against nitrosamine-induced stomach cancer. Source: National Research Council, *Diet and Health* (Washington, DC: National Academy Press, 1989).

• In a case-control study of Hawaiian men of Japanese ancestry, researchers reported in 1990 that consumption of all types of vegetables was protective against stomach cancer. Source: P. H. Chyou et al., "A Case-Cohort Study of Diet and Stomach Cancer," *Cancer Research* 60:7501–4.

• The high rate of stomach cancer in Japan caused some Japanese scientists to speculate that a diet high in soy sauce might be a factor. However, in 1991 researchers at the University of Wisconsin observed just the opposite. In laboratory tests, mice given fermented soy sauce experienced 26 percent less cancer than mice on the regular diet. Also, soy-supplemented mice averaged about one-quarter the number of tumors per mouse as the control group. Soy sauce "exhibited a pronounced anticarcinogenic effect," the researchers concluded. Source: J. Raloff, "A Soy Sauce Surprise," *Science News* 139:357.

• A number of studies have shown that a diet rich in cruciferous vegetables such as broccoli, cabbage, cauliflower, and Brussels sprouts can lower the risk for cancer of the stomach, breast, and large intestine. In 1992 researchers at Johns Hopkins University School of Medicine reported that they had identified the ingredient in broccoli that worked as a powerful anticancer compound in laboratory experiments. The chemical in broccoli, sulforaphane, boosts the production of an important enzyme known to neutralize carcinogens before they trigger tumor growth. In addition to broccoli, sulforaphane is found in bok choy, ginger, scallions, and other vegetables. Source: Paul Talalay, *Proceedings of the National Academy of Sciences*, March 16, 1992, and "Broccoli Contains Powerful Cancer Fighter, Study Shows," *Cleveland Plain Dealer*, March 15, 1992.

DIAGNOSIS

Stomach cancer is difficult to diagnose by modern medical methods. Only 18 percent of current stomach cancers are detected in the local stage before spreading to other organs of the body. Cancer of the stomach is commonly confused with other abdominal disorders, especially gastric ulcers, and the patient may feel no unusual symptoms. The normal hospital procedure is called a gastroscopy and allows direct X ray viewing of the entire stomach. A biopsy is performed if cancer is suspected, and the lining of the stomach may be brushed and washed to obtain cell samples. Follow-up chest and skeletal X rays and a liver scan are taken to determine possible metastases.

The condition of the stomach is relatively easy to diagnose by traditional Oriental medicine, and the tendency toward acidosis, ulcerations, or tumors can be monitored long before they actually develop so that preventive dietary action can be taken. To diagnose stomach problems, corresponding areas in the face can be observed: the upper lip and the bridge of the nose. The entire digestive system is reflected in the mouth as a whole, and the upper lip mirrors the upper digestive tract, especially the stomach. More specifically, the left side of the upper lip corresponds with the upper, more yin part of the stomach, while the right side shows the lower, more yang region. Swelling in the upper lip shows an expanded stomach condition caused by consumption of refined grains, sugar and other sweeteners, alcohol, and tropical fruit and juices or overeating. A contracted upper lip reflects a tightening in the stomach due to excessive intake of meat, eggs, salt, or dry baked goods. Both of these conditions reflect overacidity in the stomach, and the tendency or presence of ulcerations may be indicated by inflammation, a blister or discoloring on the upper lip.

Brown blotches or freckles on the upper part of bridge of the nose indicate chronic stomach acidosis, ulcerations, hypoglycemic and diabetic tendencies, or possible stomach cancer. In the case of stomach cancer, a slight green tinge may show up in this area. The skin as a whole also shows the condition of the stomach. A splotchy brown or dirty skin color suggests chronic acidity in the stomach as a result of excess sugar or fruit consumption. Discolorations along the stomach meridian, especially in the area below the knee or on top of the foot in the extended region of the second and third toes, are a good indicator of stomach imbalances. Again, a green shading in either of these locations indicates possible stomach cancer.

The near back of the tongue also may be examined to observe developing stomach problems. A dark red color indicates inflammation, ulcerations, and a potential development of stomach cancer. A white or yellow color or white patches indicate accumulations of fat and mucus in the stomach. Blue or purple signifies overconsumption of sugar, soft drinks, alcohol, drugs, medications, and other extreme yin substances. Small mushroomlike eruptions are signs of acidity, ulcerations, and possible nausea and regurgitation.

DIETARY RECOMMENDATIONS

The main cause of stomach cancer is the long-time consumption or overconsumption of foods and drinks that are producing alkaline or acid conditions in the body. Accordingly, it is necessary to avoid all overly expansive foods, including all refined food such as white rice, white bread, and other refined flour products, sugar, honey, chocolate, carob, and similar sweeteners; sugar-treated food and beverages; artificial soda and soft drinks; coffee, black tea, and alcohol; cold, icy beverages; all stimulants and spices, including curry, mustard, and pepper; all aromatic foods and beverages; butter, milk, and cream; chemicalized food, seasonings, and beverages; oily, greasy food; tropical fruits, juices, and vegetables of tropical origin, including potatoes, sweet potatoes, yams, tomatoes, and eggplant. In addition, all extreme yang foods, such as beef, pork, poultry, and eggs; all types of dairy food, including cheese; very salty food; hard baked flour products such as hard bread and cookies; all baked animal food; and high-protein and high-fat food are to be avoided. The following dietary guidelines should be observed.

• **Whole Grains.** Fifty to 60 percent of daily consumption, by volume, should be whole-cereal grains. The first day prepare plain pressure-cooked short-grain brown rice. On following days, alternate brown rice pressure-cooked with 20 to 30 percent millet (which is particularly beneficial to the stomach), then rice with 20 to 30 percent barley, then rice with 20 to 30 percent aduki beans or lentils, and then plain rice again. A delicious morning porridge can be made by taking leftover rice or millet, adding a little more water to soften, and seasoning with a little miso at the end and simmering for two to three minutes more. In ordinary pressure cooking, the ratio of grain to water should be about 1:2. For seasoning, cook with a postage stamp–sized piece of kombu or a pinch of sea salt, depending on the person's condition. Other grains can be used occasionally, including whole wheat berries, rye, corn, and whole oats, though oats should be avoided for the first month. Buckwheat and seitan should be minimized. Good-quality sourdough bread may be enjoyed two to three times a week, and noodles, both udon and soba, may also be taken two to three times a week. Avoid all hard baked products until the condition improves, including cookies, cake, pie, crackers, muffins, and the like.

• **Soup:** Five to 10 percent soup, consisting of one or two cups or bowls per day of soup cooked with wakame sea vegetable and various land vegetables such as onions and carrots and seasoned with miso or shoyu. Occasionally a small volume of shiitake mushroom may be added to the soup. Autumn squash, cabbage, onions, and other round, sweet vegetables may be used often. Millet-squash soup is especially beneficial for this condition. The miso used in seasoning soups may be barley miso, brown rice miso, or soybean (hatcho) miso and should be naturally aged two to three years. To satisfy a sweet tooth, millet soup with sweet vegetables such as squash, cabbage, onions, and carrots may be prepared often.

• **Vegetables:** Twenty to 30 percent vegetables, cooked in a variety of forms. Among vegetables, daikon and its greens are particularly recommended for frequent use, as are autumn squash, cabbage, onions, and other round vegetables. As a general rule, the following dishes may be prepared, though the frequency may differ from person to person: nishime-style vegetables, four times a week; squash-aduki-kombu dish, three times a week; dried daikon, one cup, three times a week; carrots and carrot tops or daikon and daikon tops, three times a week; blanched vegetables, five to seven times a week; pressed salad, five to seven times a week; raw salad and salad dressing, avoid; steamed greens, five to seven times a week; sautéed vegetables, two to three times a week, using water the first month and then a small volume of sesame oil thereafter; kinpira, two-thirds of a cup, two times a week; tofu, dried tofu, tempeh, or seitan with vegetables, two times a week.

• **Beans:** Five percent small beans, such as aduki beans, lentils, chickpeas, or black soybeans, may be used daily, cooked together with sea vegetables such as kombu or with onions and carrots. Other beans may be used altogether two to three times a month. For seasoning, a small volume of unrefined sea salt or shoyu or miso can be used. Bean products, such as tempeh, natto, and dried or cooked tofu, may be used occasionally, but in moderate volume.

• **Sea Vegetables:** Five percent or less sea vegetable dishes, including wakame and kombu, daily when cooking grain, in soup, etc. A sheet of toasted nori may also be taken daily. A small dish of hijiki or arame should be prepared two times a week. All other sea vegetables are optional. Sea vegetables can be cooked with other vegetables or sautéed with a small volume of sesame oil after softening them by soaking and boiling lightly in water.

• **Condiments:** Condiments to be available on the table are gomashio (sesame salt), on the average made with 1 part salt to 18 parts sesame seeds (reduced to 1:16 after two months); kelp or wakame powder; umeboshi plum; and tekka, though all other regular macrobiotic condiments may be used if desired. These condiments may be used daily on grains and vegetables, but the volume should be moderate to suit individual appetite and taste.

• **Pickles:** Pickles, made at home in a variety of ways, are to be eaten daily, one tablespoon in all, though salty pickles are to be minimized.

• **Animal Food:** Meat, poultry, eggs, and other strong animal food is to be avoided. A small volume of white-meat fish may be eaten once a week. The fish should be prepared steamed, boiled, or poached and garnished with grated daikon or ginger. After two months, fish may be eaten twice a week if desired. Strictly avoid blue-meat and red-meat fish and all shellfish.

• **Fruit:** None the best, the less the better, including both tropical and temperate-climate fruit, until the condition improves. If cravings develop, a small volume of cooked fruit with a pinch of sea salt or dried fruit (also preferably cooked) may be taken. Avoid all fruit juices and cider.

• **Sweets and Snacks:** Avoid all sweets and desserts, including good-quality macrobiotic desserts, until the condition improves. To satisfy a sweet tooth, use sweet vegetables every day in cooking, drink sweet vegetable drink (see special drinks below), and make sweet vegetable jam. Mochi, rice balls, vegetable sushi, and other grain-based snacks may be eaten frequently. Limit rice cakes, popcorn, and other dry or baked snacks, as they may harden the tumor. In the event of cravings, a small volume of amasake, barley malt, or rice syrup may be taken.

• **Nuts and Seeds:** Nuts and nut butters are to be avoided due to their high amount of fat and protein, except for chestnuts. Unsalted, roasted seeds such as sunflower seeds and pumpkin seeds may be consumed as a snack, up to one cup altogether per week.

• **Seasonings:** Seasonings, such as unrefined sea salt, shoyu, and miso, are to be used moderately in order to avoid unnecessary thirst. Avoid mirin and garlic. If you become particularly thirsty after the meal or between meals, you should cut back on these seasonings until the normal level of thirst returns.

• **Beverages:** Beverages and other dietary practices can follow the general recommendations in Part I, including bancha twig tea as the main beverage. Strictly avoid the beverages on the "infrequent" and "avoid" list and don't take grain coffee for the first two to three months after starting this new way of eating.

The most important thing in connection with dietary practice is chewing very well, until all food becomes liquid in the mouth and well mixed with saliva. Chew very, very well at least 50 times, preferably 100 times, per mouthful. It is also important to avoid overeating and eating within three hours of sleeping.

As noted in the introduction to Part II, persons who have received or who are currently undergoing medical treatment may need to make further dietary modifications.

SPECIAL DRINKS AND PREPARATIONS

Persons with stomach cancer may also consume some special drinks and dishes, which, taken in small volume, can strengthen blood quality. These dishes include:

• **Sweet Vegetable Drink:** Take one small cup every day for the first month, then two to three times a week the second month.

• **Carrot-Daikon Drink:** Take one small cup two to three times a week for two to four weeks, and then once every three days for one month.

• **Scallion-Miso Condiment:** Scallion-miso condiment can be used frequently in small volume as one of the regular condiments. This is made by cooking chopped scallions and an equal volume of miso with a small amount of sesame oil. However, condiments should not be used in excess, and a salty or strong taste should be avoided.

• **Brown Rice Cream:** In the event the stomach has been removed in part or whole by surgery, genuine brown rice cream can be used. Two to three bowls may be consumed per day with a small volume of condiments such as scallion-miso, gomashio (sesame salt), tekka, or umeboshi plum for the initial several days. After that period, regular brown rice and other cereal grains can be served, gradually shifting toward more complete meals, including various side dishes. During both times, it is very important to chew the food thoroughly until it assumes a liquid form, up to 100 or more times per mouthful. The removed portion of the stomach will often restore itself as time passes. Even if the amputated section is not restorable, chewing well can sufficiently serve for digestion.

• **Grated Daikon:** Grate about one half cup of fresh daikon, add a few drops of shoyu, and take two to three times a week.

HOME CARES

• **Body Scrub:** Scrubbing the whole body, including the abdominal region and the spinal region, with a towel that has been immersed in hot water and squeezed out is very helpful for better circulation of blood, lymph, and other body fluids, as well as for activating physical and mental energies.

• **Compress Guidelines:** For a small number of tumors in the female reproductive system, a compress may be needed to gradually help draw out excess mucus and fat. Please see a qualified macrobiotic teacher for guidance on the proper use and frequency of a compress or plaster. Several types are used depending on the person's condition. Precede the compress or plaster with application of a towel that has been soaked in hot water and squeezed out over the affected area for about three to five minutes to stimulate circulation.

• **Taro Plaster:** A taro potato plaster may be applied for three to four hours or overnight on the stomach region, immediately after a hot ginger compress applied for three to five minutes. They can be used daily for two to three weeks or whenever necessary to help reduce tumor development and to provide relief in the case of aches and pains.

• **Palm Healing:** Application of warmth on the stomach region as well as palm healing for one-half to one hour also can help ease pain or ache in the stomach region.

OTHER CONSIDERATIONS

• Maintaining clean, fresh air inside the home is important, and for this purpose green plants can be placed in each room. Indoor air circulation can also be maintained by frequently opening the windows.

• Wearing cotton underwear and avoiding synthetic fabrics are helpful for better skin metabolism and to facilitate energy flow through the body.

• Avoid frequent exposure to artificial radiation, including medical and dental X rays, smoke detectors, television, video terminals, and hand-held appliances, which are weakening to the stomach and digestive system.

• Try to be happy, positive, and outgoing. Singing, dancing, and playing are particularly beneficial in improving overall health and mentality and harmonizing with the rhythms of nature.

• Light exercise, including breathing fresh air outdoors and ten to fifteen minutes a day practicing long exhalations through the nostrils, will promote harmonious mental and physical metabolism and contribute to overall relaxation.

PERSONAL EXPERIENCES

Stomach Cancer

In 1983 doctors in New York told Katsuhide Kitatani that he had stomach cancer. After surgery, he was put on chemotherapy, but the cancer spread to the lymph system and he was told that he had only six to twelve months to live. Mr. Kitatani, a senior administrator at the United Nations for many years, started to wind up his affairs. Then one day at a party he ran into a friend who had been suffering from lymph cancer. Mr. Kitatani noticed that all her hair, which had fallen out during medical treatment, had been restored. He asked her how she did it.

She said, "I'm practicing macrobiotics."

"What kind of economics is that?" he asked.

The friend gave him the name of a book to read, and in the fifth or sixth bookstore he looked he finally found the book. It described how a medical doctor—the president of a large American hospital—whose body was riddled with tumors had healed his own terminal condition with the help of a macrobiotic dietary approach. "The diet looked very easy, very Japanese," Mr. Kitatani, who was born in Japan, reflected afterward. "It included plenty of rice, wakame, and miso soup." After arranging a consultation with me in Boston, he started the diet. "I bought three macrobiotic cookbooks and asked my wife to start cooking. I was a very good supervisor." His wife started the diet immediately, but his twin sons were skeptical. Mr. Kitatani's friends were encouraging but also expected him to die shortly.

As his condition improved, Mr. Kitatani looked back on his own previous way of eating and the factors that had led to his illness. "I was fifteen when World War II ended. We were starving and had lost the will to produce. We received sugar from the American GIs. Soon I was crawling around on my hands and knees and developed skin disease, but I didn't associate it with what I was eating at the time." Hot springs helped his skin condition. In a U.S. occupation forces camp where he worked, Mr. Kitatani developed a liking for catsup, ice cream, and many other highly processed foods. Later he started working for the United Nations and over the last few decades has been posted all over the world. "Wherever I went, the first question I would ask is: 'Where's the best restaurant?'"

After nine months on his new diet, Mr. Kitatani's cancer went away completely, and he had the unexpected joy of having to replan the rest of his life. He decided that the best way he could help others would be to start a macrobiotic club at the United Nations. "The pace of life is getting quicker and quicker. All around the world people now have access to modern supermarkets and industrially processed food. At the UN we arrange for fertilizers to be shipped, insecticides to be sprayed, and the symptoms of diseases to be eliminated without addressing their underlying causes. People talk till they're blue in the face but don't seem to take action.

"All around the world people are incapacitated and unproductive. UN debates are really selfish and guided by egocentric thinking. The UN has been successful on limited occasions in avoiding conflagrations. In the future, it seems to be that peace will come from individuals who are free of physical and spiritual diseases. Every one of us is an actual or potential peacemaker." For the last ten years Mr. Kitatani has been cancer-free, and he is now deputy secretary-general of the United Nations specializing in world population issues.

Source: Michio Kushi with Alex Jack, *One Peaceful World* (New York: St. Martin's Press, 1987).

16

Liver Cancer

FREQUENCY

An estimated 12,300 Americans will die of liver cancer this year. Another 15,400 new cases will develop, almost evenly divided between men and women. Accounting for about 2 percent of primary cancers in this country, the liver is a common site of metastases from other parts of the digestive system, the breast, and the lungs. There is a higher incidence of liver cancer in Asia than in North America or Europe. In China, liver cancer is one of the top three cancers, and it is also high in the Philippines, Hong Kong, and Papua New Guinea, where it is associated with aflatoxin poisoning.

Hepatomas, tumors involving the epithelial lining of both lobes of the liver, and *cholingiocarcinomas,* which began in the bile ducts and spread to the liver itself, account for half of all liver cancers in the United States. Other varieties include *hemangiosarcomas* or mixed tumors of sarcoma cells and dilated blood vessels; *mixed sarcomas,* which spread to other parts of the liver and lymph nodes in the vicinity of the lung and brain; *hepatoblastomas,* rare granular tumors found in children; and *adenocarcinomas,* glandular tumors that develop in the bile ducts.

Most liver cancer patients die from liver failure within six months of diagnosis. Only 1 percent currently survive five years or more. Current medical treatment usually calls for a total hepatic lobectomy, a surgical operation in which the tumor and part or all of the healthy tissue in one lobe around it are removed. For inoperable cancers, a chemotherapy technique called hepatic artery infusion is offered. This procedure calls for placing a catheter directly into blood vessels going to the liver in order to concentrate drugs in that organ.

STRUCTURE

The liver is situated in the right side of the abdominal cavity above the intestines and adjacent to the stomach, gallbladder, and pancreas. About the same size as the brain, it weighs approximately three pounds and governs many of the body's digestive, circulatory, and excretory functions. Its many operations include filtering toxins from the blood; making and transporting bile; controlling blood sugar levels; converting carbohydrates, fat, and protein into one another; and manufacturing hormones and enzymes. In traditional Oriental medicine, the liver is known as the body's general because of its commanding functions. Using a contemporary metaphor, we may liken it to the body's Environmental Protection Agency, which monitors the quality of the internal environment and neutralizes any harmful substances. A person cannot live without a liver. However, even if 80 percent of the organ is removed, it will continue to function, and the missing section often grows back.

CAUSE OF CANCER

When leaving the heart, part of the blood passes to the digestive organs, where oxygen is supplied to the tissues and food that has been absorbed is picked up. Rather than circulating directly through the body, this metabolized material from the intestines and stomach goes directly to the liver. There it is cleansed of impurities before being sent into the bloodstream. A healthy liver can filter a relatively large and continuous amount of toxic substances that enter the body. For instance, the liver can neutralize about one-third of an ounce of alcohol per hour. However, after years of imbalanced food and beverage intake, the liver may grow swollen or hard and lose its natural ability to function.

As a compact, active, and central body organ, the liver is yang in structure and thus particularly affected by overconsumption of beef, pork, poultry, eggs, dairy products, salt, and other strong yang foods. Though liver disorders tend to have a yang origin, the symptoms can be accelerated by expansive, yin substances such as alcohol, foods high in fat and oils, flour products, sugar, tropical fruits and vegetables, raw food, and stimulants.

A look at fat metabolism is helpful at this point to understand the mechanism of degenerative disease and tumor formation, including liver cancer, at the cellular level. Lipids are the family name for fats, oils, and fatlike substances, including fatty acids, cholesterol, and lipoproteins. Fats are solid at room temperature, while oils are fluid. Solid lipids tend to contain more saturated fatty acids. Fatty acids are long chains of carbon and hydrogen atoms including an oxygen molecule at one end. Saturated fatty acids are bonded or saturated to hydrogen atoms. Unsaturated fatty acids lack at least one pair of hydrogen atoms. Polyunsaturated fatty acids are those in which more than one pair is missing.

Fatty acids are the building blocks of fats, just as simple sugars are the fundamental units of carbohydrates. In order to help digest fats, which are insoluble in water and form large globules, the liver secretes bile, a yellowish liquid stored in the gallbladder. In the intestine, bile serves to emulsify fats and enables them to be broken down into fatty acids and glycerol by digestive enzymes.

Lipids are essential to digestion but can be harmful to the body, especially saturated acids like stearic acid, found in animal tissues, which coats the red blood cells, blocks the capillaries, and deprives the heart of oxygen. One of the main constituents of lipids is cholesterol, a naturally occurring substance in the body, which contributes to the maintenance of cell walls and serves as a precursor of bile acids and vitamin D and also as a precursor of some hormones.

Cholesterol is not found in plant foods but is contained in all animal products, especially meat, egg yolks, and dairy products. Since cholesterol is insoluble in the blood, it attaches itself to a protein that is soluble in order to be transported through the body. This combination is called a lipoprotein. However, excess cholesterol in the bloodstream tends to be deposited in artery walls and, as plaque, eventually causes constriction of the arteries and reduces the flow of blood. Normally, fat is absorbed by the lymph and enters the bloodstream near the heart. However, if excess lipids accumulate in the body, eventually some will become deposited in the liver. Such stored fat, primarily from meat and dairy products, is usually the chief source of liver disorders culminating in the development of liver cancer.

Because of increased public awareness of the connection between cholesterol, saturated fat, and heart disease, many people have switched to unsaturated fats and oils, including vegetable cooking oils, mayonnaise, margarine, salad dressings, and artificial creamers and spreads. However, unsaturated fats serve to redistribute cholesterol from the blood to the tissues and combine with oxygen to form free radicals. These are unstable and highly reactive substances that can interact with proteins and cause the loss of elasticity in tissue and general weakening of cells. Medical studies show that polyunsaturated lipids actually accelerate tumor development more than saturated fats and oils.

Whole grains also contain polyunsaturated fats, but these are naturally balanced by the right proportion of vitamin E and selenium, which are usually lost in the refining process. Similarly, unrefined cooking oils (in which the vitamin E remains) are a balanced product and, if used in moderate amounts, will contribute to proper metabolism.

The liver also regulates the amount of sugar in the blood. It turns any excess sugar into a starch called glycogen, which is stored in the liver. When blood sugar levels are low, the liver converts glycogen back into sugar and sends it into the blood to nourish body cells. If we consume our principal food as complex carbohydrates such as whole grains, these starches will be broken down into sugar molecules slowly and be properly absorbed in the intestines and sent to the liver. But if we take much of our diet in the form of simple carbohydrates such as refined grains, fruit, sucrose, or honey, decomposition occurs primarily in the stomach, resulting in the release of strong acids and the rapid transfer of sugar to the liver in large quantities. If there is too much sugar already stored as glycogen or if the liver is weak from chronic abuse, excess sugar will get into the bloodstream and contribute to the eventual weakening of the organism.

Cancer of the liver is the culmination of chronic liver illness and may be preceded by hepatitis, jaundice, or cirrhosis. As we have seen, though essentially a yang disease, liver cancer is accelerated by extreme yin substances, including alcohol, sugar, refined flour, and foods containing chemical additives, preservatives, or pesticides. It is interesting to observe that the incidence of hepatoma has risen sharply over the last thirty years. From 1907 to 1954, only sixty-seven cases were known in medical literature. During this period the Mayo Clinic had diagnosed only four cases. Hepatoma, a form of liver cancer affecting the epithelial tissue, appears to be linked with the tremendous explosion of yin foodstuffs following World War II. These include ice cream, soda pop, citrus fruits, ice-cold drinks, processed and artificial foods, white bread, and a wide range of prescription and nonprescription drugs such as aspirin, birth-control pills, and marijuana. Now each year several thousand Americans develop hepatomas.

MEDICAL EVIDENCE

• In the sixteenth century, Renaissance anatomist Gabriel Fallopius, who described the ovary and after whom the Fallopian tubes are named, associated malignant tumors with imbalanced diet and improper liver functioning. "The efficient cause of cancer, however, is a flux of atrabiliary humor, for only in the spleen and the liver can this tumor arise from congestion because it is there that this humor is generated . . . the cause of the flux is a faulty mixture of the humors due to bad food. . . ." Among the foods mentioned as possible causes of cancer were beef and salty and bitter foods. Source: L. J. Rather, *The Genesis of Cancer: A study in the History of Ideas* (Baltimore: Johns Hopkins University Press, 1978), 17.

• In 1928 in Bielefeld, Germany, Max Gerson, M.D., reported relieving a case of cancer of the bile ducts with a whole-grain–based diet that excluded meat, white flour, alcohol, coffee, tea, spices, tobacco, and medications. Dr. Gerson went on to devote his life to the nutritional approach to cancer, and in 1941 fled Nazi Germany to set up a cancer clinic in New York. Several years later he testified before a U.S. Congressional committee and called for a return to the traditional diet in order to reverse the rising cancer rate. Summing up his twenty-five years of cancer research and treatment, he wrote: "Cancer is not a local but a general disease, caused chiefly by the poisoning of our foodstuffs prepared by modern farming and [the] food industry." In treating cancer patients, he saw detoxification of the liver as the key to stimulating the body's natural immunity. "In the near future," he predicted, "hospitals and cancer clinics for chronic degenerative disease will be more or less forced to use fruits and vegetables grown by organic gardening methods. . . ." Source: Max Gerson, M.D., *A Cancer Therapy: Results in Fifty Cases* (Del Mar, CA: Totality Books, 1958).

• In 1945 Dr. Albert Tannenbaum reported that spontaneous hepatomas in male mice were affected by both caloric restriction and a high-fat diet. Mice on a low-fat diet registered 9 percent liver tumors in contrast to 35 percent on a high-fat diet. Source: A. Tannenbaum, "The Dependence of Tumor Formation on the Composition of the Calorie-restricted Diet As Well As on the Degree of Restriction," *Cancer Research* 5:616–25.

• In 1949 Dr. Tannenbaum and Herbert Silverstone reported to the NCI that spontaneous liver tumors in mice were accelerated by increasing the protein in their diet. Mice on a diet high in casein, a protein found in milk and dairy products, registered 61 percent tumors compared to 11 percent malignancies in mice fed a grain-based diet. Source: A. Tannenbaum and H. Silverstone, "Effects of Varying the Proportion of Protein (Casein) in the Diet," *Cancer Research* 9:162–73.

• In 1955 physiologist Kasper Blond described the progressive development of diseases in the digestive tract, culminating in liver cancer, as interrelated

rather than isolated phenomena, and characterized cancer as an illness resulting from incorrect nutrition, especially overconsumption of animal protein.
"The whole syndrome of metabolic disorders which we call oesophagitis, gas-
tritis, duodenitis, gastric and duodenal ulcer, cholecystitis, cholangitis, pancreatitis, proctitis, and others are considered only stages of a dynamic process,
starting with liver failure and portal hypertension, and resulting in cirrhosis of
the liver tissue and in cancer." Source: Kasper Blond, M.D., *The Liver and
Cancer* (Bristol: England: John Wright & Sons, 1955), 136.

• Chlordane and heptachlor, related chemical pesticides, caused liver cancer, aplastic anemia, and leukemia in 1969 laboratory tests. Used primarily as
corn-soil insecticides, chemical residues from these substances move up the
food chain and are found in a majority of American dairy products, meat,
poultry, and fish. In 1974 the Environmental Protection Agency suspended
their use for most crops, but they are still used in termite control and on
pineapples, strawberries, and Florida citrus fruits. In 1982, in Honolulu, heptachlor sprayed on pineapples turned up in the city's milk and ice cream supply
and in the breast milk of nursing mothers. As a result, the island of Oahu
recalled its entire supply of milk. Sources: Samuel S. Epstein, M.D., *The
Politics of Cancer* (New York: Doubleday, 1979), 271–81, and *Boston Globe*,
April 8, 1982.

• In 1972 Japanese researchers reported that wakame, a common sea vegetable eaten in Asia, suppressed the reabsorption of cholesterol in the liver and
intestine in laboratory experiments. Other studies showed that hijiki, another
sea vegetable, and shiitake mushrooms also lowered serum cholesterol and
improved fat metabolism. Source: N. Iritani and S. Nogi, "Effects of Spinach
and Wakame on Cholesterol Turnover in the Rat," *Atherosclerosis* 15:87–92.

• In 1975 researchers reported a correlation between liver cancer incidence
and per capita intake of potatoes in more than twenty countries. Source: B.
Armstrong and R. Doll, "Environmental Factors and Cancer Incidence and
Mortality in Different Countries, with Special Reference to Dietary Practices,"
International Journal of Cancer 15:617–31.

• In 1976 scientists reported more than 250 cases of liver cancer or other
tumors in women using oral contraceptives. Studies indicated the risk of developing liver adenomas increased fivefold after five years of pill use and
twenty-fivefold after nine years of use. Source: H. A. Edmondson et al., "Liver-
Cell Adenomas Associated with Use of Oral Contraceptives," *New England
Journal of Medicine* 294:470–72.

• In 1978 studies showed that test animals fed 20 percent of their caloric
intake as sucrose developed liver cancer. The mice's diet contained the same
proportion of sugar consumed by the average Briton. Source: B. Hunter et al.,
*Tumorgenicity and Carcinogenicity with Xylitol in Long-term Dietary Adjust-
ments in Mice* (Huntingdon, England: Huntingdon Research Centre).

• Excessive alcohol consumption, especially among smokers, can lead to
cancers of the mouth, esophagus, throat, larynx, and liver, according to the
director of the NCI. Source: Arthur Upton, M.D., "Hearing Before the Subcommittee on Nutrition of the Committee on Agriculture, Nutrition, and For-
estry of the U.S. Senate," Ninety-sixth Congress, October 2, 1979.

• Azo dyes, a category of artificial colorings used in foods and cosmetics, have been linked with tumors in test animals, especially liver cancer. Processed foodstuffs that contain Azo dyes include Life Savers, caramels, filled chocolates, and other penny candies; soft drinks, artificial fruit drinks, and ades; jellies, jams, and marmalades; stewed fruit sauces, fruit gelatins, and fruit yogurts; ice cream; pie fillings, puddings, and caramel custard; whips and dessert sauces; crackers, cheese puffs, chips, cake and cookie mixes, and waffle and pancake mixes; refined macaroni and spaghetti; mayonnaise and salad dressings; catsup and mustard, and some packaged and canned soups. The cancer tests were originally conducted on rabbits in 1906 and on rodents in 1924 and 1934. Source: Ruth Winter, *Cancer-causing Agents: A Preventive Guide* (New York: Crown, 1979).

• Mormons, who generally eat a well-balanced diet high in whole grains, vegetables, and fruit, moderate in meat, and low in stimulants and tobacco, have about 45 percent less liver cancer than other Americans, according to a 1980 epidemiological study. Source: J. E. Engstrom, "Health and Dietary Practices and Cancer Mortality among California Mormons," in J. Cairns et al. (eds.), *Cancer Incidence in Defined Populations, Banbury Report 4* (Cold Spring Harbor, NY: Cold Spring Harbor Laboratory) 69–90.

• In 1980 researchers reported that mice exposed to extract of black pepper developed significantly more tumors, especially of the liver, lung, and skin, than controls. The incidence in pepper-treated mice was 77 percent, versus 11 percent for controls. The authors noted that U.S. per capita human consumption of pepper is 280 milligrams per day and suggested that this was the first experiment to study the possible link between the spice and cancer. Source: J. M. Concon et al., "Black Pepper [*Pipen Nigram*] Evidence of Carcinogenicity," *Nutrition and Cancer* 1, no. 3:22–26.

• Trichloroethylene (TCE), a chemical used in decaffeinated coffee, has been linked with liver cancer in mice. The substance is also used in obstetrical anesthesia. In 1982 its replacement, methylene chloride, was discovered to cause cancer in laboratory animals. Sources: Thomas H. Corbett, M.D., *Cancer and Chemicals* (Chicago: Nelson-Hall, 1977), 182, and *Community Nutrition Institute Newsletter*, July 15, 1982.

• Toxaphene, the most widely used insecticide in the United States, causes significant increases of liver cancer in animals in NCI tests. It is used on a variety of crops, including corn, wheat, soybeans, peanuts, lettuce, and tomatoes, and on livestock. Residue of the chemical has seeped into many American lakes, rivers, and waterways, accumulating in the flesh of fish, oysters, shrimp, and other seafood. In 1982 the Environmental Protection Agency banned the pesticide for most common uses. Source: *Boston Globe*, October 19, 1982.

DIAGNOSIS

Modern medicine employs a variety of technological methods to diagnose liver cancer. These include blood tests, X rays, tomograms, CAT scan, liver scan, angiogram, and radiologic catheter invasion. If a tumor is suspected, a needle biopsy will follow these tests. An exploratory laparotomy, in which the abdominal wall is surgically opened to examine the inner organs, may also be performed to determine whether the tumor is primary or has metastasized from another area. Currently about 74 percent of liver cancers have spread from local to regional areas by the time they are detected.

The condition of the liver can be simply, safely, and accurately diagnosed by traditional Oriental medicine. The potential development of liver troubles, including cancer, can be spotted well ahead of time, allowing preventive or corrective dietary action to be taken. To begin with, the liver's relative condition can be noted by trying to place the fingers under the ribcage on the right side. If you feel pain here or are unable to place your fingers deeply under the ribs, your liver is swollen. You should be able to insert four fingers without feeling pain or tense resistance.

For more precise diagnosis, carefully observe the central region of the forehead immediately above the nose and between the eyebrows. This area corresponds to the liver in traditional Oriental physiognomy. Vertical lines or wrinkles appearing here are a sign of mucus and fat accumulating in the liver and the expansion or hardening of the organ. The deeper and longer the wrinkles, the more serious the condition. If only one or two lines show, the liver is harder and more rigid as a result of too much salt, animal food, and other yang substances as well as overconsumption of food. On the other hand, if the skin around the lines has puffed up, the cause is too much yin such as alcohol, sugar, drugs, fatty, oily food, and processed or artificial foods.

Pimples in this region above the nose show hard fat deposits in the liver or stone formation in the gallbladder due to excess intake of animal fat, including dairy products. Dry, flaky skin in this area, extending sometimes to the region over the eyebrows, indicates an overconsumption of fats and oils from either animal or vegetable sources together with flour products and a lack of adequate whole grains and cooked vegetables. If this area has white or yellow patches as well as vertical lines, development of a cyst or tumor in the liver or formation of a stone in the gallbladder is very likely.

The texture and coloring of the skin further show the condition of the inner organs. In the case of liver troubles, an oily skin condition suggests disorders in the liver, gallbladder, and general digestive system due to an overconsumption of oily foods from either animal or vegetable sources. Yellow shadings on the eyes, lips, hands, feet, or other areas of the skin show disorders of the bile function due to excessive yang food intake including meat, eggs, seafood, poultry, and salt. A blue-gray color, especially on the cheeks, indicates chronic liver hardening caused by yang animal foods aggravated by sugar, alcohol, stimulants, or other extreme yin. Tumor formation in general is indicated by green colorations on the skin. In the case of liver cancer, this hue often shows up along some area of the liver meridian, especially in the part that runs from inside the first toe up along the inside of the leg to the area below the knee. Also, a green color appearing on the fourth toe and its area extending to the front of the foot below the anklebone suggests developing liver cancer, duodenal ulcer, or gallstones.

DIETARY RECOMMENDATIONS

Liver cancer is mainly caused by overconsumption of animal food, especially that high in protein and fat, such as chicken and eggs and cheese, as well as by overconsumption of sugar, sugar-treated foods, stimulants, aromatic food and drink, alcohol, and various chemical additives. (Liver cancer caused by excessive egg consumption is more difficult to relieve.) All these foods and beverages are to be avoided. Refined flour and flour products, even though of vegetable quality, are to be eliminated in order to prevent mucus formation. Though most vegetable oils are unsaturated in quality, their use is to be limited, except for the occasional use of unrefined sesame oil, corn oil, and other good-quality oil after one month without using any oil. As a whole, overconsumption of food and drink—even though of a healthy, natural, unchemicalized quality—is to be avoided. Any foods that make the body colder, including fruit juice, soft drinks, icy beverages, and ice cream, are also to be avoided. Refrain, too, from overuse of salt and salty food, as well as overcooking vegetables. All vegetables of tropical origin, even though they are now grown in temperate zones, including potatoes, sweet potatoes, yams, tomatoes, eggplant, and avocado, are to be discontinued. Tropical fruits and juices, too, are to be avoided, as well as spices such as mustard, pepper, and curry; all stimulant seasonings and drinks, including mint, peppermint, and other herb teas; all alcoholic beverages; and coffee and black tea. The following are general guidelines, by volume of food, for daily consumption:

• **Whole Grains:** Fifty to 60 percent of daily consumption, by volume, should be whole-cereal grains. The first day prepare plain pressure-cooked short-grain brown rice. On the following days, alternate brown rice pressure-cooked with 20 to 30 percent millet, then rice with 20 to 30 percent barley, then rice with 20 to 30 percent aduki beans or lentils, and then plain rice again. A delicious morning porridge can be made by taking leftover rice, adding a little more water to soften, and seasoning with a little miso at the end and simmering for two to three minutes more. In ordinary pressure cooking, the ratio of grain to water should be about 1:2. For seasoning, cook with a postage stamp–sized piece of kombu instead of salt, though in some cases sea salt may be used, depending on the person's condition. Other grains can be used occasionally, including whole wheat berries, rye, corn, and whole oats, though avoid oats for the first month. However, buckwheat and seitan should be limited in use because they are very contracted relative to other grains and grain products. Flour products, even unrefined whole wheat bread, chapatis, pancakes, or cookies, should be totally avoided or limited in volume for a period of a few months. Whole-grain pasta and noodles may be eaten a couple times a week.

• **Soup:** Five to 10 percent soup, consisting of one or two cups or bowls per day of soup cooked with wakame sea vegetable and various vegetables, especially leafy green and white vegetables, and seasoned lightly with miso or shoyu. Occasionally a small volume of shiitake mushroom may be added to the soup. The miso may be barley miso, brown rice miso, or soybean (hatcho) miso and should be naturally aged two to three years. Grain soups, bean soups, and other soups may be taken from time to time.

• **Vegetables:** Twenty to 30 percent vegetables, cooked in a variety of forms, mainly steamed, boiled, and, after one month without oil, occasionally sautéed.

Among vegetables, broccoli, leafy green tops of carrots, turnips, daikon, and watercress are especially recommended. Root vegetables such as carrots, daikon, and burdock are also very beneficial, and cabbage, onions, pumpkin, and acorn and butternut squash may also be eaten regularly. As a rule of thumb, the following dishes may be prepared, though the frequency may differ from person to person: nishime-style vegetables, three times a week; squash-aduki-kombu dish, three times a week; dried daikon, one cup, three times a week; carrots and carrot tops or daikon and daikon tops, three times a week; blanched vegetables, five to seven times a week; pressed salad, five to seven times a week; raw salad, avoid the first month, then once in ten to fourteen days; steamed greens, five to seven times a week; sautéed vegetables, two times a week, prepared with water the first month, then with sesame or corn oil once or twice a week after that; kinpira, two-thirds cup, two times a week; dried tofu, tofu, tempeh, or seitan with vegetables, two times a week.

• **Beans:** Five percent small beans, such as aduki beans, lentils, chickpeas, or black soybeans, may be used daily, cooked together with sea vegetables such as kombu or with onions and carrots. Other beans may be used altogether two to three times a month. For seasoning, a small volume of unrefined sea salt or shoyu or miso can be used. Bean products, such as tempeh, natto, and dried or cooked tofu, may be used occasionally, but in moderate volume.

• **Sea Vegetables:** Five percent or less sea vegetable dishes, including wakame and kombu, daily when cooking grain, in soup, etc. A sheet of toasted nori may also be taken daily. A small dish of hijiki or arame should be prepared two times a week. All other sea vegetables are optional.

• **Condiments:** Condiments to be available on the table are gomashio (sesame salt), on the average made with 1 part salt to 18 parts sesame seeds; kelp or wakame powder; umeboshi plum; and tekka, though all other regular macrobiotic condiments may be used if desired. These condiments may be used daily on grains and vegetables, but the volume should be moderate to suit individual appetite and taste.

• **Pickles:** Pickles, made at home in a variety of ways, are to be eaten daily, one tablespoon in all, though salty pickles are to be minimized. Rice bran (nuka) pickles are the most suitable.

• **Animal Food:** Fish and other animal food is to be avoided. However, in the event that animal food is craved, a small volume of white-meat fish may be eaten once every ten days to two weeks. The fish should be prepared steamed, boiled, or poached and garnished with grated daikon or ginger. Strictly avoid blue-meat and red-meat fish and all shellfish.

• **Fruit:** The less the better until the condition improves. If cravings develop, a small volume of cooked fruit with a pinch of sea salt or dried fruit (also preferably cooked) may be taken. Avoid all fruit juices and cider.

• **Sweets and Snacks:** Avoid all sweets and desserts, including good-quality macrobiotic desserts, until the condition improves. To satisfy a sweet tooth, use sweet vegetables every day in cooking, drink sweet vegetable drinks (see special drinks below) and use sweet vegetable jam and amasake. Mochi, rice balls, vegetable sushi, and other grain-based snacks may be eaten frequently. Limit rice cakes, popcorn, and other dry or baked snacks, as they may harden the tumor. In the event of cravings, a small volume of barley malt or rice syrup may be taken.

• **Nuts and Seeds:** Nuts and nut butters are to be avoided due to their high amount of fat and protein, except for chestnuts. Unsalted, roasted seeds such as sunflower seeds and pumpkin seeds may be consumed as a snack, up to one cup altogether per week.

• **Seasonings:** Seasonings, such as unrefined sea salt, shoyu, and miso, are to be used moderately in order to avoid unnecessary thirst. Avoid mirin and garlic. If you become particularly thirsty after the meal or between meals, you should cut back on these seasonings until the normal level of thirst returns.

• **Beverages:** Beverages and other dietary practices can follow the general recommendations in Part I, including bancha twig tea as the main beverage. Strictly avoid the beverages on the "infrequent" and "avoid" list and don't take grain coffee for the first two to three months after starting this new way of eating.

The most important thing in connection with dietary practice is chewing very well, until all food becomes liquid in the mouth and well mixed with saliva. Chew very, very well, at least 50 times, preferably 100 times, per mouthful. It is also important to avoid overeating and eating within three hours of sleeping.

As noted in the introduction to Part II, persons who have received or who are currently undergoing medical treatment may need to make further dietary modifications.

SPECIAL DRINKS AND DISHES

Several special drinks may need to be taken, depending on the individual case. Please see a qualified macrobiotic teacher for guidance. Amounts and frequencies given here are averages; these will differ from person to person.

• **Sweet Vegetable Drink:** Take one small cup every day for the first month then every other day the second month.

• **Carrot-Daikon Drink:** Take one small cup every day or every other day for one month, then two times a week for the second month.

• **Shiitake Tea:** For liver cancer, a special daily drink of one or two cups of boiled shiitake mushroom can help relieve internal tension and improve the liver. This tea is made by soaking a dried shiitake mushroom, cut in quarters, in spring water and cooking with one to two teaspoons of grated daikon and one teaspoon of shoyu added for seasoning. Shiitake mushroom and fresh daikon may also be cooked frequently in miso soup or as a part of vegetable dishes and consumed several times per week. Shiitake is useful for helping to dissolve excessive animal fats in the body.

• **Brown Rice Cream:** In the event that appetite declines or is lost, genuine brown rice cream can be consumed with a small volume of condiments such as gomashio (sesame salt), tekka, or umeboshi plum. Lightly seasoned miso soup with scallions and nori cooked in it can also be served. As appetite returns, regular dishes can gradually be added. A dish of raw fresh salad or temperate-climate fruit in season, in moderate volume, may also help restore the appetite.

• **Grated Daikon:** Grate about one half a small cup of fresh daikon, add a few drops of shoyu, and take two to three times a week.

HOME CARES

• **Body Scrub:** Scrubbing the whole body, including the abdominal region and the spinal region, with a towel that has been immersed in hot water and squeezed out is very helpful for better circulation of blood, lymph, and other body fluids, as well as for activating physical and mental energies.

• **Compress Guidelines:** For a small number of liver tumors, one or more of the following compresses may be needed to help gradually draw out excess mucus and fat. Please see a qualified macrobiotic teacher for guidance on the proper use and frequency of a compress or plaster. Several types are used, depending on the person's condition. Precede the compress or plaster with application of a towel that has been soaked in hot water and squeezed out over the affected area for about three to five minutes to stimulate circulation.

• **Lotus-Root Plaster:** Apply lotus plaster over the affected area consisting of grated fresh lotus root, mixed with a small amount of flour and about 5 percent fresh grated ginger.

• **Lotus Root and Potato Plaster:** Apply a plaster consisting of half grated lotus root and half grated white potato, mixed with a small amount of flour and about 5 percent fresh grated ginger.

• **Taro Plaster:** A taro potato plaster can be applied on the liver region, front and back, for three to four hours or overnight, immediately after administering a hot ginger compress on the same area for three to five minutes. These compresses will ease the tumor or hardening of the liver and improve the overall condition. They are also good for reducing liver pain.

OTHER CONSIDERATIONS

• Daily physical exercise that does not produce exhaustion is recommended. Ten to fifteen minutes of daily breathing exercises, especially emphasizing long exhalation, is also beneficial. These physical and breathing exercises contribute to relaxing tensions in the body and mind as well as harmonizing physical metabolism.

• Keeping air quality clean and fresh is important for maintenance of general health. For that purpose, green leafy plants can be placed in the house and the windows periodically opened to allow circulation of fresh air.

• Avoid wearing wool and synthetic fibers. At the minimum wear cotton underwear and use cotton sheets and pillowcases.

• Avoid watching television for long stretches. Similarly, avoid other artificial sources of electromagnetic energy such as video terminals, smoke detectors, and hand-held electrical appliances, which can weaken the liver.

PERSONAL EXPERIENCE

Liver Cancer

In spring of 1979, sixty-two-year-old Hilda Sorhagen experienced a tenderness in her liver area, nausea, diarrhea, and constipation. Her color turned brownish-yellow, and her friends asked her if she had been to Florida because she appeared so dark. For several years she had been ailing and suffered from poor digestion, fatigue, and nervousness. Some years before, her husband died, and she faced mounting pressures from looking over his business and the demands of raising three teenagers. "I had seen so many doctors for one thing or another without improvement nor a positive diagnosis," she recalled of this period. "It was always 'go for X rays' or 'see a specialist.' When I did go, I knew no more than before. They found nothing and blamed it on tension."

When her children grew up, she turned over the family business to the son and entered a yoga ashram in Pennsylvania. The community followed an Indian-style vegetarian diet high in dairy foods, spices, sweets, and raw fruit.

When preliminary medical tests failed to find anything, Hilda came to see me in April 1979, and I evaluated her condition as cancerous. Subsequent examination by her family physician confirmed a hardening of the lower part of her liver, and CEA blood tests were elevated in the cancerous range. However, because of her previous unsatisfactory experience with medical diagnosis, she refused X rays and decided to begin the Cancer Prevention Diet. Although her sister died from liver cancer two years previously, Hilda's doctors and children were not convinced that she had a malignancy and opposed her decision.

Taking a week off from her yoga work, Hilda came to Boston and took some introductory classes in medicinal cooking, visual diagnosis, and shiatsu massage at the EWF. Upon her return, she found that since all the food in the ashram was prepared in a community kitchen, she could no longer fulfill her commitments to the ashram to her satisfaction. Locating an apartment nearby, she resolved to live and cook by herself. Her children were not supportive of her approach, and she did not want to burden others with taking care of her. Yet often she was so weak that she could not get out of bed but "somehow managed to drag myself into the kitchen to put up a pot of brown rice."

Looking back, she noted:

The first sign of improvement was change in energy which was immediately noticeable. I felt stronger; I wanted to be more active. I remembered feeling that I wanted to walk up the hill to the meditation room whereas before I could barely get in the car to drive, even though it was only 1,500 yards away. I wanted to walk, and when I had made it to the top I met one of the ashram members. He was surprised to see me so early in the morning. I felt such a victory and gratitude that I wept with joy. There was a time when I thought I would never be able to walk that path again.

In the summer of 1980 her condition had improved considerably, and Hilda stayed in several macrobiotic study centers in Philadelphia to develop her cooking further. I saw her again during this period and observed that the tumor had disappeared.

Commenting upon her previous way of eating, she recalled, "Michio told me to stop eating raw fruit. I argued that fruit was healthy and one meal a day consisted of fruit only. I pleaded, 'Not even an apple?' and he just looked at me. Now I understand why he looked at me the way I now look at my students when they ask the same question."

In addition to yoga, Hilda is now teaching cooking, and her relationship with her children has changed, and they have grown very close. "I have more energy now than my children," she reported in the autumn of 1982. "This lifestyle has helped me to speed up my spiritual evolution and I have become a more loving person. I will continue to live a macrobiotic way of life because I love the food, and it has saved my life."

In the fall of 1981 a group at the ashram decided to experiment with the macrobiotic diet for six weeks. The results were so remarkable that Guru Amrit Desai, the community's spiritual leader, asked the entire 150-member group to adopt the macrobiotic way of eating. He described the approach as *sattvic* or balanced, pure, and cleansing according to the traditional dietary ideals set forth in the Bhagavad Gita and other Hindu scriptures.

As grains, beans, sea vegetables, and fermented foods became the focus of meal planning, the ashram cooks replaced cheese, eggs, spices, and honey, which had been used extensively in the past. Jeffrey Magdow, M.D., a staff physician at the community's Kripalu Center for Holistic Health, reported about six months after the transition: "In addition to my own personal experience of many benefits through the practice of this diet, I have seen stabilized energy patterns, improved elimination, and a heightened awareness of the effects of foods on mental and physical well-being. . . ." Sources: Personal communication from Hilda Sorhagen, and Alex Jack and Karin Stephan, "Whole-Grain Ashram," *East West Journal,* July 1982, 8–9.

17

Kidney and Bladder Cancer

FREQUENCY

Cancers of the kidney, bladder, and other parts of the urinary tract will claim an estimated 20,200 American lives this year, and 28,100 new cases will develop. Overall, mortality from bladder cancer has fallen during the last thirty years (22 percent in men and 42 percent in women). However, kidney cancer deaths are on the rise, 35 percent among men and 22 percent among women. About one-third of all urinary cancers occurs in the kidney and two-thirds in the bladder, ureters, and urethra. Kidney cancer occurs about evenly in men and women and is found among both adults and children. Bladder cancer is much more prevalent in men, especially those in the fifty-five to seventy-five age group.

Standard medical treatment calls for surgical removal of the afflicted kidney along with adjacent lymph nodes and adrenal glands in an operation called a radical nephrectomy. In a rarer form of kidney cancer known as renal pelvis carcinoma, the ureter will be removed along with the kidney in a procedure called a nephroureterectomy. A person can survive with only one kidney. If both kidneys are removed, a kidney transplant may be performed or kidney dialysis instituted. A kidney dialysis machine performs the functions of the kidneys by filtering fluids through tubes imbedded in the patient's arms. The patient must undergo this treatment two or three times a week for three or four hours' duration each time. Radiation therapy is sometimes used prior to kidney surgery to shrink a tumor. The five-year survival rate for kidney cancer is a little above 53 percent.

In the case of bladder cancer, superficial tumors are generally removed by burning or cutting with the use of a cystoscope, a flexible tube inserted through the urethra, or an abdominal incision. Total removal of the bladder, in advanced cases, is called a cystectomy. In men the prostate is often malignant and is removed as well. An artificial bladder is then constructed, usually with a section of the small intestine, and connected to a disposable bag on the outside of the body for the elimination of urine. Radiation in the form of external voltage or internally implanted radioactive seeds is also sometimes employed before bladder surgery in order to destroy invasive tumors. Chemotherapy is not used as a primary treatment for urinary cancers but may be used to control pain following surgery. Seventy-eight percent of bladder cancer patients treated by these methods live five years or more.

STRUCTURE

The two kidneys are bean-shaped organs located in the upper part of the abdominal cavity near the spinal column. The main tasks of the kidneys are to filter impurities from the blood and to discharge excess fluid from the body in the form of urine. About a quart of blood passes through the kidneys every minute, and these organs serve to regulate the amount of salt, water, and other constituents of the bloodstream. Urine is formed in the kidney by filtration of urea and other wastes from the blood vessels and the absorption and excretion of other substances from the filtrate.

In general, urine is amber in color, forms a mildly acidic reaction, and has a slight odor and a salty taste. The quantity of urine discharged varies with the amount of fluids consumed, but usually amounts to between 1,000 and 1,500 cubic centimeters a day. The quantity of solids in the urine changes with the diet and is significantly higher following consumption of foods higher in fat and protein. People eating the modern diet excrete about forty to seventy-five grams of solid waste daily in their urine, of which 25 percent is urea, 25 percent chlorides, 25 percent sulfate and phosphates, and the rest organic acids, pigments, hormones, and so on. In unhealthy urine, high levels of albumin, sugar, blood, pus, acetone, fat, chyle, cellular material, and bacteria may be present.

The adrenal glands, attached to the upper part of the kidneys, are part of the endocrine system. They secrete hormones, including adrenalin, regulating mental and emotional stress. The ureters are long, narrow tubes that convey the urine from each kidney to the bladder by muscular action. The bladder is a hollow Y-shaped organ situated in the pelvis, which serves as a reservoir for urine. It can hold about one pint. The urethra is the canal through which the urine is discharged from the body. The urethra extends from the neck of the bladder to the genital region. In men, the urethra is divided into the prostatic portion and the penile portion. In women, the urinary system is largely separated from the reproductive system.

CAUSE OF CANCER

Kidney disorders may be divided into two groups. 1) Overly contracted, tight, and inflexible (yang) kidney conditions result in the restriction of blood flow and urination; and 2) loose or swollen (yin) kidney conditions prevent complete filtration of the blood and can lead to excessive retention or elimination of liquids. Preliminary signs of contracted and hardening kidneys are tossing and turning during sleep, insomnia, nightmares, and rising early in the morning. Tight kidneys are caused by overconsumption of extreme yang foods such as eggs, meat, other animal products, dry baked goods, and commercial salt as well as overactivity and a pressure-filled environment. Initial symptoms of overly expanded kidneys are snoring, groaning, bedwetting, lower back pain, getting up to urinate at night, and getting up late in the morning. This yin condition may be caused by a high intake of beverages (especially milk, fruit juices, and coffee) as well as foods of tropical origin, fruit, sugar, and sweets. A sedentary lifestyle contributes to weak, sluggish kidneys.

Over time, excessive consumption of a combination of extreme yin and yang foodstuffs and beverages can lead to the formation of stones, cysts, or tumors in the urinary tract. These obstructions develop when an excess of solid wastes cannot pass through the fine network of cells in the interior of the kidneys, the ureters, or the bladder. The kidneys are a frequent site of mucus and fatty-acid accumulation. In this condition, the kidneys often retain water and become chronically swollen. Since the process of elimination is impaired, excess fluid is often deposited in the legs, producing periodic swelling and weakness. At the same time, excessive perspiration will also usually develop. If someone with this swollen condition continues to consume large amounts of expansive foods, the deposited fat and mucus will crystallize into kidney stones. Stones are principally caused by long-term eating of high-fat foods combined with chilled or frozen foods, particularly ice cream, sherbet, yogurt, orange juice, soft drinks, ice water, and other beverages that make the body cold.

Over a long period of time, cysts and stones will culminate in the formation of tumors as the kidney fights back in self-defense to restrict the flow of excess waters and irritating fluids through its system. In the case of bladder cancer, excessive toxins and other irritants in the urine, especially from processed foods and chemicalized water, can ultimately give rise to cancer. Kidney cancer, affecting the more tight, compact part of the urinary system, is a relatively more yang form of cancer. Bladder cancer, affecting the expanded, hollow portion of the urinary system, is relatively more yin. To restore balance, a slightly more yin macrobiotic diet is recommended for kidney cancer, a more yang diet in the case of bladder cancer.

MEDICAL EVIDENCE

• Looking back over four decades of medical work in French Equatorial Africa, Dr. Albert Schweitzer reported that he had never had any cancer cases in his hospital and that its occurrence among the African people was very rare. He attributed the rise of degenerative diseases to the importation of European foods including condensed milk, canned butter, meat and fish preserves, white bread, and especially refined salt. "It is obvious to connect the fact of increase of cancer with the increased use of salt by the natives. In former years there was only available the little salt extracted from the ocean. . . . So it is possible that the formerly very seldom and still infrequent occurrence of cancer in this country is connected with the former very little consumption of salt and the still rare use of it." Source: Albert Schweitzer, M.D., *Briefe aus dem Lambarenespital*, 1954.

• In 1948 laboratory tests first linked saccharin, an artificial sweetener used in diet colas, toothpaste, cosmetics, and animal feed, with bladder cancer and cancer of the reproductive organs. A controversial 1977 study, published in a British medical journal, observed that men who used saccharin regularly faced a 60 percent greater risk of bladder cancer. However, other studies showed no significant relationship. Sources: G. R. Howe et al., "Artificial Sweeteners and Human Bladder Cancer," *Lancet* 2:578–81, and *Diet, Nutrition, and Cancer* (Washington, DC: National Academy of Sciences, 1982), 14:1–5.

• A 1971 study reported that women who drank coffee regularly had about 2.5 times higher risk of developing urinary cancer than nonusers. The relative risk for men was 24 percent. The test controlled for cigarette smoking and high-risk occupational exposure to chemicals known to affect the bladder and kidneys. Source: P. Cole, "Coffee-drinking and Cancer of the Lower Urinary Tract," *Lancet* 1:1335–37.

• Bottled spring water can reduce the risk of cancer, according to an Illinois experiment. Mice on a high-protein, high-sugar diet were divided into two groups. One group received bottled spring water, and the control group received Chicago tap water. The mice on spring water lived 20 percent longer. Source: Dr. Hans Kugler, *Slowing the Aging Process* (New York: Pyramid, 1973).

• A 1975 epidemiological study reported that Seventh-Day Adventists in California have 72 percent less bladder cancer than the general population. The church members avoid meat, poultry, fish, rich and refined food, coffee, tea, hot condiments, alcohol, and spices and eat proportionately more whole grains, vegetables, fresh fruit, and nuts. Source: R. L. Phillips, "Role of Life-styles and Dietary Habits in Risk of Cancer among Seventh-Day Adventists," *Cancer Research* 35:3513–22.

• A 1975 epidemiological study found a direct association of bladder cancer deaths with per capita intake of fats and oil, especially in women. The scientists also linked kidney cancer with higher intake of meat, milk, total animal protein, and coffee. Source: B. Armstrong and R. Doll, "Environmental Factors and Cancer Incidence and Mortality in Different Countries, with Special Reference to Dietary Practices," *International Journal of Cancer* 15:617–31.

• A New York study found that women in seven counties with chlorinated municipal drinking water ran a 44 percent greater chance of dying from cancer of the urinary or gastrointestinal tract than women whose water was unchlorinated. Source: *Washington Post*, May 3, 1977, A3.

• A 1979 case-control study reported an inverse association between consumption of foods high in vitamin A and bladder cancer. Source: C. Mettlin and S. Graham, "Vitamin A and Lung Cancer," *Journal of the National Cancer Institute* 62:1435–38.

• In a 1991 case-control study, men with lung cancer, bladder cancer, prostate cancer, larynx cancer, colorectal cancer, and esophagael cancer had from 10 to 24 percent lower intake of vegetables and fruits high in carotene than controls. Source: W. C. Ruth et al., "A Case-Control Study of Dietary Carotene in Men with Lung Cancer and in Men with Other Epithelial Cancers, *Nutrition and Cancer* 15, no. 1:63–68.

• In a 1991 case-control study in Hawaii, researchers reported a decreased risk for bladder cancer among women who consumed vegetables and fruits high in vitamin C, such as broccoli, cabbage, and oranges, and among men who consumed dark green vegetables, such as watercress, broccoli, and spinach. Source: A. M. Y. Nomura et al., "Dietary Factors in Cancer of the Lower Urinary Tract," *International Journal of Cancer* 48:199–205.

DIAGNOSIS

When kidney cancer is suspected, modern medicine offers the following diagnostic methods: laboratory tests, including urinalysis; X rays; an intravenous pyelogram (IVP) to locate tumors; ultrasound examination of the abdomen; a renal angiogram to determine the location and extent of tumor growth; a tomogram of the kidney to distinguish between a cyst and a tumor; and a CAT scan of the pelvis and upper abdomen. Sometimes a needle aspiration biopsy is performed, but this procedure has been implicated in spreading cancer along the path of the needle and is increasingly avoided. Many kidneys are nearly completely damaged before being diagnosed as cancerous, and one-third of patients have metastases to other locations. In the case of bladder cancer, diagnostic procedures include lab tests, IVP, cystoscopy, cystogram, bone scan, liver scan, ultrasound, lymphangiogram, and a cystourethrogram in which the bladder and urethra are observed during urination. About 82 percent of bladder cancers are diagnosed in local stages before spreading to regional areas or other organs. In men, bladder surgery can result in impotence.

Traditional visual diagnostic techniques do not rely on potentially harmful X rays or mechanical invasions of the body. Simple visual methods allow the kidneys to be monitored long before the onset of serious illness and permit corrective dietary adjustments to be made. These nutritional measures will safeguard against the development of kidney troubles in healthy individuals and offset any tendency toward urinary cancer in those who already are sick.

In physiognomy, the area under the eyes corresponds to the kidneys. Darkness or black coloring of the skin in this region signifies kidney stagnation and toxic blood due to kidney malfunction. During adulthood, but increasingly even during youth in modern society, many people develop eyebags under the lower eyelid. Eyebags may have one of two causes, though the appearance may be similar: 1) a pool of liquid and 2) pooled mucus. The first type of eyebag appears watery and swollen. Both types of eyebags show disorders of the kidney, bladder, and excretory functions. The first type, due to excess liquid, indicates swelling of the kidney tissues and frequent urination. Excessive intake of any kind of liquid, including all kinds of beverages, fruits, and juices, may cause this condition. The second type of eyebag does not necessarily accompany frequent urination but shows mucus and fat accumulation in the kidney tissue. If small pimples or dark spots appear on these mucous-caused eyebags, accumulated mucus and fat in the kidney tissues may be forming kidney stones. If these eyebags are chronic, mucous accumulation is developing in the ureter, the wall of the bladder, and the reproductive organs (ovaries, Fallopian tubes, and uterus in women and prostate gland in men), creating bacterial activity, inflammation, itching, vaginal discharge, ovarian cysts, and eventually the growth of tumors and cancers in these areas.

Both types of eyebags also indicate the decline of physical and mental vitality as a natural result of the above conditions. Overloaded body systems, fatigue, laziness, forgetfulness, indecisiveness, and loss of clear judgment are developing. The water-caused eyebag is easily corrected by the restriction of liquid intake, while the mucous-caused eyebag can be corrected by the restriction of all mucous- and fat-forming food, including dairy products, meat, poultry, sugar, refined flour, and all sorts of oil. This type of eyebag takes longer than the watery eyebag to clear up. In visual diagnosis, the right eye and its surrounding area corresponds to the right kidney, the left eye to the left kidney. Relative darkness, swelling, tightness, or other markings indicate which kidney is more affected.

The ears, which are shaped like kidneys, also mirror the internal condition of the urinary tract and should be checked carefully. Redness around the edge of the ear indicates an overly yin condition of the kidneys caused by excessive consumption of sugar, dairy food, fruit, and juices. Overconsumption of oil, fat, and other strong yin items will also overburden the kidneys and show up in ears that are oily to the touch. Moles or warts on the ears show deposits of mucus in the kidneys caused by an accumulation of animal protein. The left ear shows the left kidney, the right ear, the right kidney, and the location of these abnormalities indicates precisely where troubles in the kidneys are occurring. Bumps or pimples on the ears show deposits of fat and developing kidney stones. Deafness is often connected with buildup of fat in the kidney. Excessive wax in the ears indicates fatty deposits in the ureter.

The kidneys can be aggravated by too much fluid consumption, and this shows up in generally wet or damp hands and feet. Kidney disorders, including cancer, are indicated by pain or hardness on the initial point of the kidney meridian at the bottom of the foot. Calluses here represent an effort on the part of the kidneys to discharge excess mucus, protein, and fat through the meridian or energy channel in the foot. Flour products, fats and oils, and sugar and sweets especially give rise to this condition.

Urine itself can be inspected for general clues to the condition of the kidneys and bladder. Urine that is healthy is light gold or yellow in color. Too much salt will turn the urine darker, and too little salt or too yin a diet will result in urine that is much lighter in color. If too much fluid is consumed, urination will become very frequent. Normally, we should urinate about three or four times a day. More than this indicates that too much fluid is being consumed, while less means that not enough is being consumed.

The upper part of the forehead corresponds with the bladder, and lines or ridges in this area indicate trouble in this organ.

Posture is a further clue to kidney condition. Leaning forward while sitting, standing, or walking indicates overly contracted kidneys. This yang condition may also be shown by a stiff back, walking brusquely, or running, or wearing shoes with elevated heels. On the other hand, leaning backward, leaning against things, and slouching, as well as wearing shoes with elevated toes, are all signs of overly expanded (yin) kidneys.

DIETARY RECOMMENDATIONS

Cancer of the kidney is caused mainly by overconsumption of dairy food and animal food rich in saturated fats, together with sugar, chemicals, and artificial beverages. Cheese, eggs, and chicken are a typical combination. Cancer of the bladder is largely caused by overconsumption of dairy foods, sugar products, chemicals, stimulants, fruits, juices, and food that produces fat and mucus. All these foods are to be avoided. The kidneys govern salt metabolism, and use of salt should be minimized in the case of kidney cancer for the first several months. Overconsumption of salt tends to solidify the mass of cancer cells.

Kombu, which is rich in minerals, may be used for seasoning instead. The use of miso and shoyu should also be light. All oily and greasy food as well as all refined flour products, including bread, pancakes, and cookies, are to be avoided. Food and beverages that lower the body temperature, including fruits, icy drinks, and artificial beverages, are to be discontinued. For improvement of urinary cancer, eating baked flour products is not advisable. All spices, including mustard, peppers, and curry, and any fragrant, aromatic condiments and supplements are to be avoided. Following are the general dietary guidelines, by daily volume, for urinary cancer, including cancer of the kidney and bladder:

• **Whole Grains:** Fifty to 60 percent of daily consumption by volume, should be whole-cereal grains. The first day prepare plain pressure-cooked short-grain brown rice. On following days, alternate brown rice pressure-cooked with 20 to 30 percent millet, then rice with 20 to 30 percent barley, then rice with 20 to 30 percent aduki beans or lentils, and then plain rice again. A delicious morning porridge can be made by taking leftover rice, adding a little more water to soften, and seasoning with a little miso at the end and simmering for two to three minutes more. In daily pressure cooking, the ratio of grain to water should be about 1:2. For seasoning, cook with a postage stamp–sized piece of kombu instead of salt. Other grains can be used occasionally, including whole wheat berries, rye, corn, and whole oats, though oats should be avoided for the first month. Avoid buckwheat and limit seitan for either one of these conditions for the first three months. Flour products, even unrefined whole wheat bread, chapatis, pancakes, or cookies, should be totally avoided or limited in volume for a period of a few months. Whole-grain pasta and noodles may be eaten a couple times a week.

• **Soup:** Five to 10 percent soup, consisting of one or two cups or bowls per day of soup cooked with wakame sea vegetable and various vegetables, especially leafy green and white vegetables, and seasoned lightly with miso or shoyu. Occasionally a small volume of shiitake mushroom may be added to the soup. The miso may be barley miso, brown rice miso, or soybean (hatcho) miso and should be naturally aged two to three years. Grain soups, bean soups, and other soups may be taken from time to time.

• **Vegetables:** Twenty to 30 percent vegetables, cooked in a variety of forms, mainly steamed, boiled, and, after one month without oil, occasionally sautéed. Among vegetables, green vegetables are needed to help recover from kidney or bladder cancer, especially quickly sautéed greens. As a rule of thumb, the following dishes may be prepared, though the frequency may differ from person to person: nishime-style vegetables, three times a week; squash-aduki-kombu dish, three times a week; dried daikon, one cup, three times a week; carrots and carrot tops or daikon and daikon tops, three times a week; blanched vegetables, five to seven times a week; pressed salad, five to seven times a week; raw salad, avoid the first month, then once in seven to ten days; steamed greens, five to seven times a week; sautéed vegetables, two times a week prepared with water the first month, then with sesame or corn oil once or twice a week after that; kinpira, two-thirds of a cup, two times a week; dried tofu, tofu, tempeh, or seitan with vegetables, two times a week.

• **Beans:** Five percent small beans, such as aduki beans, lentils, chickpeas, or black soybeans, may be used daily, cooked together with sea vegetables such as kombu or with onions and carrots. Other beans may be used altogether two to three times a month. For seasoning, a small volume of unrefined sea salt or shoyu or miso can be used. Bean products, such as tempeh, natto, and dried or cooked tofu, may be used occasionally, but in moderate volume. Dried tofu is better for this condition than fresh tofu.

• **Sea Vegetables:** Five percent or less sea vegetable dishes, including wakame and kombu, daily when cooking grain, in soup, etc. A sheet of toasted nori may also be taken daily. This is especially good for the bladder. A small dish of hijiki or arame should be prepared two times a week. All other sea vegetables are optional.

• **Condiments:** Condiments to be available on the table are gomashio (sesame salt), on the average made with 1 part salt to 18 parts sesame seeds; kelp or wakame powder; umeboshi plum; and tekka, though all other regular macrobiotic condiments may be used if desired. These condiments may be used daily on grains and vegetables, but the volume should be moderate to suit individual appetite and taste. Shiso leaf powder and green nori flakes are especially good for bladder and kidney troubles.

• **Pickles:** Pickles, made at home in a variety of ways, are to be eaten daily, one tablespoon in all, though salty pickles are to be minimized.

• **Animal Food:** Fish and other animal food is to be avoided. However, in the event that animal food is craved, a small volume of white-meat fish may be eaten once every seven to ten days. The fish should be prepared steamed, boiled, or poached and garnished with grated daikon or ginger. Strictly avoid blue-meat and red-meat fish and all shellfish.

• **Fruit:** The less the better until the condition improves. If cravings develop, a small volume of cooked fruit with a pinch of sea salt or dried fruit (also preferably cooked) may be taken. Avoid all fruit juices and cider.

• **Sweets and Snacks:** Avoid all sweets and desserts, including good-quality macrobiotic desserts, until the condition improves. To satisfy a sweet tooth, use sweet vegetables every day in cooking, drink sweet vegetable drink (see special drinks below), and use sweet vegetable jam and amasake. Mochi, rice balls, vegetable sushi, and other grain-based snacks may be eaten frequently. Limit rice cakes, popcorn, and other dry or baked snacks, as they may harden the tumor. In the event of cravings, a small volume of barley malt or rice syrup may be taken.

• **Nuts and Seeds:** Nuts and nut butters are to be avoided due to their high amount of fat and protein, except for chestnuts. Unsalted, roasted seeds such as sunflower seeds and pumpkin seeds may be consumed as a snack, up to one cup altogether per week.

• **Seasonings:** Seasonings, such as unrefined sea salt, shoyu, and miso, are to be used moderately in order to avoid unnecessary thirst. Avoid mirin and garlic. If you become particularly thirsty after the meal or between meals, you should cut back on these seasonings until the normal level of thirst returns.

• **Beverages:** Beverages and other dietary practices can follow the general recommendations in Part I, including bancha twig tea as the main beverage. Strictly avoid the beverages on the "infrequent" and "avoid" list and don't take grain coffee for the first two to three months after starting this new way of eating. All beverages are to be warm or hot. Cold beverages are to be avoided. All liquid intake should be limited to actual thirst. Water quality is especially important with this kind of cancer. Be sure that you are using good-quality spring or well water for cooking and drinking and avoiding tap water, distilled water, and water either too high or too low in minerals.

The most important thing in connection with dietary practice is chewing very well, until all food becomes liquid in the mouth and well mixed with saliva. Chew very, very well, at least 50 times, preferably 100 times, per mouthful. It is also important to avoid overeating and eating within three hours of sleeping.

As noted in the introduction to Part II, persons who have received or who are currently undergoing medical treatment may need to make further dietary modifications.

SPECIAL DRINKS AND DISHES

One or more of several special drinks or side dishes may need to be taken, depending on the individual case. Please see a qualified macrobiotic teacher for guidance. Amounts and frequencies given here are averages; these will differ from person to person.

• **Sweet Vegetable Drink:** Take one small cup every day for the first month, then every other day the second month.

• **Carrot-Daikon Drink:** For kidney cancer, take one small cup every day for five days, then every other day for two weeks, then every three days for one month. For bladder cancer, take every third day for six weeks; this will help induce urination.

• **Shiitake-Daikon Tea:** Cook a small volume of shiitake mushroom in 1 cup of water. After five minutes, add one-third cup grated daikon, a little grated ginger, and a few drops of shoyu. Drink one small cup once every three days for one month.

• **Kombu-Lotus Tea:** For bladder cancer, prepare a tea with one-third kombu and two-thirds lotus root, using about four times the volume of water and cooking for fifteen to twenty minutes. Take one-half to one cup every day for six weeks.

• **Aduki Juice:** One or two cups of aduki bean juice cooked with a little sea salt or a piece of kombu may be used often to help kidney functions and restore smooth urination.

• **Rice Juice:** Rice juice, which rises to the surface while cooking brown rice, can be used daily or frequently as a beverage. Also, hot bancha tea may occasionally be poured over leftover grain and be eaten with a small volume of condiments.

• **Daikon-Nori-Ginger Tea:** Drinking one or two cups of hot water in which two tablespoons of grated daikon (or red radish), one roasted crushed nori sheet, and one-half teaspoon of grated ginger (seasoned with one teaspoon of shoyu) have boiled for three to five minutes is helpful for stimulating the bladder and proper urinary passage.

• **Ume-Sho-Kuzu:** In case of weakness, in connection with bladder cancer especially, take a cup of this tea or ume-sho-bancha once every three days for four to six weeks.

• **Grated Daikon:** Grate about one-half a small cup of fresh daikon, add a few drops of shoyu, and take two to three times a week.

HOME CARES

• **Body Scrub:** Scrubbing the whole body, including the abdominal region and the spinal region, with a towel that has been immersed in hot water and squeezed out is very helpful for better circulation of blood, lymph, and other body fluids, as well as for activating physical and mental energies.

• **Compress Guidelines:** For a small number of tumors in the kidney or bladder, a compress may be needed to help gradually draw out excess mucus and fat. Please see a qualified macrobiotic teacher for guidance on the proper use and frequency of a compress or plaster. Several types are used, depending on the person's condition. Precede the compress or plaster with application of a towel that has been soaked in hot water and squeezed out over the affected area for about three to five minutes to stimulate circulation.

• **Taro Plaster:** In case of pain on the kidney, apply a taro plaster for three hours, preceded for three to five minutes with a ginger compress. Then do again the next day or twice a day, altogether for several days.

• **Lotus-Taro Plaster:** A plaster combining an equal volume of grated fresh lotus root and taro potato (mixed with a little white flour for consistency and 5 to 10 percent grated ginger) applied from the back on the area of the kidneys for three to four hours is helpful for kidney cancer if used daily for two to three weeks. This should be preceded by a ginger compress for three to five minutes.

• **Ginger Compress:** A ginger compress applied for ten to fifteen minutes once a day on the abdomen (but not over the tumor) helps reduce blockage of the urethra. This compress should be repeated for several days.

• **Other Remedies:** Massage, acupuncture, or moxibustion (burning an herb on the skin) can help to relieve pain. A ginger compress on the painful area for three to five minutes can also help, together with the use of all the above home cares.

OTHER CONSIDERATIONS

• Avoid wearing wool and synthetic fibers. Nylon is particularly irritating to the bladder. At the minimum wear cotton underwear and use cotton sheets and pillowcases.

• Avoid watching television for long stretches. Radiation weakens the kidneys. Similarly, avoid other artificial sources of electromagnetic energy such as video terminals, smoke detectors, and hand-held electrical appliances, which can weaken the kidney and bladder.

• A daily hot bath or shower should be quick and not frequent (i.e., not two to three times a day).

• Psychologically, keeping a positive mind and a strong will is important. Also, any comfortably manageable exercise, including walking outdoors, contributes to improvement. Visualization, prayer, meditation, and other spiritual practices, performed daily, will also be beneficial.

• The kidneys and bladder are particularly susceptible to cold weather and chills. Keep these organs protected and warm at all times, especially during the winter. In the Far East, a cotton band is commonly worn around the abdomen and back to keep these organs warm.

18

Pancreatic Cancer

FREQUENCY

Nearly 25,000 Americans will die from pancreatic cancer this year, and 28,300 new cases will arise. The illness is found in men about 50 percent more often than women, but it is rising more rapidly among women, and overall slightly more women than men die from this disease. About 90 percent of pancreatic cancers are *adenocarcinomas*, affecting the tissue of the organs, and most of these are accompanied by pancreatitis and obstruction of the ducts. The other 10 percent are *tumors of the islet cells*. Pancreatic cancer may spread to the liver or small intestine.

Modern medical treatment calls for surgery, but because the disease is difficult to diagnose in early stages, many tumors have already metastasized and are considered inoperable. If operable, a partial or total pancreatectomy is performed. The first procedure calls for removal of part of the organ, adjacent lymph nodes, the duodenum, part of the stomach, and the common bile duct. A total pancreatomy involves removing the whole pancreas. Radiation and chemotherapy may be given after surgery to control pain. The survival rate for pancreatic cancer is 3 percent. Many patients die within a few months of diagnosis.

STRUCTURE

The pancreas is six to eight inches in length and weighs about three ounces. It is situated behind the stomach and is connected to the duodenum through a common bile duct with the liver and gallbladder. The sections of the pancreas are known as the head, body, and tail. The head secretes pancreatic juice into the duodenum, and this juice aids in the digestion of carbohydrates, fats, and protein. The body of the pancreas produces enzymes and hormones, including insulin, which regulate sugar levels in the blood. These hormones are secreted by the islets of Langerhans, a network of cells scattered throughout the pancreas, which vary in number from 200,000 to 1,800,000. They are most numerous in the tail portion of the pancreas, which touches the spleen.

CAUSE OF CANCER

Diabetes and hyperinsulinism are the two major degenerative diseases associated with the pancreas and are related to the rise of tumors in this organ. To understand the progressive development of pancreatic disorders, it is necessary to consider the effects of the three different forms of sugar on the body. Simple sugars or *monosaccharides* are found in fruits and honey and include glucose and fructose. Double sugars or *disaccharides* are found in cane sugar and milk and include sucrose and lactose. Complex sugars or *polysaccharides* are found in grains, beans, and vegetables and include cellulose.

In the normal digestive process, complex sugars are decomposed gradually and at a nearly even rate by various enzymes in the mouth, stomach, pancreas, and intestines. Complex sugars enter the bloodstream slowly after being broken down into smaller saccharide units. During the process, the pH of the blood remains slightly alkaline.

In contrast, simple and double sugars are metabolized quickly, causing the blood to become overacidic. To compensate for this extreme yin condition, the pancreas secretes a yang hormone, insulin, which allows excess sugar in the blood to be removed and enter the cells of the body. This produces a burst of energy as the glucose (the end product of all sugar metabolism) is oxidized and carbon dioxide and water are given off as wastes. Diabetes is a disease characterized by the failure of the pancreas to produce enough insulin to neutralize excess blood sugar. After years of excessive consumption of refined sugar, fruit, dairy products, chemicals, and other highly yin substances, the islet cells in the pancreas become expanded and lose their ability to secret insulin. Sugar begins to appear in the urine, the body loses water, and reserve minerals are depleted. To offset these symptoms, modern medicine treats diabetes with artificial injections of insulin.

Much of the sugar that enters the bloodstream is originally stored in the liver in the form of glycogen until needed, when it is again changed into glucose. When the amount of glycogen exceeds the liver's storage capacity of about fifty grams, it is released into the bloodstream in the form of fatty acid. This fatty acid is stored first in the more inactive places of the body, such as the buttocks, thighs, and midsection. Then, if refined sugars continue to be eaten, fatty acid becomes attracted to more yang organs such as the heart and kidney, which gradually become encased in a layer of fat and mucus.

This accumulation can also penetrate the inner tissues, weakening the normal functioning of the organs and causing their eventual stoppage such as in atherosclerosis. The buildup of fat can also lead to various forms of cancer, including tumors of the breast, colon, and reproductive organs. Still another form of degeneration may occur when the body's internal supply of minerals is mobilized to offset the debilitating effects of simple sugar consumption. For example, calcium from the bones and teeth may be depleted to balance the effects of excessive intake of candy and soft drinks.

As a small, compact organ, the pancreas is yang in structure. Pancreatic cancer results primarily from the long-time consumption of eggs, meat, seafood, poultry, refined salt, and other strong yang animal foods high in protein and saturated fat, in combination with refined sugars and other strong yin foods and beverages, chemicals, and drugs. Tumors in the pancreas may follow the development of pancreatitis (the acute or chronic inflammation of the organ) and hyperinsulinism (an overly contractive condition in which blood sugar levels are abnormally low from secretion of too much insulin). The overproduction of insulin attracts fatty acids and coagulates into tumors in the bile duct or the islets of Langerhans. Diabetes may be treated and relieved by adopting a slightly more yang macrobiotic diet consisting of whole grains and vegetables, prepared with a slightly longer cooking time and heavier taste, while cancer of the pancreas can be reversed by a slightly more yin diet consisting primarily of whole grains and vegetables prepared with a little bit less cooking and a lighter taste.

MEDICAL EVIDENCE

• A 1968 Japanese study of mortality in men found a direct association between high meat consumption and pancreatic cancer. High vegetable intake was found to be inversely associated with the disease. Source: K. Ishii et al., "Epidemiological Problems of Pancreas Cancer," *Japan Journal of Clinical Medicine* 26:1839–42.

• A 1975 epidemiological study found a direct correlation between sugar intake and pancreatic cancer mortality among women in thirty-two countries. Source: B. Armstrong and R. Doll, "Environmental Factors and Cancer Incidence and Mortality in Different Countries, with Special Reference to Dietary Practices," *International Journal of Cancer* 15:617–31.

• A 1977 Japanese study reported that men who ate meat daily risked pancreatic cancer 2.5 times more than those who did not. Source: T. Hirayama, "Changing Patterns of Cancer in Japan with Special Reference to the Decrease in Stomach Cancer Mortality," in H. H. Hiatt et al. (eds.), *Origins of Human Cancer, Book A, Incidence of Cancer in Humans* (Cold Spring Harbor, NY: Cold Spring Harbor Laboratory, 1977), 55–75.

• In 1979 the American Diabetes Association revised its dietary recommendations, stating that "carbohydrate intake should usually account for 50–60 percent of total energy intake," with "glucose and glucose containing disaccharides (sucrose, lactose) . . . restricted." In addition, the guidelines recommended that "whenever acceptable to the patient, natural foods containing unrefined carbohydrate with fiber should be substituted for highly refined carbohydrates, which are low in fiber" and "dietary sources of fat that are high in saturated fatty acids and foods containing cholesterol should be restricted." Source: "Principles of Nutrition and Dietary Recommendations for Individuals with Diabetes Mellitus: 1979," *Journal of the American Dietetic Association* 75:527–30.

• Mormons, whose diet is high in whole grains, vegetables, and fruits, moderate in meat, and low in stimulants, alcohol, and tobacco, have substantially less pancreatic cancer than the general population, according to a 1980 epidemiological survey. Male Mormons have 36 percent less and females 19 percent less. High church officials, who adhere more faithfully to the group's dietary recommendations, have 53 percent less pancreatic cancer. Source: J. E. Engstrom, "Health and Dietary Practices and Cancer Mortality among California Mormons," in J. Cairns et al. (eds.), *Cancer Incidence in Defined Populations, Banbury Report 4* (Cold Spring Harbor, NY: Cold Spring Harbor Laboratory), 69–90.

• People who drink a cup of coffee a day are nearly twice as likely to develop cancer of the pancreas as non–coffee drinkers, according to a 1981 study by the Harvard School of Public Health. Source: B. MacMahon et al., "Coffee and Cancer of the Pancreas," *New England Journal of Medicine* 304:630–33.

• The per capita intake of several foods has been associated with pancreatic cancer in a number of international studies. Analyses of mortality data have produced direct associations with intake of fats and oils, sugar, animal products, eggs, milk, and coffee. Source: *Diet, Nutrition, and Cancer* (Washington, DC: National Academy of Sciences, 1982), 17:12–13.

• In a study of twenty-four patients with pancreatic cancer who adopted a macrobiotic diet, Tulane University researchers found that their mean length of survival was 17.3 months, compared with 6.0 months for matched controls from a national tumor registry diagnosed during the same time period (1984–85). The one-year survival rate was 54.2 percent in the macrobiotic patients versus 10.0 percent in the controls. All comparisons were statistically significant. Source: Gordon Saxe, "A Retrospective Study of Diet and Cancer of the Pancreas," in Ann Fawcett and the East West Foundation, *Cancer-free: 30 Who Triumphed Naturally over Cancer* (Tokyo and New York: Japan Publications, 1991).

• In a 1991 case-control study in Poland, researchers reported a strong positive association between intake of foods high in cholesterol and pancreatic cancer and an inverse association with foods high in vitamin C, retinol, and fiber. Source: W. Zatonski, "Nutritional Factors and Pancreatic Cancer: A Case-Control Study from South-west Poland," *International Journal of Cancer* 48:390–94.

• In a case-control study carried out in Australia in the mid-1980s, researchers examined the diets of 104 patients with pancreatic cancer and found that they ate more boiled eggs and omelets as well as other sweet and fatty foods than controls. "This study contributes further support to the emerging view that fruit and vegetables have an important role to play in the minimization of the risk of cancer of the pancreas," the scientists concluded. Source: P. Baghurst et al., "A Case-Control Study of Diet and Cancer of the Pancreas," *American Journal of Epidemiology* 134 (1991):167–79.

• In a study of the dietary habits of French Canadians, researchers reported in 1991 that pancreatic cancer was associated with total fat intake, particularly saturated fat, and cholesterol intake. Source: P. Ghadirian et al., "Nutritional Factors and Pancreatic Cancer in the Francophone Community in Montreal, Canada," *International Journal of Cancer* 47:1–6.

DIAGNOSIS

In the hospital, pancreatic cancer is diagnosed by a variety of means, including lab tests, a fasting blood sugar test, liver scans, upper and lower GI series, CAT scan, ultrasound, and an ERCP (endoscopic retrograde cholangiopancreatography). The ERCP is a kind of endoscope or tube, which is swallowed and woven into the duodenum. It contains a tiny catheter, which is inserted into the duct of the pancreas. X rays may then be taken of a dye injected into the pancreas. If a tumor is indicated, cell and tissue samples will be taken in a biopsy or a major surgical procedure called a laparotomy, in which the abdominal wall is opened and the inner organs palpated by the surgeon.

Oriental medicine relies on simpler, visual cues to ascertain the condition of the pancreas. In facial diagnosis, two major areas correspond with the pancreas: 1) the upper bridge of the nose, and 2) the outside of the temples. Swellings, discolorations, or other abnormal markings in these locations indicate pancreatic and sometimes also spleen disorders. For instance, a dark color shows overburdening of the pancreas and elimination of excessive sugars, including cane sugar, honey, syrups, chocolate, fruit, and milk. Red pimples and patches in these regions are caused by excess sugar, sweets, juice, and fruits. Whitish-yellow pimples are caused by fats and oils from both animal and vegetable sources, including dairy foods. Dark patches and pimples are caused by excessive sweets or by salt and flour products. Moles here are caused by excess animal-quality protein and fat and show an overactive spleen and pancreas. A light green color appearing together with whitish, reddish, or dark fatty, oily skin textures in either of these areas indicates possible pancreatic cancer.

Blisters on the eyes may also reflect tumor development in the pancreas. A reddish-yellow color in the pink area inside the lower eyelid is caused by consumption of excess yang animal food together with excess yin. A blue-gray color in the middle regions of the white of the eye further suggests cancer in the pancreas.

Above the bridge of the nose, hair growing between the eyebrows shows that the person's mother ate a high amount of dairy food and fatty animal food during the third and fourth months of pregnancy. A person with this type of eyebrows is particularly susceptible to pancreatic, spleen, and liver disorders and should be careful to avoid meat, poultry, eggs, dairy foods, and oil and fatty foods.

Oily skin in general shows disorders in fat metabolism, including pancreatic troubles. A yellowish color to the skin from excess yang foods also shows bile troubles and probable pancreatic malfunctioning.

Finally, cancer of the pancreas, spleen, or lymph is indicated by the presence of a light green color along the spleen meridian. Observe especially the area of the foot below the anklebone extending to the outside of the big toe.

Oriental diagnosis allows us to quickly scan these and other areas and accurately determine the condition of the pancreas and other internal organs. A propensity to cancer can be identified long before it develops and corrective dietary adjustments taken.

DIETARY RECOMMENDATIONS

The primary cause of pancreatic cancer is the long-time overconsumption of animal food, especially chicken, eggs, cheese, and shellfish such as shrimp, crabmeat, and lobster, which gradually gather in the pancreas and create a tumor. All animal food should be avoided, including meat, dairy food, and fish and seafood, all of which are high in fat and cholesterol. Pancreatic cancer is also accelerated by the overconsumption of salty food, hard baked food, and roasted food, as well as sugar and sugar-treated food, soft drinks, spices, stimulants, tropical fruits and fruit juices, and chemicals used in various ways for food production and processing. All these foods and beverages are to be avoided. Though not the cause of pancreatic cancer, refined flour and flour products easily tend to produce mucus and should therefore also be avoided. Commercial seasonings, sauces, and dressings, in which artificial chemical processing is involved, should also be discontinued. It is especially important to avoid all foods and drinks that make organs, muscles, and tissues tight, including a high amount of salty food. The following are general guidelines for dietary practice, by volume of daily food consumption:

• **Whole Grains:** Fifty to 60 percent of daily consumption, by volume, should be whole-cereal grains. The first day prepare plain pressure-cooked short-grain brown rice. On subsequent days, alternate brown rice pressure-cooked with 20 to 30 percent millet, then rice with 20 to 30 percent barley, then rice with 20 to 30 percent aduki beans or lentils, and then plain rice again. A delicious morning porridge can be made by taking leftover rice, adding a little more water to soften, and seasoning with a little miso at the end and simmering for two to three minutes more. In daily pressure cooking, the ratio of grain to water should be about 1:2. For seasoning, cook with a small postage stamp–sized piece of kombu instead of salt. Other grains can be used occasionally, including whole wheat berries, rye, corn, and whole oats, though oats should be avoided for the first month. However, buckwheat should be avoided for about six months, because it is very contractive and may harden the tumor. Seitan is also very yang and should be minimized. Flour products, even unrefined whole wheat bread, chapatis, pancakes, and cookies, should be totally avoided or limited in volume for a period of a few months. Whole-grain pasta and noodles may be eaten a couple times a week.

• **Soup:** Five to 10 percent soup, consisting of one or two cups or bowls per day of soup cooked with wakame sea vegetable and various vegetables, especially sweet, round vegetables such as squash, onions, and cabbage, and seasoned lightly with miso or shoyu. Occasionally a small volume of shiitake mushroom may be added to the soup. The miso may be barley miso, brown rice miso, or soybean (hatcho) miso and should be naturally aged two to three years. Grain soups, bean soups, and other soups may be taken from time to time.

• **Vegetables:** Twenty to 30 percent vegetables, cooked in a variety of forms, mainly steamed, boiled, and, after one month without oil, occasionally sautéed. Among vegetables, round vegetables such as squash, pumpkin, onions, and cabbage may be prepared proportionately more, though leafy green vegetables and root vegetables should also be consumed frequently. Lighter cooking, which leaves some freshness and crispness, is recommended. Prepare at least one dish every day in this way. As a rule of thumb, the following dishes may be prepared, though the frequency may differ from person to person: nishime-style vegetables, three times a week; squash-aduki-kombu dish, three times a week; dried daikon, one cup, three times a week; carrots and carrot tops or daikon and daikon tops, three times a week; blanched vegetables, five to seven times a week; pressed salad, five to seven times a week; raw salad, avoid; steamed greens, five to seven times a week; sautéed vegetables, prepared with sesame oil lightly brushed on the pan once or twice a week; kinpira, two-thirds of a cup, two times a week; dried tofu, tofu, tempeh, or seitan with vegetables, 2 times a week.

• **Beans:** Five percent small beans, such as aduki beans, lentils, chickpeas, or black soybeans, may be used daily, cooked together with sea vegetables such as kombu or with onions and carrots. Other beans may be used altogether two to three times a month. For seasoning, a small volume of unrefined sea salt or shoyu or miso can be used. Bean products, such as tempeh, natto, and dried or cooked tofu, may be used occasionally, but in moderate volume.

• **Sea Vegetables:** Five percent or less sea vegetable dishes, including wakame and kombu, daily when cooking grain, in soup, etc. A sheet of toasted nori may also be taken daily. A small dish of hijiki or arame should be prepared two times a week. All other sea vegetables are optional.

• **Condiments:** Condiments to be available on the table are gomashio (sesame salt), on the average made with 1 part salt to 18 to 20 parts sesame seeds; kelp or wakame powder; umeboshi plum; and tekka, though all other regular macrobiotic condiments may be used if desired. These condiments may be used daily on grains and vegetables, but the volume should be moderate to suit individual appetite and taste.

• **Pickles:** Pickles, made at home in a variety of ways, are to be eaten daily, one tablespoon in all, though salty pickles are to be minimized. Rice bran (nuka) pickles are the most suitable.

• **Animal Food:** Fish and other animal food is to be avoided. However, in the event that animal food is craved, a small volume of white-meat fish may be eaten once every ten days to two weeks. The fish should be prepared steamed, boiled, or poached and garnished with grated daikon or ginger. Strictly avoid blue-meat and red-meat fish and all shellfish.

• **Fruit:** The less the better until the condition improves. If cravings develop, a small volume of cooked fruit with a pinch of sea salt or dried fruit (also preferably cooked) may be taken. Avoid all fruit juices and cider.

• **Sweets and Snacks:** Overuse of sweets is connected with pancreatic disorders, so it is very important to avoid all sweets and desserts, including good-quality macrobiotic desserts, until the condition improves. To satisfy a sweet tooth, use sweet vegetables every day in cooking, drink sweet vegetable drinks, or prepare sweet vegetable jam. If cravings arise, a small volume of amasake, barley malt, or rice syrup may be taken. If cravings persist, a little cider, apple juice, or chestnut may be prepared. Mochi, rice balls, vegetable sushi, and other grain based snacks may be eaten frequently. Limit rice cakes, popcorn, and other dry or baked snacks, as they may harden the tumor.

• **Nuts and Seeds:** Nuts and nut butters are to be avoided due to their high amount of fat and protein, except for chestnuts. Unsalted, roasted seeds such as sunflower seeds and pumpkin seeds may be consumed as a snack, up to one cup altogether per week.

• **Seasonings:** Seasonings, such as unrefined sea salt, shoyu, and miso, are to be used moderately in order to avoid unnecessary thirst. Avoid mirin and garlic. If you become particularly thirsty after a meal or between meals, you should cut back on these seasonings until the normal level of thirst returns.

• **Beverages:** Beverages and other dietary practices can follow the general recommendations in Part I including bancha twig tea as the main beverage. Strictly avoid the beverage on the "infrequent" and "avoid" list and don't take grain coffee for the first two to three months after starting this new way of eating.

The most important thing in connection with dietary practice is chewing very well, until all food becomes liquid in the mouth and well mixed with saliva. Chew very, very well at least 50 times, preferably 100 times, per mouthful. It is also important to avoid overeating and eating within three hours of sleeping.

As noted in the introduction to Part II, persons who have received or who are currently undergoing medical treatment may need to make further dietary modifications.

SPECIAL DRINKS AND DISHES

Several special drinks may need to be taken, depending in the individual case. Please see a qualified macrobiotic teacher for guidance. Amounts of frequencies given here are averages; these will differ from person to person.

• **Sweet Vegetable Drink:** Take one to one and one-half small cups every day for the first month, then every other day the second month.

• **Carrot-Daikon Drink:** Take one to one and one-half small cups every day for two to four weeks, then once every three days for one month.

• **Lotus-Shiitake-Kombu Tea:** Combine finely chopped lotus root (50 percent), kombu (25 percent), shiitake mushroom (25 percent) with four times as much water. Boil and simmer for 20 minutes, adding three to four drops of shoyu at the end. Drink one small cup every day for two weeks, then twice a week for another month.

• **Shiitake-Seaweed Tea:** In the event that pain arises, a cup or two of boiled dried shiitake mushroom and nori or wakame kombu may be consumed for several days. The taro potato plaster and ginger compress, as mentioned below, are also helpful to reduce pains.

• **Carrot Juice:** To relax the pancreas in case of pain, a small volume of fresh carrot juice may be taken. Simmer for three minutes and take one small cup for four to five days.

• **Grated Daikon:** Grate about one-half small cup of fresh daikon, add a few drops of shoyu, and take two to three times a week.

HOME CARES

• **Body Scrub:** Scrubbing the whole body, including the abdominal region and the spinal region, with a towel that has been immersed in hot water and squeezed out is very helpful for better circulation of blood, lymph, and other body fluids, as well as for activating physical and mental energies.

• **Compress Guidelines:** For a small number of pancreatic tumors, a compress may be needed to help gradually draw out excess mucus and fat. Please see a qualified macrobiotic teacher for guidance on the proper use and frequency of a compress or plaster. Several types are used depending on the person's condition. Precede the compress or plaster with application of a towel that has been soaked in hot water and squeezed out over the affected area for about three to five minutes to stimulate circulation.

• **Taro Plaster:** A taro potato plaster can be applied on the area every day for three to four hours, immediately following a hot ginger compress applied for three to five minutes. This application may be continued for the initial two- to three-week period and thereafter occasionally two to three times per week.

• **Buckwheat Plaster:** In the event of swelling from fluid retention in the pancreatic and abdominal regions or from gas formation, which quite often arises (both during the period of cancer development and/or during the period of recovery), a buckwheat plaster can be applied for one to two hours daily for several days. (A kombu plaster may be used instead of a buckwheat plaster to relieve gas formation.) Full-body shiatsu massage or palm healing to the abdominal region, one-half to one hour daily, can also be helpful.

OTHER CONSIDERATIONS

• Daily physical exercise that does not produce exhaustion is recommended. Ten to fifteen minutes of daily breathing exercises, especially emphasizing long exhalation, is also beneficial. These physical and breathing exercises contribute to relaxing tensions in the body and mind as well as harmonizing physical metabolism.

• Keeping air quality clean and fresh is important for maintenance of general health. For that purpose, green leafy plants can be placed in the house and the windows periodically opened to allow circulation of fresh air.

• Avoid wearing wool and synthetic fibers. At the minimum wear cotton underwear and use cotton sheets and pillowcases.

• Avoid watching television for long stretches. Radiation weakens the chest area. Similarly, avoid other artificial sources of electromagnetic energy such as video terminals, smoke detectors, and hand-held electrical appliances.

PERSONAL EXPERIENCE

Pancreatic Cancer

On August 21, 1973, Jean Kohler, a professor of music at Ball State University in Muncie, Indiana, underwent exploratory surgery at Indiana University Medical Center. The fifty-six-year-old pianist had always been healthy and kept fit by gardening and lifting weights. During the summer he had experienced an itching spreading from his leg and thought he had contracted poison oak. Initial medical tests turned up nothing. However, chief surgeon John Jesseph discovered a tumor the size of a fist on the head of Kohler's pancreas. Moreover, the cancer had spread to the duodenum. Like most other pancreatic cancer patients, Kohler's condition was discovered too late to operate. Dr.

Phillip Christiansen, the other doctor in the case, concluded pessimistically, "I know nothing coming out of research in the next ten years that could possibly help him." Kohler was told he would live anywhere from one month to three years and was advised to take chemotherapy to control the pain.

After five days of drug treatment, Kohler suffered badly swollen hands and arms as well as a cough, chills, and general stress. With the help of his wife, Mary Alice, he decided to search for an alternative treatment. An Indiana nutritionist referred him to me, and the Kohlers arrived in Boston for a consultation on September 25. Visual diagnosis, especially the presence of a small blister on Jean's right eye, confirmed the presence of pancreatic cancer.

Kohler expressed a sincere desire to follow the Cancer Prevention Diet for pancreatic tumors outlined above, and I told him that he would be out of danger within three to six months. Prior to this time, Jean had consumed meat twice a day, eaten much canned and packaged food, and had a well-developed sweet tooth. He especially enjoyed milk, cocoa, soft drinks, milkshakes, and desserts topped with whipped cream. A threat of diabetes several years earlier made him switch to diet sodas and saccharin and sucaryl instead of sugar.

In Boston the Kohlers spent a few days learning to cook according to yin and yang. "One of the most amazing, and totally unexpected, benefits for us personally was that after only five days of macrobiotic food, Jean's hands were suddenly much more flexible," Mary Alice later recalled. "He could reach farther on the keyboard than ever before! This condition has remained to the present time."

On April 7, 1974, after following the diet faithfully for about six months, Kohler returned to Boston. Visual diagnosis indicated that all signs of cancer activity had disappeared. There was a small tumor, the size of a walnut, but it was no longer malignant. Back home Jean continued the Cancer Prevention Diet for another three months and in July was healthy enough to add a little maple syrup to his way of eating. He continued to improve steadily over the next two years, and his medical tests, including the CEA, which tests for cancer cells in the bloodstream, returned to normal.

For seven years from initial discovery of the tumor, Kohler led a completely normal, active life. In addition to continuing his academic duties and performing musical concerts, he tirelessly wrote letters to scientists around the country about his medical case, delivered hundreds of speeches, and published a book on his recovery. Many thousands of people were helped by his example. As he often said, "The best thing ever to happen to me was having so-called terminal cancer."

The medical world, however, tended to discount his case even though he had compelling scientific documentation. He was often told that only an autopsy would show whether his surgeon's original diagnosis of cancer was accurate and whether it had truly disappeared. In September 1980 Kohler suddenly became ill and checked into Boston's Beth Israel Hospital. Doctors, looking at his medical records, suspected that the pancreatic cancer had come back and asked permission to perform exploratory surgery. Kohler's friends and relatives strongly opposed it, but Jean consented, saying, "I'm too weak to explain, but I have to do this."

On September 14 Kohler died in the hospital. According to Dr. Michael

Sobel, the surgeon who performed two operations on him and examined the autopsy, Jean's death had "nothing to do with cancer." Microscopic signs of previous cancer were discovered showing that the diagnosis of his original doctors in Indiana was correct. However, no current cancer activity was found. "For someone to survive seven years with cancer of the pancreas without being treated is extremely rare, if not unheard of," Dr. Sobel commented. Kohler's death was attributed to a liver infection and complications resulting from hemorrhaging following surgery.

In death, as in life, Jean Kohler showed that cancer is not incurable and can be reversed by a balanced diet centered around whole grains and vegetables, accompanied by faith in nature and a strong will to live. Sources: Jean and Mary Alice Kohler, *Healing Miracles from Macrobiotics* (West Nyack, NY: Parker, 1979), and Tom Monte, "The Legacy of Jean Kohler," *East West Journal*, March 1981, 14–18.

Pancreatic Cancer

Norman J. Arnold, fifty-two, a resident of Columbia, South Carolina, was in the prime of life. President and chief executive officer of the Ben Arnold Company, he directed the largest wholesaler of wine and alcoholic beverages in the Southeast and among the ten largest in the nation. Active in community affairs, he headed up local chapters of the Boys Club, the Zoological Society, and the Heart Fund. Appointed to several state commissions, he served as the committee chairman for the Governor's Economic Task Force. With his wife and family he was active in educational, philanthropic, and synagogue activities.

On July 28, 1982, Arnold underwent routine gallbladder surgery at Providence Hospital in Columbia. During the surgery, it was discovered that he had a primary cancer in the head of the pancreas, which had metastasized to the liver. In the consultations with his surgeon, and gastroenterologist, he was told that he had from three to nine months to live. Even though the prospects of surviving pancreatic cancer are about null, the doctors advised him to start chemotherapy and/or radiation as a way of "possibly gaining more time." A doctor at Lombardi Cancer Center at Georgetown University recommended a very potent chemotherapy treatment, involving three chemicals, for "as long as my body could take it."

Arnold had always been an active, energetic, and above-average amateur athlete, and a very optimistic and positive person. The chemotherapy treatment made him weak and tired, and gave him a deep feeling of helplessness and hopelessness. "This debilitated feeling was more painful to me than the actual pain which I endured," he later recalled. "This miserable existence combined with the fact that I did not want my growing incapacity to be a physical and psychological burden to my three sons [twins, thirteen, and an older boy, sixteen] and my wife. I also did not want their last memory of me to be that of an invalid."

During the eight-week period in which he took five chemotherapy treatments, Arnold learned about macrobiotics, made inquiries through a medical doctor who had relieved his own cancer on the diet, and arranged to meet with me. "I had heard there were those who promoted certain nonconventional cancer treatments in order to financially exploit cancer victims," Arnold noted later. "I was therefore very skeptical of Mr. Kushi at the outset, but my concern proved to be totally unfounded."

Arnold started eating a macrobiotic regimen, modified for his particular condition, in August 1982. In October he received his fifth and final chemotherapy treatment. On his own initiative, Arnold decided to discontinue the chemical injections because he "preferred a more acceptable quality of life, even if that meant less time alive, rather than a questionably longer existence as a cripple. "On the macrobiotic diet, he gradually began to recover his vigor and energy and positive, cheerful attitude.

"In time, I found that I had more energy and vitality than I had had for twenty years. My wife, who also had adhered strictly to the macrobiotic diet with me, had positive results both physically and psychologically. My sixteen-year-old son, who plays first-string center on his high school basketball team, discovered that the macrobiotic diet greatly increased his strength and especially his endurance. My thirteen-year-old twin boys demonstrated more concentration, mental agility, and stamina in their schoolwork when eating macrobiotically, as they do alternate with the 'standard teenage junk food' diet outside our home."

In the nine months following his last chemotherapy treatment, the various CAT scans and ultrasound tests showed the pancreas tumor and the "spots" on the liver decreasing in size. In the six months since then, further CAT scans, ultrasound, and blood tests showed no evidence of disease.

Having already outlived his original prognosis by almost two years, Arnold says he is mentally and physically relaxed and functioning better than he has for many years. "I play vigorous, singles tennis matches almost every day and find that I have much more strength and endurance than I have had for a very long time. Last month I beat my forty-one-year-old gastroenterologist in a 6–4, 7–5, 6–8, 8–6 match!" Nine years later, he is still in excellent health and cancer-free. Source: Letters from Norman Arnold to Congressman Claude Pepper, Chairman of the U.S. House Subcommittee on Health and Long-term Care, January 18, 1984.

Pancreatic Cancer

Hugh Faulkner had never been happier. He had completed a successful career as a general practitioner in London and retired to a beautiful old farmhouse in Italy. After returning to the countryside outside of Florence with his wife, Marian, the former London doctor learned he had cancer of the pancreas.

"We both knew the diagnosis was more or less a death sentence," he recalled in an interview with the Independent, a British newspaper.

After her husband was referred to a surgeon who wanted to operate immediately, Marian asked, "What happens if he doesn't have surgery?" She was told: "He'll certainly obstruct." Bowel obstruction or difficulties with food absorption are common with pancreatic cancer, and Dr. Faulkner started to experience both. He underwent surgery to relieve the obstruction, but surgeons made no attempt to remove the cancer. In the hospital, after several days on liquids, he was put on solid foods again. "That day the lady from the kitchens came to see me," he recalls. " 'Would you like steak and kidney pudding, dear?' she asked. I noticed we were given no advice at all on diet."

Meanwhile, a young woman who had given the Faulkners shiatsu treatments for back pain recommended macrobiotics. Dr. Faulkner recalled that during his career he had not been a conventional physician. "I used to refer my patients to people I thought could help them even if I thought they were 'alternative.' But I hadn't referred cases of incurable cancer. And I hadn't any real contact with alternative medicine. I'm not a believer; I'm congenitally skeptical."

After reading several books, Dr. Faulkner decided that macrobiotics might "help improve the quality of the months remaining to me." The usual rate of survival after diagnosis for pancreatic cancer is two to four months. It is rare to live even a year. "All our medical friends naturally assumed that I would die," Dr. Faulkner explained. "But by this time I'd decided that what I was afraid of was not death itself. It was the pain, the incontinence, the loss of autonomy when I became helpless that I dreaded."

Back in England, the Faulkners checked into a hospice—a center for the dying. While awaiting the end, they went to the Community Health Foundation, the macrobiotic center in London. A macrobiotic teacher who was visiting from Boston advised them on diet and encouraged them to see me for additional recommendations.

About six weeks later they met me during one of my European seminars. "Mr. Kushi was a small, slim, very modest man, with considerable charisma," Dr. Faulkner recalled. "It was all very warm and friendly and unmedical. Kushi spent a long time examining my skin texture—its appearance, elasticity, and color. Then I said,"Well, can macrobiotics heal my cancer?' "

" 'No,' said Kushi, 'but your body can. What we can do is advise you on a diet and way of life that will almost certainly make you feel much better, and give your body a chance to reject the cancer. We can't give you any guarantees—but we have plenty of evidence from cases like yours that it can work.' "

Although Dr. Faulkner was a little skeptical, Marian was enthusiastic, and they decided to try it. Returning to their farmhouse in Italy, the couple started cooking for themselves. The diet I recommended was a modified version of the standard macrobiotic diet. For breakfast, there was whole-grain porridge and occasionally whole-grain bread. Lunch included vegetable soup and tofu, tempeh, or another protein dish. Dinner consisted of pressure-cooked brown rice and vegetables and, occasionally, stewed fruit.

Dr. Faulkner's diarrhea went away, and he began to feel better. Marian also experienced improvement—she began to feel more energetic and confident. Visitors who came by to say farewell to the dying doctor were amazed to find him chopping wood and full of energy.

By the autumn of 1988, medical tests showed "no evidence of cancer, no evidence of abnormality of any kind." In London some doctors questioned the initial diagnosis of cancer. Dr. Faulkner showed them his biopsy report and introduced them to his surgeon. They didn't want to believe and labeled his recovery "spontaneous regression."

Now, five years after his initial diagnosis. Dr. Faulkner continues to thrive.

He eats and sleeps well, entertains many visitors, and swims several times a week. He has also learned to read music, play the jazz harmonica, and use a word processor. "I have a lot more energy than I've had in years."

"As an orthodox doctor, I myself wouldn't have thought of diet influencing the course of disease," Dr. Faulkner admits. "I'm now quite sure that we can learn a great deal from alternative medicine.

"The big change in macrobiotics was hope, however implausible. That and the feeling that I was regaining control of my destiny."

Source: "A Doctor Heals Himself of Terminal Cancer," *One Peaceful World Newsletter*, Autumn 1989, and Hugh Faulkner, *Physician, Heal Thyself* (Becket, MA: One Peaceful World Press, 1992).

19

Female Reproductive Cancers: Ovary, Uterus, Cervix, and Vagina

FREQUENCY

Cancer of the reproductive organs is the third most common form of cancer in American women (after lung and breast). This year, an estimated 24,000 women will die of cancers of the ovary, uterus (endometrium), cervix, vagina, and other reproductive organs, and 71,500 new cases will develop, as well as 55,000 new cases of noninvasive cancer of the cervix.

Ovarian cancer, which will claim 13,000 lives this year, is rarely detected early and kills most patients in less than a year. There are many varieties of ovarian tumors, both benign and malignant, and precancerous conditions, including dermoid cysts. Standard treatment for ovarian cancer is a *hysterectomy* (surgical removal of the uterus) and a *salpingo-oophorectomy* (removal of the ovary and Fallopian tubes). This operation may be done through the vagina or the abdomen, and the woman will no longer have menstrual periods or be able to conceive children. An *omentectomy* is also often performed as a preventive measure, and this operation involves removing a fold of abdominal membrane, which is often the site of metastases. Internal or external radiation treatment may follow surgery, and chemotherapy may be used for maintenance. The current five-year survival rate for ovarian cancer is 39 percent.

Cancer of the uterus, especially the endometrium, comprises 4 percent of all cancers in the United States and will account for 45,500 new cases this year and 10,000 deaths. In some parts of the country it is growing at the rate of 10 percent a year. This dramatic rise, almost unparalleled in the history of cancer, has been associated with use of the birth-control pill by women of child-bearing age and estrogen additive therapy in menopausal women over fifty. Usual treatment is a total abdominal hysterectomy. The ovaries, Fallopian tubes, and pelvic lymph nodes may also be taken out depending on the individual case. Radiation treatment and chemotherapy commonly follow, along with hormone therapy, especially large doses of progesterone. The remission rate is 83 percent.

Cancer of the cervix appears primarily in women over forty. However, it is on the increase in younger women, and cervical dysplasia and sometimes herpes type 2 virus are considered precancerous conditions. Cervical cancer can spread to other reproductive sites as well as the rectum, bladder, liver, lymph, and bones. It is treated with a hysterectomy, radium implants, or experimental chemotherapy. Cervical dysplasia is often treated with cryosurgery, a procedure in which nitrous oxide or other gas is used to freeze and kill affected cells. This year about 4,400 American women will die of cervical cancer, and 13,500 new cases will develop. The five-year survival rate is 66 percent.

Cancers of the vagina and vulva are rarer, accounting for about 1,000 deaths this year and 5,000 new cases. They affected women mostly over fifty, but are increasingly found in younger women as well. Vaginal tumors tend to spread quickly to the pelvic lymph nodes, and vulvar tumors may spread to the vagina, lungs, liver, or bones. Depending on the stage and type, the patient may receive a hysterectomy, a vaginectomy (removal of the vagina), or a vulvectomy (removal of the vulva). Internal radiation implants and external pelvic irradiation may be used to supplement surgery. Survival rates range from 8 to 75 percent.

STRUCTURE

The ovaries are the primary organs of the female reproductive system. Each of these tiny paired organs is about the size of an almond and the production of eggs (ova) takes place in the follicles. A follicle consists of an ovum surrounded by one or several layers of follicle cells. At birth, the ovaries contain about 800,000 follicles. This number decreases until, at menopause, few, if any, follicles remain. When a follicle has reached maturity, it will either rupture and release its ovum or collapse and decompose. The former process is known as ovulation. The latter process is called atresia and involves the natural degeneration and discharge of follicles from the body during menstruation.

Following ovulation, the egg enters a fingerlike end of the Fallopian tube and begins its movement into the uterus. If intercourse has taken place, the egg has the possibility of being fertilized. The union of egg and sperm occurs in the fimbriated end of the uterine tube. If an ovum is fertilized, it begins to develop as it passes through the uterine tube and into the uterus. Implantation of the fertilized ovum in the uterus takes place after about seven to ten days. The uterus or womb averages two and a half inches in length and weighs approximately fifty grams. It has a capacity of two to five cubic centimeters and is tightly constructed. During pregnancy it increases substantially and at full term reaches a length of about twenty inches. The uterus returns to its original condition following delivery

The lining of the uterus, which is shed during menstruation and is regenerated after about two days, is called the endometrium. The neck of the uterus, connecting the womb with the vagina, is called the cervix. The chief organs of intercourse are the vagina and the vulva, consisting of the major and minor lips, and the clitoris.

CAUSE OF CANCER

Female sexual disorders have risen sharply in recent years. In 1988 approximately 600,000 American women had hysterectomies. The variety of sexual disorders ranges from menstrual cramps and irregularities to vaginal discharge,

blocked Fallopian tubes, ovarian cysts, fibroid tumors, and cancer. To understand the origin and development of these illnesses, we must examine the
menstrual cycle.

The cycle of menstruation correlates with the process of ovulation. During
the first half of the menstrual cycle, between the woman's period and ovulation,
the hormone estrogen reaches its peak. During the second half of the menstrual
cycle, between ovulation and onset of the period, the hormone progesterone
predominates. The length of time for each stage in the cycle is largely dependent on the types of food that a woman eats. If a woman eats primarily whole
grains and cooked vegetables, menstruation usually takes only three days.
However, among women who eat a diet high in meat, sugar, and dairy products, five or six days is the norm. The next phase, in which the endometrium
regenerates itself, usually takes two days. However, with proper eating, this
can be accomplished in only one day. The following stage, in which the follicle
matures, lasts about eight days, and ovulation should occur in the part of the
cycle that is exactly opposite to the onset of menstruation or, ideally, fourteen
days. In healthy women, conception usually arises at this time or four to five
days after ovulation. During this phase, the yellow endocrine body (corpus
luteum) found in the ovary in the site of the ruptured follicle matures and
secretes progesterone. This hormone influences the changes that take place in
the uterine wall during the second half of the menstrual cycle. The follicle and
corpus luteum eventually decompose during this phase if not fertilized and are
discharged during menstruation.

If a woman is eating properly, her menstrual cycle should correlate with the
monthly lunar cycle, of about twenty-eight days. During the full moon, the
atmosphere becomes brighter and charged with energy. A woman who regularly eats grains, cooked vegetables, and other yang foods and is physically
active will usually menstruate at this time. The condition of the atmosphere will
cause her to become more energized, necessitating the discharge during her
period. During the new moon, the atmosphere is darker or more yin. Women
who menstruate at this time are usually consuming a more expansive diet. After
eating properly for some period a woman begins to menstruate at the time of
either the full or new moon, indicating that her condition is in harmony with
the natural atmospheric and lunar cycle.

During the first half of the menstrual cycle, women quickly regain balance
and can readily follow a more centered diet of whole grains, cooked vegetables,
and seasonal fresh fruit. Immediately prior to ovulation, fertility is expressed
with general feelings of joy, contentment, and bliss. The woman feels wonderful and exudes cheerfulness and confidence, and her eating remains centered
during the few days of ovulation.

During the second half of the cycle, as menstruation approaches, some
women experience dissatisfaction, irritability, and constant hunger. Overcooked foods, animal food, and other heavier substances may become unap-
pealing and if taken in too great a quantity frequently lead to excessive intake
of sweets, fruits, salad, and liquid. In such cases, just prior to menstruation,
some women may experience swelling of the breasts and a general bloated
feeling. The woman may continue to crave strong foods in the yin category and
to feel impatient and melancholy.

In order to have a smooth menstrual cycle, it is important for the woman to adjust her diet during the two halves of her month. During the first two weeks, between menstruation and ovulation, she should eat plenty of dark, leafy green vegetables along with whole grains and other more substantial foods to which she will be naturally attracted. During the last two weeks, between ovulation and menstruation, she will feel more comfortable if she reduces her intake of overcooked foods and avoids animal food altogether. Otherwise they will produce an increased craving for sweets, fruit, juices, salads, and lighter foods. To prevent this compulsion from arising, the woman can eat more lightly cooked vegetables at this time along with lighter seasonings and less salt. Special dishes, such as mochi, turnip or radish tops, or amasake, are very helpful and will reduce cravings for more extreme foods.

An irregular menstrual cycle results if the diet is imbalanced too much in one direction or the other. For example, if it totals less than twenty-eight days, this usually indicates an overly yang condition from eating excessive animal and overly energizing foods. A cycle longer than average, up to thirty-two or thirty-five days, shows that a woman may well be consuming too many foods in the yin category such as sweets, fruits, and dairy food. Both conditions can be corrected by eating a more central diet of grains and vegetables.

Menstrual cramps are usually caused by an excessive intake of animal products, especially meat, fish, eggs, and dairy food, in combination with too many expansive foods such as sugar, soft drinks, refined flour, and chemically processed foods. Cramps can be eliminated in two to three months on a balanced standard macrobiotic diet.

Excessive menstrual flow can result from overconsuming either too many foods from the yin or yang category. In the case of too many contractive foods, including animal foods rich in protein and fat, the blood thickens and the flow lasts longer. This is often accompanied by an unpleasant odor. When too many expansive foods, including foods that slow down the body metabolism, are consumed, the blood becomes thinner than normal, and menstruation is prolonged. When a woman eats a more balanced diet, menstruation will be of shorter duration and the flow will be lighter.

Biologically, women need not eat any animal food, except occasional consumption, if desired, of very light white fish or shellfish. Imbalanced diet can give rise to headaches, depression, and emotional outbursts prior to menstruation. This condition has recently been recognized by medical science under the name Premenstrual Syndrome (PMS). It can be corrected by centering the diet, especially avoiding extremes of meat and sugar and chemicalized food.

Deposits of fat and mucus, coming largely from animal foods, dairy foods, sugar, and refined flour products, often accumulate in the inner organs if an imbalanced way of eating continues over several years. In women this buildup tends to concentrate in the breasts and in the uterus, the ovaries, the Fallopian tubes, and the vagina. The solidification of mucus or fat around these organs can result in the development of cysts. Those that occur in the comparatively tight ovaries are saturated in quality, or yang, whereas those in the more expanded vagina or vulva contain more grease and mucus—their quality is yin. Most cysts are soft when they begin to form, but with the continuation of an improper diet they harden and often calcify. This type of cyst is something like a stone and is very difficult to dissolve. Some varieties of cysts contain fat and protein and can become extremely hard, in which case they are called dermoid cysts. Tumors represent the final stage in this process as the body attempts to localize the continuing influx of unhealthy nutrients by creating blockages and obstructions in various organs and sites of the body. The accumulation of fat and mucus can also block the Fallopian tubes, preventing the passage of egg and sperm and resulting in the inability to conceive.

Foods that, when overconsumed, create cysts and tumors in the reproductive organs include varied combinations of milk, cheese, ice cream, and other dairy products; sugar, soft drinks, chocolate, and other sweeteners; fruit and fruit juices; nut butters; greasy and oily foods; refined flour and pastries such as croissants, doughnuts, and sweet rolls; and hamburgers and other animal foods. Once again, serious reproductive illnesses may be relieved by eliminating extreme foods and centering the diet on whole grains, beans, vegetables, sea vegetables, and small volumes of fruit and seeds.

Recently some cancer specialists have linked the spread of herpes type 2 virus with cancer of the cervix. This type of herpes can be considered a precancerous condition, but it is not caused by a virus introduced from the outside. Herpes is the effect of poor eating, especially foods high in fat and sugar. A multitude of viruses and other microorganisms live in symbiosis with the human organism and usually will not give rise to disease unless the blood quality is weakened. If the blood quality is strong, the body's immune system will neutralize and destroy any harmful bacteria, or other organisms. The current epidemic of herpes is the result of degenerating blood quality. Widespread consumption of synthetic and artificial foods, on top of meat and sugar, has created a weakened condition in which harmful viruses can thrive. People who eat a balanced diet and over time have strengthened their blood and immune system need have no fear of getting infected with herpes.

MEDICAL EVIDENCE

• In 1674 an English physician named Wiseman associated cancer with the effects of faulty nutrition on the blood and sexual organs. "This disease might arise from an error in diet, a great acrimony in the meats and drinks meeting with a fault in the first concoction, which, not being afterwards corrected in the intestines, suffered the acrimonious matter to ascend into the blood, where, if it found vent either in the menstrua in women, or by the hemorrhoids or urine in men, the mischief might have been prevented." Source: Frederick Hoffman, *Cancer and Diet* (Baltimore: Williams & Wilkins, 1937), 6.

• In 1896 Robert Bell, M.D., senior staff member at the Glasgow Hospital for Women, adopted a nutritional approach to tumors of the uterus and breast after twenty years as a cancer surgeon. "I had been taught that this [surgery] was the only method by which malignant disease could be successfully treated, and, at the time, believed this to be true. But failure after failure following each other, without a single break, inclined me to alter my opinion. . . . The disease invariably recurred with renewed virulence, suffering was intensified, and the life of the patient shortened. . . . That cancer is a curable disease, if its local development is recognized in its early stage, and if rational dietetic and therapeutic measures are adopted and rigidly adhered to, there can be no doubt whatever." Source: Robert Bell, M.D., *Ten Years' Record of the Treatment of Cancer without Operation* (London: Dean & Son, 1906), 6, 14–15.

• As early as 1938, when it was synthesized, laboratory tests associated DES (diethylstilbestrol) with breast cancer. From 1945 to 1970 the drug was widely used to prevent miscarriage, control menstrual disorders and estrogen deficiencies, serve as a "morning after" birth-control pill, and act as a chemotherapeutic agent for prostate cancer in men and for breast cancer in postmenopausal women. In 1954 DES was approved by the U.S. Department of Agriculture as a feed additive for poultry, cattle, and hogs, and by 1970, 75 percent of all beef in the United States had been fattened with DES. In the early 1970s epidemiological studies associated the use of DES during pregnancy with an increase in vaginal and cervical cancer among the daughters of DES users, primarily between the ages of ten and thirty. DES was discontinued in 1979. Sources: Samuel S. Epstein, M.D., *The Politics of Cancer* (New York: Doubleday, 1979), 214–33, and *Diet, Nutrition, and Cancer* (Washington, DC: National Academy of Sciences, 1982), 14:13–14.

• In 1974 epidemiological data associated ovarian cancer with a high-fat diet. Source: C. H. Lingeman, "Etiology of Cancer in the Human Ovary," *Journal of the National Cancer Institute* 53:1603–18.

• In 1975 researchers reported a direct correlation between per capita intake of total fat and incidence of cancer of the uterus and mortality from ovarian cancer. They also linked total protein consumption with endometrial cancer and total protein and fruit consumption with cervical cancer. Source: B. Armstrong and R. Doll, "Environmental Factors and Cancer Incidence and Mortality in Different Countries with Special Reference to Dietary Practices," *International Journal of Cancer* 15:617–31.

• Seventh-Day Adventist women in California ages thirty-five to fifty-four have 84 percent less cervical cancer and 12 percent less ovarian cancer than the national average, according to a 1975 epidemiological study. Female church members over fifty-five have 36 percent less cervical cancer and 47 percent less ovarian cancer. Together both age groups have 40 percent fewer uterine tumors of other kinds. The Seventy-Day Adventists, about half of whom are vegetarian, eat 25 percent less fat and 50 percent more fiber, especially whole grains, vegetables, and fruit, than the general population. Source: R. L. Phillips, "Role of Life-styles and Dietary Habits in Risk of Cancer among Seventh-Day Adventists," *Cancer Research* 35:3513–22.

• "Worldwide use of birth control pills, in spite of conclusive evidence of carcinoginicity of estrogens in experimental animals," warned Samuel S. Epstein, M.D., "constitutes the largest uncontrolled experiment in human carcinogenesis ever undertaken." The cancer specialist cited studies estimating that oral contraceptives could cause 10,000 fatalities a year, especially from ovarian cancer. Source: Samuel S. Epstein, M.D., *The Politics of Cancer* (New York: Doubleday, 1979), 222.

• Endometrial cancer increased sharply during the early 1970s. Researchers associated this with excessive use of synthetic estrogens by women at the time of menopause. In 1976, following publicity about the hazards of oral contraceptives and synthetic hormones, the use of estrogens partially diminished and endometrial cancer rates began to fall. Source: H. Jick et al., "The Epidemic of Endometrial Cancer," *American Journal of Public Health* 70 (1980):264–67.

• A 1981 epidemiological study in Hawaii found a direct association between ethnic patterns of total fat consumption (including animal fat, saturated fat, and unsaturated fat) and uterine cancer. Source: L. N. Kolonel et al., "Nutrient Intakes in Relation to Cancer Incidence in Hawaii," *British Journal of Cancer* 44:332–39.

• Writing in an American Cancer Society journal for clinicians in 1982, David Schottenfeld, M.D., chief of epidemiology and director of cancer control of Memorial Sloan-Kettering Cancer Center in New York, asserted that "some evidence suggests that the risk of uterine cervical dysplasia and carcinoma in situ may be increased by the long-term use of oral contraceptives." He stated that among women using Oracon®, the risk of endometrial cancer was 7.3 times that of nonusers. There is also a risk for liver cancer among users of oral contraceptives, though recent studies show a lowered risk for ovarian cancer in pill users. Discussing iatrogenesis, or doctor-caused disease, he concluded: "The risk-benefit evaluation of a drug should take into account the likely outcome of the disease if untreated, and whether or not alternative therapies are available." Source: David Schottenfeld, M.D., "Cancer Risks of Medical Treatment," *Ca—a Cancer Journal for Clinicians* 32:258–79.

• A 1984 case-control study found that women with ovarian cancer consumed greater amounts of foods high in animal fats and significantly less vegetable fat compared with controls. There was a significant trend toward increased risk of ovarian cancer with increasing animal fat consumption. The risk was 1.8 times greater for those with high intake. Source: D. W. Cramer et al., "Dietary Animal Fat in Relation to Ovarian Cancer Risk," *Obstetrics and Gynecology* 63:833–38.

• In a 1988 study in Italy, dietary intake of beta-carotene was inversely associated with risk of invasive cervical cancer. Source: C. La Vecchia et al., "Dietary Vitamin A and the Risk of Intraepithelial and Invasive Cervical Neoplasia," *Gynecology and Oncology* 30:187–95.

• In 1988 researchers at Johns Hopkins University reported that taxol, a compound developed from the bark of the Pacific yew tree, may benefit women with severe ovarian cancer. In 1991 researchers at the M. D. Anderson Cancer Center in Houston suggested that taxol may benefit women with breast cancer as well. In studies of twenty-five women with advanced breast cancer who had failed to respond to chemotherapy, a majority of the women experienced some tumor shrinkage after nine months' experimental treatment. Source: E. K. Rowinsky and R. C. Donehower, *Journal of the National Cancer Institute* 83:1778–82, and Kathy A. Fackelmann, "The Adjuvant Advantage," *Science News*, February 22, 1992.

• In 1989 MIT researchers reported that women consuming a diet high in complex carbohydrates and low in protein showed "improved depression, tension, anger, confusion, sadness, fatigue, alertness, and calmness" before the onset of menstruation, in comparison to women with severe PMS eating the usual diet high in refined carbohydrates and fat. Besides sweets, the women suffering from PMS consumed more calories and more snack foods. Source: Judith J. Wurtman et al., "Effect of Nutrient Intake on Premenstrual Depression," *American Journal of Obstetrics and Gynecology* 161:1228–34.

• Dairy food consumption was linked with ovarian cancer by researchers at Harvard in 1989. The scientists noted that women with ovarian cancer had low blood levels of transferase, an enzyme involved in the metabolism of dairy foods. The researchers theorized that women with low levels of transferase who eat dairy foods, especially yogurt and cottage cheese, could increase their risk of ovarian cancer by as much as three times. The researchers estimated that women who consume large amounts of yogurt and cottage cheese increased their risk of ovarian cancer up to three times. "Yogurt was consumed at least monthly by 49 percent of cases and 36 percent of controls," researchers reported. "Worldwide, ovarian cancer risk is strongly correlated with lactose persistence and per capita milk consumption, further epidemiological evidence that lactose rather than fat is the key dietary variable for ovarian cancer . . . [A]voidance of lactose-rich food by adults may be a way of primary prevention of ovarian cancer . . ." Source: Daniel W. Cramer et al., "Galactose Consumption and Metabolism in Relation to the Risk of Ovarian Cancer," *Lancet* 2:66–71.

• A new medical textbook on reproductive health and disorders recommended a high-fiber, low-fat diet to help prevent or reduce PMS. "Diet throughout the month, and especially during the premenstrual interval, should be high in complex carbohydrates and moderate in protein (emphasizing alternatives to red meat), but low in refined sugar and salt (sodium), with regular, small meals throughout the day." The authors further recommended that "women should reduce or eliminate their consumption of tea, coffee, caffeine-containing beverages, chocolate, and alcohol, and stop smoking." Source: Robert A. Hatcher et al., "Menstrual Problems," *Contraceptive Technology 1990–1992* (New York: Irvington, 1990).

DIAGNOSIS

Ovarian cancer is generally diagnosed by gynecologists on the basis of a pelvic examination, a Pap smear, and a parancentesis or cul-de-sac aspiration, in which fluid from between the vagina and rectum is drained out by needle for examination under a microscope. A needle biopsy will be taken if a malignancy is suspected, and metastases will be detected through a mammogram, GI series, or intravenous pyelogram (IVP). Uterine cancer is commonly observed following a pelvic examination and a D and C (dilatation and curettage) in which a small amount of tissue is scraped from the inside of the uterus. Metastases will be checked out with X rays to the chest, IVP, bone and liver scans, and endoscopy of the lower colon and bladder. Cervical, vaginal, and vulver cancers are diagnosed with a pelvic examination, a Pap smear, and a colposcopy, in which a viewing scope transmits a magnified area of the sex organs to a television monitor.

The condition of the reproductive system can be observed directly without technological intervention or potentially harmful X rays. If the woman has a vaginal discharge, for example, its color can help locate the site and extent of the swelling. If the discharge is yellowish in color, a cyst is developing. A white discharge is less serious, but usually leads to development of a soft type of cyst unless the woman changes her way of eating. A green discharge signifies tumorous growth, especially if the color has been occurring for any length of time.

Vaginal discharges, ovarian cysts, and fibroid tumors are frequently indicated by a yellow coating in the lower part of the whites of the eyes. Dark spots in the whites of the eye indicate ovarian cysts or tumors or kidney stones.

The eyelashes also correspond with reproductive functions. Eyelashes that curve outward show degeneration of the sex organs due to consumption of excessive yin foods, especially fruits, juices, and dairy products during early childhood. Eyelashes that curve inward indicate excess intake of strong foods in the yang category, including eggs and meat. In this case, there may be menstrual cramps or lack of menstruation due to contraction of the ovaries. Menstrual cramps are also indicated when a woman smiles by the presence of a horizontal line or ridge appearing between the upper lip and nose.

Split fingernails and abnormal colors on the fingertips, resulting from a chaotic way of eating, indicate malfunctions in the reproductive system as well. If one thumbnail or thumb tip shows these conditions and the other is normal, it indicates that the ovary corresponding to the abnormal side is malfunctioning.

Pimples in the center of the cheeks with a fatty appearance may reflect the formation of cysts in the ovarian region.

Along the bladder meridian, a green shade appearing around either ankle on the outside of the leg indicates developing cancer in the uterus or bladder. Also, a fatty swelling along the ankle region indicates mucous and fat accumulation in the uterine region and may be a sign of a precancerous condition.

DIETARY RECOMMENDATIONS

Cancer in the ovary is largely caused by overconsumption of eggs and other food rich in protein and rich in fat. Uterine cancer is caused more by meat and chicken. Hard dairy food, as well as too much salty, baked, and roasted foods, which make the muscles and tissues tight, also contribute to both ovarian and uterine cancer and should be avoided. Cancer in the cervix or vagina is caused by fat- and cholesterol-rich foods like those in the case of ovarian and uterine tumors, but also by proportionately more consumption of light dairy food, fruits, and flour products. Cancer in the reproductive region as a whole is accelerated by the intake of synthetic chemicals, including various kinds of drugs and estrogen replacements, as well as artificial birth-control methods and other unnatural regulation of reproductive and menstrual functions. Accordingly, all these things should be avoided. Sugar, sugar-treated foods, and other sweeteners, including artificial ones, also should be avoided. Flour products such as white bread, pancakes, and cookies tend to form mucus and fat and should not be eaten. Food and beverages that possess stimulant, aromatic, and fragrant characteristics, including seasonings such as curry, mustard, and pepper, coffee, alcohol, soft drinks, and herb teas should also be avoided. Oils, even unsaturated vegetable oils, should be minimized. All oily or greasy cooking methods, including deep frying, are to be avoided for some period until the condition improves. Salad dressings, mayonnaise (dairy or soy), and other oily dressings and spreads are to be avoided. All chemicalized foods and beverages are to be avoided, while those of more organic and natural quality are recommended. Following are general guidelines for daily food consumption:

• **Whole Grains:** Fifty to 60 percent of daily consumption, by volume, should be whole-cereal grains. The first day prepare plain pressure-cooked short-grain brown rice. On following days, alternate brown rice pressure-cooked with 20 to 30 percent millet, then rice with 20 to 30 percent barley, then rice with 20 to 30 percent aduki beans or lentils and then plain rice again. A delicious morning porridge can be made by taking leftover rice, adding a little more water to soften, and seasoning with a little miso at the end and simmering for two to three minutes more. In daily pressure cooking, the ratio of grain to water should be about 1:2. For seasoning, cook with a small postage stamp–sized piece of kombu instead of salt. Other grains can be used occasionally, including whole wheat berries, rye, corn, and whole oats, though oats should be avoided for the first month. However, buckwheat should not be eaten for about six months because it is very contractive and may harden the tumor. Seitan is also very yang and should be minimized. Flour products, even unrefined whole wheat bread, chapatis, pancakes, and cookies, should be totally avoided or limited in volume for a period of a few months, though people with ovarian and other female problems typically like roasted, baked, or crunchy foods. Whole-grain pasta and noodles may be eaten a couple times a week.

• **Soup:** Five to 10 percent soup, consisting of one or two cups or bowls per day of soup cooked with wakame sea vegetable and various vegetables, especially daikon and daikon leaves and other green leafy vegetables, and seasoned lightly with miso or shoyu. Occasionally a small volume of shiitake mushroom may be added to the soup. The miso may be barley miso, brown rice miso, or soybean (hatcho) miso and should be naturally aged two to three years. Grain soups, bean soups, and other soups may be taken from time to time.

• **Vegetables:** Twenty to 30 percent vegetables, cooked in a variety of forms, mainly steamed, boiled, and, after four to six weeks without oil, occasionally sautéed. Various type of leafy vegetables—green, yellow, and white—can be cooked in different styles, as can various root vegetables such as carrots, turnips, daikon, radishes, lotus root, and burdock roots, though burdock should be used much less frequently than other root vegetables. Round vegetables such as acorn and butternut squash, cabbage, and onions can also be frequently used. Daikon and daikon greens are especially recommended for these conditions. As a rule of thumb, the following dishes may be prepared, though the frequency may differ from person to person: nishime-style vegetables, three times a week; squash-aduki-kombu dish, three times a week; dried daikon, one cup, three times a week; carrots and carrot tops or daikon and daikon tops, three times a week; blanched vegetables, five to seven times a week; pressed salad, five to seven times a week; raw salad, one to two times a week for ovarian cancer and temporarily avoid for the others; steamed greens, five to seven times a week; sautéed vegetables, prepared with water the first month, then with sesame oil lightly brushed on the pan once or twice a week after that; kinpira, two-thirds of a cup, two times a week; dried tofu, tofu, tempeh, or seitan with vegetables, two times a week.

• **Beans:** Five percent small beans, such as aduki beans, lentils, chickpeas, or black soybeans, may be used daily, cooked together with sea vegetables such as kombu or with onions and carrots. Other beans may be used altogether two to three times a month. For seasoning, a small volume of unrefined sea salt or shoyu or miso can be used, and frequently beans can be made with a sweet taste rather than a salty one by adding a little barley malt. Bean products, such as tempeh, natto, and dried or cooked tofu, may be used occasionally, but in moderate volume.

• **Sea Vegetables:** Five percent or less sea vegetable dishes, including wakame and kombu, daily when cooking grain, in soup, etc. A sheet of toasted nori may also be taken daily. A small dish of hijiki or arame should be prepared two times a week. All other sea vegetables are optional.

• **Condiments:** Condiments to be available on the table are gomashio (sesame salt), on the average made with 1 part salt to 18 to 20 parts sesame seeds; kelp or wakame powder; umeboshi plum; and tekka, though all other regular macrobiotic condiments may be used if desired. These condiments may be used daily on grains and vegetables, but the volume should be moderate to suit individual appetite and taste.

• **Pickles:** Pickles, made at home in a variety of ways, are to be eaten daily, one tablespoon in all, though salty pickles are to be minimized. Wash off the salt if too salty.

• **Animal Food:** Fish and other animal food is to be avoided. However, in the event that animal food is craved, a small volume of white-meat fish may be eaten once every ten days to two weeks. The fish should be prepared steamed, boiled, or poached and garnished with grated daikon or ginger. Strictly avoid blue-meat and red-meat fish and all shellfish.

• **Fruit:** The less the better until the condition improves. If cravings develop, a small volume of cooked fruit with a pinch of sea salt or dried fruit (also preferably cooked) may be taken. Women with ovarian cancer may take a little more fruit, including fresh fruit, than the others. Avoid all fruit juices and cider.

• **Sweets and Snacks:** Overuse of sweets is associated with these disorders, so it is very important to avoid all sweets and desserts, including good-quality macrobiotic desserts, until the condition improves. To satisfy a sweet tooth, use sweet vegetables every day in cooking, drink sweet vegetable drinks, or prepare sweet vegetable jam. If cravings arise, a small volume of amasake, barley malt, or rice syrup may be taken. If cravings persist, a little cider, apple juice, or chestnut may be prepared. Mochi, rice balls, vegetable sushi, and other grain-based snacks may be eaten frequently. Limit rice cakes, popcorn, and other dry or baked snacks, as they may harden the tumor.

• **Nuts and Seeds:** Nuts and nut butters are to be avoided due to their high amount of fat and protein, except for chestnuts. Unsalted, steamed or boiled seeds such as sunflower seeds and pumpkin seeds may be consumed as a snack, up to one cup altogether per week. Minimize roasted seeds.

• **Seasonings:** Seasonings, such as unrefined sea salt, shoyu, and miso, are to be used moderately in order to avoid unnecessary thirst. Avoid mirin and garlic. If you become particularly thirsty after the meal or between meals, you should cut back on these seasonings until the normal level of thirst returns.

• **Beverages:** Beverages and other dietary practices can follow the general recommendations in Part I, including bancha twig tea as the main beverage. *Mu* tea is highly recommended if consumed for a period of a few months or occasionally. *Mu* is a medicinal tea made from either nine or sixteen different herbs that serve to warm the body and strengthen weak female organs. Strictly avoid the beverages on the "infrequent" and "avoid" list and don't take grain coffee for the first two or three months after starting this new way of eating.

The most important thing in connection with dietary practice is chewing very well, until all food becomes liquid in the mouth and well mixed with saliva. Chew very, very well, at least 50 times, preferably 100 times, per mouthful. It is also important to avoid overeating and eating within three hours of sleeping.

As noted in the introduction to Part II, persons who have received or who are currently undergoing medical treatment may need to make further dietary modifications.

SPECIAL DRINKS AND DISHES

Several special drinks or dishes may need to be taken, depending on the individual case. Please see a qualified macrobiotic teacher for guidance. Amounts and frequencies given here are averages; these will differ from person to person.

• **Sweet Vegetable Drink:** Take one to one and one-half small cups every day for the first month, then every other day the second month.
• **Carrot-Daikon Drink:** Take one small cup every day for four to six weeks, then once every three days for one month.
• **Sea Vegetable Juice:** Drinking one or two small cups of sea vegetable juice every day is recommended. Simply boil the sea vegetable in water for ten minutes and consume the liquid. Arame is especially helpful.
• **Shiitake Mushrooms:** In the event of a hard cyst or tumor, a small portion of dried shiitake mushrooms may be consumed every day cooked in soup or with vegetables. Prepare by cooking with daikon and seasoning moderately with miso or shoyu. Shiitake mushrooms may also be cooked with winter melon (obtainable in Chinese or Oriental grocery stores) and seasoned with miso.
• **Grated Daikon:** For some cases of blocked Fallopian tubes or obstructions in other passages of the reproductive area, one to two cups of grated daikon, cooked with nori sea vegetable, seasoned with shoyu or miso, can be eaten daily. Occasional consumption of grated daikon, with a few drops of shoyu, is also beneficial for all cases of female reproductive cancer.

HOME CARES

• **Body Scrub:** Scrubbing the whole body, including the abdominal region and the spinal region, with a towel that has been immersed in hot water and squeezed out is very helpful for better circulation of blood, lymph, and other body fluids, as well as for activating physical and mental energies.

• **Compress Guidelines:** For a small number of tumors in the female reproductive system, a compress may be needed to help gradually draw out excess mucus and fat. Please see a qualified macrobiotic teacher for guidance on the proper use and frequency of a compress or plaster. Several types are used, depending on the person's condition. Precede the compress or plaster with application of a towel that has been soaked in hot water and squeezed out over the affected area for about three to five minutes to stimulate circulation.

• **Daikon Hip Bath:** In the event of frequent vaginal discharges, a hip bath will facilitate the elimination of accumulated fat and mucus. Ideally, the water for the hip bath should contain dried leafy greens such as daikon or turnip greens. To prepare this bath, hang several dozen bunches of these leaves to dry, either near a window or outside, but not under direct sunlight. The leaves will first turn yellow and then brown, at which time they are suitable for use. Boil two or three bunches of dried leaves for each evening's bath for ten to twenty minutes in several quarts of water to which a handful of sea salt or kombu sea vegetable can be added. The water will turn brownish in color. Then run hot water in the bathtub, add the mixture along with another handful of sea salt, and get in. The water should cover your hips. Wrap a thick cotton towel around your upper body to avoid chills and to absorb perspiration. As the water begins to cool, add more hot water, and stay in the tub for ten to fifteen minutes.

If dried leaves are not available for this bath, use sea vegetables, especially arame. If these cannot be obtained or are too expensive, add two handfuls of sea salt to the bathwater and proceed as above.

In the bath, your lower body will become very red as circulation in that area increases and the stagnated fat and mucus inside the sex organs start to loosen. Immediately following the hip bath, douche with a preparation made with one teaspoon of sea salt, two teaspoons of rice vinegar or lemon juice, and one quart of warm bancha tea. This hip bath and douche can be taken every evening or every other evening for five to ten days and thereafter once every five days or once a week, until mucus and fatty substances are generally eliminated from the uterus and vaginal regions.

• **Taro Plaster:** In the case of a cyst, tumor (including fibroid tumor) or cancerous condition, it is helpful to apply a taro potato plaster for three to four hours on the lower abdominal region. This should be preceded by a ginger compress for three to five minutes to warm the area and accelerate circulation. The taro application may be repeated every day for two to four weeks until substantial improvement is made.

• **Green Vegetable Plaster:** To relieve pain, it is also helpful in some cases to apply a paste of mashed green leafy vegetables mixed with flour for one to two hours, after warming the area with a hot towel. This green leafy plaster should be kept warm during the application by placing roasted sea salt wrapped with cotton cloth above the plaster. It is also helpful to apply a very hot compress, for example, a ginger compress, repeatedly on the base of the spine.

OTHER CONSIDERATIONS

• Daily physical exercise that does not produce exhaustion is recommended. Ten to fifteen minutes of daily breathing exercises, especially emphasizing long exhalation, is also beneficial. These physical and breathing exercises contribute to relaxing tensions in the body and mind as well as harmonizing physical metabolism.

• Keeping air quality clean and fresh is important for maintenance of general health. For that purpose, green leafy plants can be placed in the house and the windows periodically opened to allow circulation of fresh air. Don't smoke, as this will tighten the ovaries.

• Avoid watching television for long stretches. Radiation weakens the reproductive area. Similarly, avoid other artificial sources of electromagnetic energy such as video terminals, smoke detectors, and hand-held electrical appliances, which can weaken the ovaries and reproductive system.

• Though cancer is naturally accompanied by a decline in energy and vitality, normal sexual practice is not harmful if it does not lead to exhaustion.

• Avoid artificial methods of regulating your period, especially birth-control pills, estrogens, and tubal ligation, which severs the flow of electromagnetic energy through the body. As your eating improves, your menstrual cycle will become more regular and tuned to the lunar cycle, and you can gradually begin natural birth-control methods.

• Avoid abortion and cesarean section if possible. Study natural methods of delivery and, if you are in good health, consider home birth with the assistance of a midwife or other experienced medical person. Breast-feeding will help protect you and your child against future illnesses, including cancer.

• Avoid synthetic underwear and stockings, artificial tampons, chemical douches or toiletries, talcum powder, and other synthetic products that may be irritating or harmful to the reproductive system.

• During the menstrual period, a woman's excess is discharged through the skin as well as through the menstrual flow. It is recommended that a woman not take cold showers or wash her hair with cold water, since both of these tend to draw this excess away from its normal course of discharge. To clean yourself, use a wet towel or sponge.

• Deep relaxation exercises, including Do-in or shiatsu acupressure massage, around the lower back prior to menstruation, can help reduce physical and emotional discomfort. Active physical exercises are also important for healthy living.

• In the case of pain, one half hour of palm healing is helpful. This is done simply by placing one hand on a piece of cotton over the affected area, synchronizing the breath, keeping a peaceful mind, and allowing the natural energy of the environment to flow through the hand. Palm healing is more effective when a second person performs the healing, but it can be done alone.

PERSONAL EXPERIENCES

Uterine Tumor

In 1947 film star Gloria Swanson learned that she had a tumor in her uterus. She went to three gynecologists, and each one recommended an immediate hysterectomy. Finally she went to see a specialist who was considered to be the top woman's doctor in the country. "After examining me," she later recalled in an article for *East West Journal*, "he didn't say exactly what the first three had, but he did say, 'Well, you know this has to come out by Christmas'—which was about five months away."

Instead, Miss Swanson went to California to see Dr. Bieler, a physician who treated illness with diet. He said to her, "Now, Gloria, what is the function of a protein?" She said, "It's a cell builder, Dr. Bieler." He asked her, "Are you fully grown?" She said, "Dr. Bieler, don't pull my leg. You know I'm forty-seven." He said, "Well, maybe you're a ditchdigger. Or are you a tennis pro? A football player?" She said, "What are you trying to tell me?"

Dr. Bieler went on to remind Gloria Swanson that she had had a hard time with the birth of her child in 1920. He also reminded her that cancer doesn't develop overnight but can sometimes take twenty years to develop.

"Have you been eating a lot of protein?" he asked her. "Well, I guess I have," she replied. "Well, now, what are you going to do about that, if it's a cell builder?" he inquired. "Do you really think I can starve this to death?" she said. The doctor smiled and said, "You get enough protein, you don't need all that animal protein." Gloria responded, "All right. As of this moment I shall not eat any more animal protein. How long do you think it will take?" The physician replied, "I don't know: a year, two years, maybe three."

For the next two years, despite a heavy travel schedule and demanding routine. Gloria carried around her own food, consisting primarily of whole grains and vegetables and a little bit of fruit. Two and a half years had elapsed by the time she went back to see the famous specialist. "I had a feeling the tumor was gone," she wrote. "He hadn't heard from me since the time he told me what was going to happen around Christmastime (that would have been a nice Christmas present for somebody—a pathologist, I guess). I hopped up on his table, and he started hunting. Oh, it was fascinating to watch his face. I said, 'It isn't there, is it, Doctor?' 'No'—reluctantly. I said, 'Don't you want to know what I did?' 'What do you mean, what you did?' 'Well,' I said, 'I went on a diet.'"

The doctor threw his head back and laughed. "He thought it was very funny," she continued. "A diet: ha-ha-ha. I said, 'It was a non–animal protein diet, Doctor.' He laughed even harder. I said, 'Well, you can laugh; I don't think it's a laughing matter. I'm still a woman, and what's more, I'm very happy about it. But I'm not laughing about it, and I don't think you should laugh either. I'd hoped you might learn something, because I have. And I don't really think you ought to send me a bill.' And I hopped off and went home, and he never did."

In the more than thirty years since, until dying of old age, Gloria had been extremely active in promoting natural foods and macrobiotics. Several years ago she and her husband, Bill Dufty, author of *Sugar Blues*, joined my wife, Aveline, and me on a visit and speaking tour of Japan. "You're responsible for your own health," Gloria told people who asked her how she maintained her health and beauty for over eighty years. "It's quite true. There's nobody who can chew your food for you. And so if you really want to be well, you have to do it yourself." Source: Gloria Swanson, "I'm Still a Woman," *East West Journal*, March 1977, 34–35.

Uterine Cancer with Metastases to the Bone and Lungs

In April 1980 Elaine Nussbaum had a diagnostic procedure to determine the cause of excessive and prolonged menstrual bleeding. The doctor found a tumor in the connective tissue on the wall of her uterus. She was given twenty radiation treatments, a radium implant, hormone medication, and both oral and intravenous chemotherapy. In August 1980 physicians performed a radical hysterectomy and a bilateral salpingo-oophorectomy, removing her ovaries.

Elaine continued to take chemotherapy. In May 1982 she experienced pain in the lower back that continued to worsen despite medication. She could neither sit nor lie down. In August, after several days standing up for twenty-four hours, sleeping only on her husband's shoulder in a standing position, she went to an orthopedist. He diagnosed a compression fracture and found that her vertebrae were partially collapsed. To prevent complete collapse of her backbone, she was put in a brace that extended from above the chest to the lower pelvic region.

Elaine's pain continued to worsen and spread to her legs. Eventually she could no longer stand. Her husband put her in a recliner and gave her strong painkillers night and day, but the pain continued.

In September she was taken to the hospital for more X rays and tests. Bone scans showed that the cancer had spread to the lumbar spine and the thoracic spine and there were malignancies in both lungs.

Elaine received five radiation treatments, followed by chemotherapy, followed by another series of radiation treatments and more chemotherapy. The usual treatment was ten rounds of chemotherapy over intervals of three to four weeks. She felt exhausted, with low vitality, and experienced nausea and pain.

In January 1983, after four cycles of chemo, medical tests showed an increase of activity and progression of the tumor in the spine and no change in Elaine's lungs.

Toward the end of January, Elaine cut her finger opening an envelope in the mail. Infection set in because of her weakness following chemo, and she was unable to ward off the infection. Over the next ten days, she received four blood transfusions in the hospital, as well as massive doses of intravenous antibiotics. The doctors decided to put her on less toxic treatment, and it was then that she knew conventional medicine would not work for her.

After researching the alternatives, Elaine decided to start macrobiotics. She weaned herself from meat, dairy food, fruit, and sugar and, eventually, all thirty-eight pills she had been taking daily.

Beginning the diet in a hospital bed, and still using a wheelchair and a brace, Elaine was able to start using a walker relatively quickly and then a cane. In April a chronic urinary disorder disappeared. In mid-May the brace came off, and on May 22 she walked up and down the street by herself.

In June, Elaine put away her wig. As a result of chemotherapy, all of her hair had fallen out, but it now had grown back. Returning the hospital bed to the hospital, she started driving again and resumed her studies. "In six months,

I changed from a sick, depressed, pill-popping invalid to a happy, optimistic, and very grateful pain-free person," she recalled.

For the last nine years Elaine has been cancer-free. She completed a master of science degree in nutrition and has taught, lectured, and offered cooking classes around the country. "I attribute the reversal of my cancer solely to macrobiotics," she concluded, "and I hope that my story will be a source of hope and inspiration to others."

Source: Elaine Nussbaum, *Recovery: From Cancer to Health through Macrobiotics* (Garden City Park, NY: Avery Publishing Group, 1991).

Ovarian and Lymphatic Cancer

The Dobics seemed like a typical happy modern family. Milenka had two wonderful children and a challenging career as a program director for one of the largest radio stations in Belgrade. Her husband, Bosko, was in the import/export field handling agricultural machinery. In 1986, however, tragedy struck. After Milenka experienced migraine headaches, chronic tiredness, and pressure on her head, medical tests showed that she had ovarian cancer, which had already spread to the lymphatic system. Doctors operated and advised chemotherapy and radiation but were not hopeful.

In the hospital, a friend, who happened to be a doctor, gave Milenka a copy of *The Cancer Prevention Diet*, and she began to associate her condition with her past way of eating high in animal foods, especially meat, dairy, and oily dishes. Declining further medication, she left the hospital, even though her doctors told her she could expect to live only two months.

At home, Milenka told her husband and family that she would try to combat her malignancy with diet and wanted to go to the United States to study macrobiotics. With the help of friends and associates at work, funds were raised, and she and Bosko came to America in February 1987. In Boston, they attended a seminar on diet and degenerative disease at the Kushi Institute and saw me for a personal guidance session. I explained that the primary cause of her condition was past intake of cheese and dairy food, but that with proper cooking she could overcome her cancer. "At that moment," Milenka looked back, "I felt like my journey was really starting. I had hope now."

Back in Yugoslavia, Milenka started cooking macrobiotically, as well as doing self-massage and a daily body scrub, singing songs, and practicing meditation and visualization. Medical tests confirmed that she was improving, and within five months the tumor had disappeared: "To the doctors, it seemed like a miracle. They could not understand."

Milenka, Bosko, and their family studied at the Kushi Institute in Becket for several years. They helped organize seminars in their native Yugoslavia and have had a beneficial impact on the health of many people.

Source: Liliane Papin, Ph.D., "Life Is a Phoenix: A Yugoslavian Family's Triumph over Cancer," *One Peaceful World Newsletter*, Spring 1989.

20

Male Reproductive Cancers: Prostate and Testes

FREQUENCY

Prostate cancer—the most common cancer among American men—will cause 34,000 deaths in the next twelve months, and 132,000 new cases will arise. It is one of the fastest-rising cancers, increasing 79 percent in the last decade. Cancer of the testes and other male reproductive organs will claim 350 lives, and doctors will detect 6,300 new instances of the disease. Prostate cancer is the second most common cancer in men over sixty, and the incidence is higher among blacks than whites. Americans have one of the highest prostate cancer rates in the world, about ten times higher, for instance, than the Japanese.

A variety of disorders can affect the prostate gland, including both benign and malignant tumors. Depending on the particular case, the illness is treated with surgery, radiation, and hormone therapy. Techniques include a *transurethral resection* (TUR), in which a resectoscope is inserted through the penis to kill tumor cells with an electric wire loop; a *suprapubic prostectomy*, in which the bladder is opened and the prostate removed by the surgeon through the urethra; a *retropubic prostectomy*, in which the prostate and seminal vesicles are removed without going through the bladder; and a *perineal prostectomy*, in which the surgeon enters between the legs in front of the rectum. Radioactive seeds may be implanted in the prostate to reduce the tumor or external megavoltage radiation administered. Finally, to control hormone levels and retard tumor growth, estrogens in the form of DES or cortisone may be given orally. In some instances the testicles, adrenal glands, and pituitary gland may be removed to limit the spread of malignancy. Hormone therapy can result in impotence, enlarged breasts, and heart problems. Surgery may result in impotence and sterility. The current survival rate for these forms of treatment is 57 percent.

Testicular cancer is on the rise in younger American men and is the leading cause of cancer deaths among those aged twenty-nine to thirty-five. It usually affects the right testicle more than the left, seldom both, and tends to spread to the lungs. A radical orchiectomy, involving removal of one or both testicles, is the standard form of treatment. If both testicles are removed, the operation will render the patient sterile, but not impotent. If cancer has spread to the lymph nodes, radiation or chemotherapy will also be administered. If the malignancy is spreading through the blood, a lymphadenectomy may be performed, in which all the lymph nodes on one or both sides of the abdomen up to the kidneys will be removed. The survival rate for testicular cancer has greatly increased in recent years.

STRUCTURE

The testes, located in a sac called the scrotum, are the primary organs of the male reproductive system. They produce sperm and male sex hormones. The peripheral layer of the testes contains about 250 lobules or chambers. Each chamber holds from one to three minute seminiferous tubules in which spermatozoa are formed. Sperm are discharged from each tubule, floating upward to the first portion of the duct system, called the epididymis, where they are stored for weeks, months, or even years. The seminal fluid, or semen, is a mixture of sperm from the testes and fluid from several accessory reproductive organs. The main accessory organ is the prostate gland. The prostate is situated below the bladder and surrounds the urethra, connecting the bladder and penis. The prostate secretes enzymes, lipids, and other substances, which enter the seminal fluid and are deposited in the female reproductive tract by the penis during intercourse.

CAUSE OF CANCER

In structure, the prostate is classified as yang because of its relative compactness, location deep inside the body, and the alkaline fluid it secretes, which serves to neutralize the extremely yin acids of the vagina. About 30 percent of men over fifty in the United States have enlarged prostates. As this organ presses against the upper portion of the bladder and urethra, urination becomes difficult and painful. Of these cases, about one in five develops into prostate cancer; however, any enlargement of the prostate should be suspected as a precancerous condition.

Prostate enlargement and blockage of the other semen ducts arise in the same way as hardening of the arteries. They are caused principally by the overconsumption of foods rich in fat and protein in the yang category, including eggs, meat, and dairy products, all of which contain saturated fats, as well as by excessive intake of foods in the extreme yin category such as sugar, fruits, and refined flour products, which produce fat and mucus. Over time, these deposits accumulate and can turn into cysts or tumors. The blockages resulting from a high-fat diet can also contribute to impotence. However, the inability to achieve an erection is often caused by intake of too much expansive food, which causes the muscles of the reproductive system to become loose and expanded. Infertility is also caused largely from excessive intake of yin type foods, which weaken the quality of the blood, lymph, and other bodily fluids and secretions that determine the quality of the sperm. Prostate problems can be relieved by adopting a cancer prevention diet that emphasizes slightly more yin foods and style of cooking and avoids animal foods.

The testes, too, are extremely yang (compact) is structure. Tumors here also arise primarily from excessive animal foods, especially eggs, heavily salted meats, condensed dairy foods such as cheese, and high-fat and high-protein fish and seafood. A more centered way of eating will help relieve this condition.

MEDICAL EVIDENCE

• An international study completed in 1970 linked prostate cancer mortality directly with per capita coffee consumption. Source: P. Stocks, "Cancer Mortality in Relation to National Consumption of Cigarettes, Solid Fuel, Tea, and Coffee," *British Journal of Cancer* 24:215–25.

• In 1974 an epidemiologist found a high direct correlation between mortality from prostate cancer in forty-one countries and per capita intake of fats, milk, and meats, especially beef. Research also disclosed that people who regularly consumed rice had less incidence of the disease. Source: M. A. Howell, "Factor Analysis of International Cancer Mortality Data and *Per Capita* Food Consumption," *British Journal of Cancer* 29:328–36.

• Seventh-Day Adventist men in California have 55 percent less prostate cancer than other males, according to a 1975 study. The church members tend to avoid meat, poultry, fish, refined foods, alcohol, stimulants, and spices and consume whole grains, vegetables, and fresh fruits. Source: R. L. Phillips, "Role of Life-styles and Dietary Habits in risk of Cancer among Seventh-Day Adventists," *Cancer Research* 35:3513–22.

• A 1977 study based on 111 cases with prostate cancer and 111 hospital controls showed that the cancer patients consumed more high-fat foods, including beef, pork, eggs, cheeses, milk, creams, butter, and margarine. Source: I. D. Rotkin, "Studies in the Epidemiology of Prostatic Cancer: Expanded Sampling," *Cancer Treatment Reports* 61:173–80.

• A 1978 report found that U.S. counties with the highest death rates from prostate cancer also had the highest per capita intake of high-fat foods, including beef, milk and dairy products, fats and oils, pork, and eggs. Source: A. Blair and J. F. Fraumeni, Jr., "Geographic Patterns of Prostate Cancer in the U.S.," *Journal of the National Cancer Institute* 61:1379–84.

• A ten-year study of 122,261 Japanese men over forty found less prostate cancer death among those who regularly consumed green or yellow vegetables. The 1979 study also reported that vegetarian men had a lower incidence of prostate cancer than nonvegetarians. Source: T. Hirayama, "Epidemiology of Prostate Cancer with Special Reference to the Role of Diet," *National Cancer Institute Monograph* 53:149–54.

• In 1981 researchers found that the incidence of prostate cancer in four ethnic groups in Hawaii was highly correlated with consumption of animal fat and saturated fat and with total protein, especially animal protein. Source: L. N. Kolonel et al., "Nutrient Intakes in Relation to Cancer Incidence in Hawaii," *British Journal of Cancer* 44:332–39.

• A 1981 study suggested that lactose (milk sugar) fed laboratory animals tended to promote tumor growth, especially stones in the male reproductive glands and bladder. Source: S. N. Gershoff and R. B. McGandy, "The Effects of Vitamin A–deficient Diets Containing Lactose in Producing Bladder Calculi and Tumors in Rats," *American Journal of Clinical Nutrition* 34:483–89.

• A 1982 case-control study reported that prostate cancer patients consumed less foods high in vitamin A and beta-carotene, such as carrots. Source: L. M. Schuman et al., "Some Selected Features of the Epidemiology of Prostatic Cancer," in K. Magnus (ed.), *Trends in Cancer Incidence* (New York: Hemisphere), 345–54.

• After reviewing current medical evidence, the National Academy of Sciences concluded in its 1982 on cancer and diet: "In summary, the incidence of prostate cancer is correlated with other cancers associated with diet, e.g., breast cancer. There is good evidence that an increased risk of prostate cancer is associated with certain dietary factors, especially the intake of high fat and high protein foods, which usually occur together in the diet. There is some evidence that foods rich in Vitamin A or its precursors and vegetarian diets are associated with a lower risk." *Diet, Nutrition, and Cancer* (Washington, DC: National Academy of Sciences), 17:21.

• In a follow-up of nearly 7,000 Seventh-Day Adventists who had filled out dietary questionnaires in 1960, researchers found positive associations between death from prostate cancer and consumption of milk, cheese, eggs, and meat. Those who consumed all four products heavily died of this disease 3.6 times more than usual. Source: D. A. Snowdon et al., "Diet, Obesity, and Risk of Fatal Prostate Cancer," *American Journal of Epidemiology* 120:244–50.

• Based on data from the International Food and Agricultural Organization in thirty-six countries, researchers reported in 1991 that a significant correlation was found between consumption of dairy food and animal fat and the incidence of prostate cancer, colorectal cancer, lung cancer, and breast cancer. Source: Hugo Kesteloot et al., "Dairy Fat, Saturated Animal Fat, and Cancer Risk," *Preventive Medicine* 20:226–36.

• In a 1991 case-control study, men with lung cancer, bladder cancer, prostate cancer, larynx cancer, colorectal cancer, and esophagael cancer had from 10 to 24 percent lower intake of vegetables and fruits high in carotene than controls. Source: W. C. Ruth et al., "A Case-Control Study of Dietary Carotene in Men with Lung Cancer and in Men with Other Epithelial Cancers, *Nutrition and Cancer* 15, no. 1:63–68.

• In 1992, Swedish researchers reported that men with early prostate cancer may recover better without treatment compared to those who have surgery or radiation treatment. Source: *Journal of the American Medical Association*, April 22, 1992, and "Study Suggests Early Prostate Cancer May Be Best Left Alone," *New York Times*, April 22, 1992.

• In 1993, two large National Institute of Health studies reported that a vasectomy could increase a man's risk of developing prostate cancer. The studies found that men who had a vasectomy—a common surgical procedure for birth control—more than twenty years earlier had up to an 89 percent greater risk, than men who did not have the operation, of developing prostate cancer. Source: "New Studies Link Vasectomy to Higher Prostate Cancer," *New York Times*, February 17, 1993.

DIAGNOSIS

Prostate cancer is usually diagnosed by a rectal examination as well as a battery of laboratory tests, enzyme and hormone assays, and a needle biopsy if a malignancy is suspected. Skeletal and chest X rays, bone scans, and intravenous pyelogram (IVP) will be used to check for metastases. About 60 percent of prostate tumors are currently detected before spreading to other sites. In the case of testicular cancer, many of these same diagnostic methods are used, as well as an angiogram, lymphangiogram, CAT scan of chest or abdomen, and ultrasound examination of the abdomen.

Oriental medicine diagnoses potential male reproductive cancers with a variety of simple visual observations. According to physiognomy, the mouth and lower face correspond with the sex organs, and discolorations, swellings, or other abnormalities in this region may indicate improper functioning of the reproductive system. For instance, vertical wrinkles appearing on the lips show a recession of hormonal function, especially of the gonad hormones, indicating a decline in sexual function. These wrinkles may also appear in case of dehydration from lack of liquid or overconsumption of dry foods and salt, so other signs must also be observed. Generally, fatty wrinkles or sagging in the chin and upper neck indicate prostate problems in men or uterine and ovarian problems in women. Pimples that appear in the center of the cheeks and have a fatty appearance also show the formation of cysts in and around the reproductive organs.

Fat or mucous buildup in the prostate is further indicated by a yellow and white coating of mucus on the lower part of the whites of the eyes. Along the bladder meridian, cancer of the prostate shows up as a light green coloration on the fifth toe and its extended area at the outside of the foot, below the anklebone and behind the Achilles' tendon, with fatty swelling along the Achilles' tendon.

On the hands, split or uneven nails show disorders in the circulatory, nervous, and reproductive systems caused by chaotic eating habits. If one thumbnail shows this condition and the other thumbnail is normal, the testicle (or ovary in women) corresponding to the abnormal side is malfunctioning. Red, purple, and other abnormal colors appearing on the tips of the fingers also indicate disorders in the gonad region, including possible cancer or precancerous conditions.

From a combination of these and other factors, the condition of the reproductive system can be determined and appropriate corrective nutritional action taken.

DIETARY RECOMMENDATIONS

The main cause of prostate cancer is food high in protein and fat, especially chicken, turkey, beef, pork, eggs, cheese, and other dairy foods, along with salted foods, baked foods, and roasted foods, which make the muscles and tissues tight. All these should be avoided, including fish and seafood, until the condition improves. The main cause of testicular cancer is eggs, meat, cheese, and other foods high in saturated fat and cholesterol. Not only animal food, but also sugar, honey, chocolate, carob, and all sugar-treated food and beverages are to be discontinued for both conditions. Flour products, which have the potential to create mucus, such as refined white bread, pancakes, and cookies, are to be avoided also. All stimulants, including mustard, pepper, curry, mint, peppermint, and other aromatic herbs and spices, all alcoholic beverages, and coffee are to be avoided because they enhance tumor growth, though they are not the direct cause of the cancer. All chemicals artificially added or treated during food production and processing should also be avoided. Excessive consumption of oil, even of vegetable, unsaturated quality, is to be avoided, as is excessive consumption of salts and salty food and beverages. Fruit and fruit juices, if consumed frequently, can increase the swelling of the tumor, though they can neutralize animal protein and fat. Accordingly, they should be limited. All vegetables of historically tropical origin, such as potatoes, tomatoes, and eggplant, and tropical and subtropical fruits should be avoided. General dietary guidelines by volume of food consumption are as follows:

• **Whole Grains:** Fifty to 60 percent of daily consumption, by volume, should be whole-cereal grains. The first day prepare plain pressure-cooked short-grain brown rice. On subsequent days, prepare brown rice pressure-cooked with 20 to 30 percent millet, then rice with 20 to 30 percent barley, then rice with 20 to 30 percent aduki beans or lentils, and then plain rice again. A delicious morning porridge can be made by taking leftover rice, adding a little more water to soften, and seasoning with a little miso at the end and simmering for two to three minutes more. In daily pressure cooking, the ratio of grain to water should be about 1:2. For seasoning, cook with a small postage stamp–sized piece of kombu instead of salt. Other grains can be used occasionally, including whole wheat berries, rye, corn, and whole oats, though oats should be avoided for the first month. However, buckwheat should be avoided for about six months because it is very contractive and may harden the tumor. Seitan is also very yang and should be minimized. Flour products, even unrefined whole wheat bread, chapatis, pancakes, and cookies, should be totally avoided or limited in volume for a period of a few months, though people with prostate problems typically like roasted, baked, or crunchy foods. Whole-grain pasta and noodles may be eaten a couple times a week.

• **Soup:** Five to 10 percent soup, consisting of one or two cups or bowls per day of soup cooked with wakame sea vegetable and various vegetables, especially daikon and daikon leaves and other green leafy vegetables, and seasoned lightly with miso or shoyu. Occasionally a small volume of shiitake mushroom may be added to the soup. The miso may be barley miso, brown rice miso, or soybean (hatcho) miso and should be naturally aged two to three years. Grain soups, bean soups, and other soups may be taken from time to time.

• **Vegetables:** Twenty to 30 percent vegetables, cooked in a variety of forms, mainly steamed, boiled, and, after four to six weeks without oil, occasionally sautéed. Various type of leafy vegetables—green, yellow, and white—can be cooked in different styles, as can various root vegetables such as carrots, turnips, daikon, radishes, lotus root, and burdock roots, though burdock should be used much less frequently than other root vegetables. Round vegetables such as acorn and butternut squash, cabbage, and onions can also be frequently used. Daikon and daikon greens are especially recommended for these conditions. As a rule of thumb, the following dishes may be prepared, though the frequency may differ from person to person: nishime-style vegetables, three times a week; squash-aduki-kombu dish, three times a week; dried daikon, one cup, three times a week; carrots and carrot tops or daikon and daikon tops, three times a week; blanched vegetables, five to seven times a week; pressed salad, five to seven times a week; raw salad, one to two times a week; steamed greens, five to seven times a week; sautéed vegetables, prepared with water the first month, then with sesame oil lightly brushed on the pan once or twice a week after that; kinpira, two-thirds of a cup, two times a week; dried tofu, tofu, tempeh, or seitan with vegetables, two times a week.

• **Beans:** Five percent small beans, such as aduki beans, lentils, chickpeas, or black soybeans, may be used daily, cooked together with sea vegetables such as kombu or with onions and carrots. Other beans may be used altogether two to three times a month. For seasoning, a small volume of unrefined sea salt or shoyu or miso can be used. Bean products, such as tempeh, natto, and dried or cooked tofu, may be used occasionally, but in moderate volume.

• **Sea Vegetables:** Five percent or less sea vegetable dishes, including wakame and kombu, daily when cooking grain, in soup, etc. A sheet of toasted nori may also be taken daily. A small dish of hijiki or arame should be prepared two times a week. All other teas vegetables are optional.

• **Condiments:** Condiments to be available on the table are gomashio (sesame salt), on the average made with 1 part salt to 18 to 20 parts sesame seeds; kelp or wakame powder; umeboshi plum; and tekka, though all other regular macrobiotic condiments may be used if desired. These condiments may be used daily on grains and vegetables, but the volume should be moderate to suit individual appetite and taste.

• **Pickles:** Pickles, made at home in a variety of ways, are to be eaten daily, one tablespoon in all, though salty pickles are to be minimized. Rice bran (nuka) pickles are the most suitable.

• **Animal Food:** Fish and other animal food is to be avoided. However, in the event that animal food is craved, a small volume of white-meat fish may be eaten once every ten days to two weeks. The fish should be prepared steamed, boiled, or poached and garnished with grated daikon or ginger. Strictly avoid blue-meat and red-meat fish and all shellfish.

• **Fruit:** The less the better until the condition improves. If cravings develop, a small volume of fresh fruit or cooked fruit with a pinch of sea salt or dried fruit (also preferably cooked) may be taken. Tree fruits such as apples, peaches, and pears are better than ground fruits like strawberries and watermelons. Avoid all fruit juices and cider.

• **Sweets and Snacks:** Overuse of sweets is connected with prostate disorders, so it is very important to avoid all sweets and desserts, including good-quality macrobiotic desserts, until the condition improves. To satisfy a sweet tooth, use sweet vegetables every day in cooking, drink sweet vegetable drink, or prepare sweet vegetable jam. If cravings arise, a small volume of amasake, barley malt, or rice syrup may be taken. If cravings persist, a little cider, apple juice, or chestnut may be prepared. Mochi, rice balls, vegetable sushi, and other grain-based snacks may be eaten frequently. Limit rice cakes, popcorn, and other dry or baked snacks, as they may harden the tumor.

• **Nuts and Seeds:** Nuts and nut butters are to be avoided due to their high amount of fat and protein, except for chestnuts. Unsalted, steamed or boiled seeds such as sunflower seeds and pumpkin seeds may be consumed as a snack, up to one cup altogether per week. Minimize use of roasted seeds.

• **Seasonings:** Seasonings, such as unrefined sea salt, shoyu, and miso, are to be used moderately in order to avoid unnecessary thirst. Avoid mirin and garlic. If you become particularly thirsty after the meal or between meals, you should cut back on these seasonings until the normal level of thirst returns.

• **Beverages:** Beverages and other dietary practices can follow the general recommendations in Part I, including bancha twig tea as the main beverage. Strictly avoid the beverages on the "infrequent" and "avoid" list and don't take grain coffee for the first two to three months after starting this new way of eating.

The most important thing in connection with dietary practice is chewing very well, until all food becomes liquid in the mouth and well mixed with saliva. Chew very, very well, at least 50 times, preferably 100 times, per mouthful. It is also important to avoid overeating and eating within three hours of sleeping.

As noted in the introduction to Part II, persons who have received or who are currently undergoing medical treatment may need to make further dietary modifications.

SPECIAL DRINKS AND DISHES

Several special drinks may need to be taken, depending on the individual case. Please see a qualified macrobiotic teacher for guidance. Amounts and frequencies given here are averages; these will differ from person to person.

• **Sweet Vegetable Drink:** Take one small cup every day for the first month; then every other day the second month.

• **Carrot-Daikon Drink:** Take one small cup every day for four to six weeks, then once every three days for one month.

• **Lotus–Green Vegetable Drink:** Chop one-half cup dry lotus root; add two cups chopped green leafy vegetables and four times as much water. Cook fifteen to twenty minutes. Drink that juice every day or every other day, one to two cups, for two months.

• **Grated Daikon:** Take one-half to two-thirds cup garnished with nori or scallion and a few drops of shoyu twice a week to help melt fat deposits.

• **Dried Shiitake Mushroom:** This mushroom is very good in occasional soups and dishes for dissolving old fat and for calming.

• **Grated Carrots:** A small dish of grated carrots cooked with one-half teaspoon of grated ginger or a few slices of garlic is sometimes helpful for this type of cancer, if taken daily for a period of several days.

• **Ume-Sho-Bancha Tea:** Aches and pains in the prostate or testicular region usually disappear after a few weeks of proper dietary practice. However, in the meantime it is sometimes helpful to relieve pain by drinking one or two cups of hot ume-sho-bancha tea. A kuzu drink may be served instead, using the same ingredients but substituting kuzu for bancha twigs.

HOME CARES

• **Body Scrub:** Scrubbing the whole body, including the abdominal region and the spinal region, with a towel that has been immersed in hot water and squeezed out is very helpful for better circulation of blood, lymph, and other body fluids, as well as for activating physical and mental energies.

• **Compress Guidelines:** For a small number of tumors in the male reproductive system, a compress may be needed to help gradually draw out excess mucous and fat. Please see a qualified macrobiotic teacher for guidance on the proper use and frequency of a compress or plaster. Several types are used depending on the person's condition. Precede the compress or plaster with application of a towel that has been soaked in hot water and squeezed out over the affected area for about three to five minutes to stimulate circulation.

• **Taro Plaster:** For prostate cancer and enlarged prostate, a taro potato plaster may be applied for three to four hours on the lower abdomen immediately following a ginger compress for three to five minutes. This application can be repeated daily for two to three weeks.

• **Buckwheat Plaster:** For swelling of the abdominal region due to prostate cancer, it is helpful to apply a buckwheat plaster for about one hour. The plaster should be kept warm by placing roasted hot sea salt wrapped in cotton towels above it. (For ease in handling, the hot salt may be placed in a pouch made from a cotton towel, then wrapped with another towel.) This application may be repeated daily for several days.

OTHER CONSIDERATIONS

• Daily physical exercise that does not produce exhaustion is recommended. Ten to fifteen minutes of daily breathing exercises, especially emphasizing long exhalation, is also beneficial. These physical and breathing exercises contribute to relaxing tensions in the body and mind as well as harmonizing physical metabolism.

• Keeping air quality clean and fresh is important for maintenance of general health. For that purpose, green leafy plants can be placed in the house and the windows periodically opened to allow circulation of fresh air. Don't smoke, as this will tighten the prostate.

• Avoid wearing wool and synthetic fibers. At the minimum wear cotton underwear and use cotton sheets and pillowcases.

• Avoid watching television for long stretches. Radiation weakens the reproductive area. Similarly, avoid other artificial sources of electromagnetic energy such as video terminals, smoke detectors, and hand-held electrical appliances.

• Though cancer is naturally accompanied by a decline in energy and vitality, normal sexual practice is not harmful if it does not lead to exhaustion.

• Vasectomy and other artificial birth-control methods, as well as the use of drugs or medications to control sexual performance, are to be avoided in order to prevent stagnation, interruption of energy flow, or other abnormal functions.

PERSONAL EXPERIENCES

Prostate Cancer

At age sixty-three Herb Walley was diagnosed with a prostate tumor. Doctors recommended hormone treatment and put him on stilbesterol. "The side effects are pretty awful for a man who wants to remain masculine," Herb recalled. "Some of the more depressing transformations are breast and nipple enlargement with extreme tenderness, fluid retention throughout the body— the legs in particular—with resulting inconvenience of hourly toilet trips, both day and night. Also, loss of fingernail substance results in painful split and torn nails. There are many other less obvious effects which are equally annoying."

Herb finally persuaded his urologist to diminish the dosage by half. However, the effects didn't appreciably diminish. Though under control, Herb's tumor still remained malignant six years later, when a friend introduced him to a book on macrobiotics. Herb read it avidly and met with a macrobiotic teacher at the Kushi Institute who provided more specific guidelines for his condition. "After one month I felt more alive and much less depressed," Herb looked back. "I stopped taking all medications and vitamins and made monthly visits to my general practitioner for checkups." Altogether he lost sixty-five pounds of old fat from all over his body.

Ten months later, medical tests showed that the cancer was gone. To be certain, Herb checked into the Dana Farber Cancer Center in Boston, one of the nation's top cancer clinics. After many more tests and a complete bone scan, he was told that he was "clean."

Today, Herb is almost eighty. With his wife, Virginia, he operates a macrobiotic bed and breakfast in Newton, Massachusetts. "I am still 'clean,' with almost unlimited energy," Herb reports. "I can eat all I want without gaining weight, and look forward to another twenty or thirty years of excitement and happiness."

Source: Ann Fawcett and the East West Foundation, *Cancer-free: 30 Who Triumphed over Cancer Naturally* (New York and Tokyo: Japan Publications, 1991).

Testicular Cancer

In 1977 John Jodziewicz, a twenty-year-old college student from Henningsville, Pennsylvania, noted a pea-sized hardness in his left testicle. During the winter of 1979 to 1980, it increased in size and a lump appeared in his neck. On March 20, 1980, doctors at Sacred Heart Hospital discovered that he had advanced (fourth-stage) choriocarcinoma and surgically removed his left testicle. Two oncologists and a resident physician told him that this particularly malignant form of testicular cancer had spread to his left kidney, both lungs, and neck and that he had "a 1 percent chance to live out the year, even with chemotherapy."

The findings came as a shock to John and his fiancée, Ingrid Koch. John had observed a vegetarian diet for a few years, kept active physically, and felt that he was in good health. "I was sure that my 'anything goes but meat' diet, megadoses of vitamins and supplements, and rugged outdoor activities, protected me from disease," he later recalled. "But here Ingrid and I sat, being told that I would most probably die before my twenty-fourth birthday."

During the next four months, John underwent chemical therapy, including receiving intravenous injections for seven days at a stretch at two-week intervals. During the period that he received drugs he suffered fevers, nosebleeds, constipation, difficulty breathing, a persistent cough, total hair loss, chills, lack of appetite, headaches, fatigue, severe mouth ulcers, nausea, vomiting, bone-marrow depression, total body arthritis pain, dizziness, hypersensitivity of the scalp, ringing in the ears, and loosening teeth. "This was the most horrible time in my life; and these symptoms were not as a result of the cancer, but of the treatment."

After two cycles of chemotherapy, the tumors remained, and doctors began administering cis-platinum, an experimental drug, in high dosages. John's prognosis was reduced to two months, and after a series of wretchings and convulsions he was given last rites by a priest.

Two events, however, coincided to change the course of John's life and forestall imminent death. First, just before the last round with drugs, a friend introduced Ingrid's mother to macrobiotics and later encouraged John and Ingrid to visit the EWF in Philadelphia. There John met director Denny Waxman, who explained the yin/yang approach to cancer and gave him several books to read. The second turning point came in the hospital. One night John had a dream in which his mother, who had died seven years earlier, told him to go to St. Joseph's Cathedral in Montreal and pray. As a child, John, with his family, had often visited the shrine where Brother André reportedly performed many healing miracles until his death in 1937. (He was proposed for sainthood by the Vatican in 1982). At St. Joseph's, pilgrims from around the world came to crawl up the long flight of steps to the top on their knees in hope that God would reward their humility and relieve their illness.

On June 16, 1980, Ingrid and John arrived in Montreal. There were throngs of tourists, but for some reason no pilgrims that time of day. Nevertheless, John determined to climb the steps alone. As he placed his knees on the first step, he experienced what he described as a transcendent moment of illumination and felt that he had become united with the mountain on which the cathedral rested. As he ascended each step, John prayed for others whom he knew also to be in need of help and he felt his mother's spirit close by. At the top, he got up and walked into the cathedral. A priest was holding up a wafer at the altar as if in anticipation of his arrival, and John took communion. He knew that if he changed his way of life and began eating macrobiotically he would live.

Returning to Pennsylvania, John and Ingrid attended the EWF's summer camp. I met them there for the first time and assured John that he would recover completely if he followed the Cancer Prevention Diet faithfully. Back home, John and Ingrid drove three times a week to Philadelphia, seventy miles away, for macrobiotic cooking classes and other instruction in Oriental medicine and philosophy. In two weeks John's pain had entirely disappeared, and in two months the tumor in his neck had shrunk to half its previous size. In August, John went on a strenuous thirty-eight-mile hike in the woods, alone except for his dog.

In May 1981 blood tests confirmed that his body no longer had any signs of cancer. John had been off medication, including chemotherapy, for a year. Reviewing his case, John listed five reasons why he survived:

1. Total support form his family and friends.

2. Correct macrobiotic practice, including cooking classes and discipline in avoiding extreme foods.

3. A strong natural immune system.

4. The will to get better.

5. Faith in God and willingness to accept life's difficulties as opportunities for personal growth and understanding.

"I'm not only physically healthy, but I feel spiritually healthy as well," John explained in 1982, two years after his remission. "The clean, macrobiotic diet and way of life has enhanced and broadened my perspective of the Catholic tradition in which I was raised. Ingrid and I plan to study and teach macrobiotics for the rest of our lives and have a large family."

John and Ingrid were married in the summer of 1982 and are implementing their dream. Sources: Tom Monte, "Triumph over Cancer: A Young Man's Journey Back to Life," *East West Journal*, April 1982, 32–40, and "Choriocarcinoma," *Cancer and Heart Disease: The Macrobiotic Approach to Degenerative Disorders* (New York: Japan Publications, 1982), 157–59.

21

Skin Cancer and Melanoma

FREQUENCY

About 600,000 new cases of skin cancer are diagnosed each year in the United States, and about 2,100 people die annually of this disease. Because detection is comparatively easy, tumors are slow to spread, and survival is high, skin cancer is not included in many cancer statistics. However, there is a more deadly form of skin cancer, called malignant melanoma, which comprises about 3 percent of all cancers in the United States and is one of the fastest-rising malignancies in modern society. This year it will take 6,700 lives, and an estimated 32,000 new cases will arise. This represents an increase of 55 percent in women and 126 percent in men in the last generation.

Eighty percent of common skin cancers are classified as basal-cell carcinomas and occur primarily on the face or back of the hands. They do not metastasize but spread by invasion to bone and tissue. Skin cancer is often treated by surgery in a doctor's office under local anesthesia. Methods include electrosurgery with a small electric needle and curette, surgical excision with a scalpel, or chemosurgery with zinc chloride or other chemicals to remove the tumor and a portion of normal tissue around it. Radiation is sometimes used, especially on the face, where surgery would result in disfigurement. Chemotherapy and immunotherapy may also be employed.

Melanoma usually appears initially on an existing mole under the skin and spreads quickly through the lymph or blood to the lungs, brain, liver, eye, intestines, reproductive organs, or other sites. Standard treatment is surgery. Melanoma tends to recur, and patients may have many operations, supplemented with chemotherapy. Surgeons say that 80 to 90 percent of persons who have malignant melanomas removed in the early stages of the disease will survive five years or more. For melanoma that has spread to distant lymph nodes, the remission rate is 14 percent.

STRUCTURE

The main function of the skin, the body's largest organ, is to control adjustment between the external environment and the internal body condition. The skin protects the body's surface, helps regulate body temperature, and excretes waste material and water through sweat glands. Sweat glands come in two types. The exocrine glands, which are located over the entire surface of the body, serve to cool the body and guard against infection. They secrete a watery solution consisting of various fats, sugar, salts, proteins, and toxins. The second type of gland is called apocrine and is found only in certain areas, such as under the arms, the nipples, the abdomen, and reproductive areas. The apocrine glands secrete stronger solutions and give rise to body odors.

The color of the skin is regulated by melanin, a pigment that varies from brown to black in color. The less melanin in the skin, the lighter the skin color. Such factors as climate, exposure to sunlight, and daily diet influence the production of melanin.

CAUSE OF CANCER

Normally the body is able to eliminate wastes through such normal functions as urination, bowel movements, respiration, and perspiration. Imbalanced foods or beverages will trigger a variety of abnormal discharge mechanisms in the body such as diarrhea, frequent urination, fever, coughing, or sneezing. Chronic discharges are the next step in this process, and continued poor eating will usually take the form of some kind of skin disease. These are common in cases where the kidneys have lost their ability to properly clean the bloodstream. For example, hard, dry skin arises after the bloodstream fills with fat and oil, eventually causing blockage of the pores, hair follicles, and sweat glands.

Over the last ten years, the depletion of the ozone layer has contributed to an increase in skin cancer and melanoma. Ordinarily, the layer of ozone above the Earth screens out harmful ultraviolet rays of the sun. In most traditional societies around the world, where people are eating primarily grains and vegetables, skin cancer and melanoma are nonexistent. People have lived and worked in the hot sun for thousands of years without ever getting cancer.

However, among people in modern industrialized countries eating meat and sugar, refined and highly processed food, these forms of cancer were prevalent and associated with exposure to sunlight even before the ozone started to thin. The reason for this is that overall the sun is more yang—bright, hot, and intense. Exposure to the yang stimulus of the sun draws excess yin—such as fats and oils—to the body's surface. Thus natural sunlight is not the cause of cancer, but the catalyst for the body to begin discharging toxic excess to the surface through the skin. This is what we call skin cancer.

The thinning of the ozone layer has complicated this process. Sunlight naturally polarizes into yin and yang wavelengths. The more yang form is called infrared, the more yin ultraviolet. In between is visible light. Ozone—which is a light form of oxygen—is classified as more yin and serves to repel the incoming yin, ultraviolet light of the sun. With the depletion of the ozone layer, more harmful ultraviolet radiation is reaching the earth than previously. Thus people eating the modern diet may be at even greater risk for developing skin cancer or melanoma when exposed to the sun. It is advisable for such people to avoid direct sunlight and wear a hat or stay in the shade. However, for those eating in a macrobiotic direction, avoiding dairy food, fatty foods, simple sugars, stimulants, and alcohol, as well as all sorts of oily, greasy foods, the risk is minimal. Such persons may continue to enjoy natural sunlight without undue worry.

Coincidentally, one of the main causes of ozone depletion is modern agriculture and food processing, especially the processing of animal food. CFCs (chlorofluorocarbons), the main chemical responsible for ozone depletion, are associated with refrigeration and air-conditioning. The modern diet, high in perishable animal food and tropical vegetables, requires refrigeration, while most foods in the macrobiotic way of eating, including whole grains, beans, seeds, nuts, sea vegetables, and others, do not require refrigeration and can be stored naturally in a pantry. Vegetables can be kept in a root cellar or in the garden until used. Still some refrigeration may be needed, but it could be a small unit in contrast to the large modern units with gigantic freezers for ice cream and frozen foods.

Similarly, overreliance on air-conditioning is related to the modern diet. Animals foods cause the body to heat up, and people eating meat, poultry, chicken, eggs, cheese, and similar foods find hot weather uncomfortable (yang repels yang). The demand for air-conditioning would be substantially reduced if people began to shift toward a more natural way of eating, and the planet, as well as personal, health would improve. Melanoma, while classified as a skin cancer, is actually more like a muscular disorder, falling in structure between yin skin-surface tumors, occurring on the periphery of the body, and yang bone tumors, occurring in the deep, compact region of the body. Melanoma usually begins to manifest on existing moles. These are tiny dark brown mounds under the skin, which serve to eliminate excess protein and fat from the body. This protein and fat does not necessarily come from the consumption of protein itself, but is produced by a combination of consuming too many extreme yin foods such as sugar, fruits, and chemicals and general overconsumption of yang foods, including animal foods, especially poultry, eggs, heavy dairy foods, and other high-protein and high-fat foods. Skin cancer can be relieved by adopting a more yang cancer prevention diet, while a centrally balanced way of daily eating is recommended for malignant melanoma.

MEDICAL EVIDENCE

• In 1930 researchers reported that dietary fat could influence tumor growth in laboratory animals. Increasing the amount of butter in the diet from 12.5 to 25 percent increased induced skin cancer incidence from 34 to 57 percent. Source: A. F. Watson and E. Mellanby, "Tar Cancer in Mice; Condition of Skin When Modified by External Treatment or Diet, as Factors in Influencing Cancerous Reaction," *British Journal of Experimental Pathology* 11:311–22.

• In 1931 a cancer study with male rats suggested a direct relationship between the amount of protein in the diet and skin tumors. Source: J. R. Slonaker, "The Effect of Different Per Cents of Protein in the Diet," *American Journal of Physiology* 98:266–75.

• In 1941 and 1943 mice fed a diet supplemented with 15 percent corn oil, coconut oil, or lard experienced a rise in induced skin tumors from 12 to 83 percent. Source: P. S. Lavik and C. A. Baumann, "Dietary Fat and Tumor Formation," *Cancer Research* 1:181–87, and "Further Studies on Tumor Promoting Action of Fat," *Cancer Research* 3:749–56.

• In 1966 a medical doctor reported that a special protein-restricted diet helped regress melanoma. Dr. Harry B. Demopoulos put five of his patients with advanced malignant melanoma on a diet high in vegetables and fruits and a supplement that decreased serum levels of several amino acids thought to promote tumor growth. In addition, patients were not allowed to eat high-protein foods such as meat and dairy products, nuts and nut butters, as well as potatoes, bread, and flour products. However, they were allowed to eat oils, stimulants, sugar, and syrups. In three of five patients he reported an "abrupt cessation of tumor growth" and "in all three cases one or more tumors completely regressed." The fourth patient improved while on the diet, but the cancer spread when she discontinued it. The fifth patient showed no change. Source: H. B. Demopoulos, "Effects of Reducing the Phenylalanine-Tyrosine Intake of Patients with Advanced Malignant Melanoma," *Cancer* 19:657–64.

• Methylchloromethylether, a corrosive liquid used in refining cane sugar and in gelatin production, causes skin and lung cancer in laboratory animals. Source: *Carcinogens, Job Health Hazards Series* (Washington, DC: Occupational Safety and Health Administration, 1975), 7–8.

• PCBs (polychlorinated biphenyls), industrial chemicals used in such things as heavy-duty electrical equipment, air-conditioning, microwave ovens, and fluorescent lighting, have become assimilated into the North American food chain and are associated with cancer of the skin and liver. In foods PCBs are found only in animal products, especially fish, milk, eggs, and cheese, and when eaten accumulate in the adipose tissue of humans, in breast milk, and in the blood. Studies in 1976 and 1977 reported higher incidences of melanoma in workers exposed to these chemicals. Source: *Diet, Nutrition, and Cancer* (Washington, DC: National Academy of Sciences, 1982), 14:22–23.

• In 1980 investigators reported that soybeans contain substances called protease inhibitors, which retard the growth of tumors. In laboratory experiments with mice, skin tumors were blocked when soybeans, lima beans, or other seeds and beans containing this factor were added to the diet. Source: W. Troll, "Blocking of Tumor Promotion by Protease Inhibitors," in J. H. Burchenal and H. F. Oettgen (eds.), *Cancer: Achievement, Challenges, and Prospects for the 1980s* (New York: Grune and Stratton), 1:549–55.

• In a study published in the *Lancet*, researchers in Australia reported that fluorescent lighting in the office was associated with a two to two and a half times higher incidence of melanoma in females and a nearly four and a half higher incidence among males for exposure of ten years or more compared to regular lighting. Source: J. A. Treichel, *Science News* 122, August 28, 1982.

• Vitamin C can protect against sunlight-induced skin cancer in animal studies. Cornell University researchers reported that beta-carotene can help prevent impairment of the human immune system induced by ultraviolet light. Source: "3 Promising Weapons against Disease," *New York Times*, September 25, 1991.

• Worldwide skin cancer rates could increase by 26 percent by the year 2000 if the Earth's ozone layer continues to deplete at current rates, the UN

Environment Program estimated. The study predicted an annual 1.6 to 1.75 million additional cases of cataracts if the ozone layer diminishes another 10 percent by the end of the decade. UN researchers singled out the production and release of CFCs, which trigger the chemical breakdown of ozone, as the main factor in the environmental crisis. CFCs are used primarily as coolants in air conditioners and refrigerators and as propellants in the production of foam plastics. Source: *Boston Globe,* October 23, 1991, and December 2, 1991.

• Halogen lights may increase the risk of skin cancer, according to researchers at the University of Genoa in Italy. Halogen lamps emit large amounts of far-ultraviolet radiation, a type associated with skin cancer. Halogen lights are found extensively in street lighting as well as in household fixtures, including popular desk lamps. Source: Warren Leary, "New Study Offers More Evidence Linking Cancer to Halogen Lamps," *New York Times*, April 16, 1992.

DIAGNOSIS

Precancerous skin conditions include a variety of lesions and leukoplakia, the growth of white patches on the mucous membranes. Modern medicine distinguishes skin cancer from these conditions by taking a biopsy. In testing for melanoma, patients will also usually be administered a lymphangiogram, chest X rays, brain and liver scans, and sometimes a cardiac catheterization.

Oriental medicine tends to look at all skin ailments on a spectrum and focuses on three major characteristics: condition of the skin, skin color, and skin marks. Normal, healthy skin should be clean, smooth, slightly shining, and slightly moist. Wet skin indicates an overconsumption of liquid, sugar, and other sweets and results in a thin quality to the blood, rapid metabolism, a faster pulse, and excessive perspiration and urination. Wet skin can accompany a variety of disorders ranging from diarrhea, fatigue, hair loss, and aches and pains to epilepsy and various hyperactive psychological disorders.

Normal skin is slightly oily, but excessively oily skin—showing up on peripheral parts of the body such as the forehead, nose, cheeks, hair, or palms—shows overconsumption of oil and fats or disorders in fat metabolism. Dry skin also results from overconsumption of fats and oils and is caused by a formation of fat layers under the skin, preventing the elimination of moisture toward the surface. Depending on other related symptoms, dry or oily skin accompanies a wide variety of chronic and degenerative conditions.

Rough skin reflects an overconsumption of protein and heavy fats or excess intake of sugar, fruit, and drugs. The second, more yin cause is accompanied by more open sweat glands and a slightly red color. People with hardening of the arteries and accumulations of fat and cholesterol around the organs often have rough skin. Doughy skin, which appears white and flabby and lacking in elasticity, indicates overconsumption of dairy products, sugar, and white flour. A variety of illnesses are connected with this condition, affecting primarily the breasts and reproductive organs.

Aside from natural skin colors, many abnormal colors may appear on the skin. In the case of cancer, a light green color, reddish-white color, or pinkish-red color from excessive yin or yang food reflects decomposition of tissues and cells and development of cysts and tumors.

Abnormal markings on the skin may also reflect a chronic or degenerative condition. Freckles are the elimination of refined carbohydrates, especially sugar, honey, fruit sugar, and milk sugar. Moles are eliminations of excess protein and fat and appear along the corresponding meridians of the organs affected or muscle areas. Warts signify the elimination of a mixture of protein and fat and indicate developing skin diseases and possible future tumors of the breast, colon, or sex organs. White patches, the result of excess milk, ice cream, and other dairy products, indicate accumulation of fat and mucus throughout the respiratory and reproductive systems. Eczema, dry, hard, raised areas of skin, show a massive elimination of excess fats, especially from dairy foods, more particularly from cheese and eggs cooked with butter.

According to traditional iridology, clogged skin is indicated by a dark circle on the periphery of the iris of the eye. The color, intensity, and width of the ring varies in each case.

DIETARY RECOMMENDATION

Skin cancer is caused primarily by consumption of extreme yin foods and beverages. For skin cancer, avoid all extremes in the yin category of food, including refined sugar and foods and beverages treated with sugar such as soft drinks; artificial and chemicalized food; oily and greasy food; all dairy foods, including cheese, milk, butter, cream, and yogurt; all foods having stimulant and aromatic qualities, including curries, mustard, peppers, and various fragrant beverages and teas; all sorts of alcohol; fruits and fruit juices; nuts; and raw vegetables. It is also necessary to avoid extreme foods in the yang category, especially all sorts of fatty, greasy animal food, including meat, poultry, eggs, and oily fishes. In cooking, all foods are to be cooked, and the use of oil should be either avoided or minimized. Fried foods and oily salad dressings are to be avoided. In addition, it is necessary to avoid all flour products, including breads, pancakes, cookies, and cream-of-wheat type cereals, except for the occasional use of whole-grain flours baked without yeast. Avoid vegetables that originally came from tropical climates and are too expansive (yin) for regular use. These included potatoes, sweet potatoes, tomatoes, eggplant, beets, green peppers, and avocado.

The primary cause of melanoma is chicken and eggs and cheese and other dairy food, in combination with sugar and sweets, stimulants, and baked flour products, which accelerate its spread. Avoid all these foods, as well as those listed above for skin cancer in general.

For both skin cancer and melanoma, all foods are to be cooked and not eaten raw. The use of sea salt, shoyu, miso and various condiments should be moderate.

For Kaposi's sarcoma, see the dietary recommendations in the chapter on AIDS-related cancer.

Recommended daily food for these forms of cancer, by volume of daily intake, should consist of:

• **Whole Grains:** Fifty to 60 percent of daily consumption, by volume, should be whole-cereal grains. The first day prepare plain pressure-cooked short-grain brown rice. On following days, prepare brown rice pressure-cooked with 20 to 30 percent millet, then rice with 20 to 30 percent barley, then rice with 20 to 30 percent aduki beans or lentils, and then plain rice again. A delicious morning porridge can be made by taking leftover rice, adding a little more water to soften, and seasoning with a little miso at the end and simmering for two three minutes more. In ordinary pressure-cooking, the ratio of grain to water should be about 1:2. For seasoning, cook with a postage stamp–sized piece of kombu or a pinch of sea salt, depending on the person's condition. Other grains can be used occasionally, including whole wheat berries, rye, corn, buckwheat, and whole oats, though oats should be avoided for the first month. Good-quality sourdough bread may be enjoyed two to three times a week and noodles, both udon and soba, may also be taken two to three times a week. Avoid all hard baked products until the condition improves, including cookies, cake, pie, crackers, muffins, and the like.

• **Soup:** Five to 10 percent soup, consisting of one or two cups or bowls per day of soup cooked with wakame sea vegetable and various land vegetables such as onions and carrots and seasoned with miso or shoyu. Occasionally a small volume of shiitake mushroom may be added to the soup. Millet soup made with sweet vegetables is especially beneficial for this condition. The miso used in seasoning soups may be barley miso, brown rice miso, or soybean (hatcho) miso and should be naturally aged two to three years.

• **Vegetables:** Twenty to 30 percent vegetables, cooked in a variety of forms. Among vegetables, round vegetables such as cabbage, onions, pumpkin, and acorn and butternut squash are especially recommended, as well as root vegetables such as burdock, carrots, and daikon. Many other hard, leafy green vegetables are also to be used.

As a general rule, the following dishes may be prepared, though the frequency may differ from person to person: nishime-style vegetables, four times a week; squash-aduki-kombu dish, three times a week; dried daikon, one cup, three times a week; carrots and carrot tops or daikon and daikon tops, three times a week; blanched vegetables, five to seven times a week; pressed salad, five to seven times a week; raw salad and salad dressing, avoid; steamed greens, five to seven times a week; sautéed vegetables, two to three times a week, using water the first one to two months and then a small volume of sesame oil thereafter; kinpira, two-thirds of a cup, two times a week; tofu, dried tofu, tempeh, or seitan with vegetables, two times a week.

• **Beans:** Five percent small beans, such as aduki beans, lentils, chickpeas, or black soybeans, may be used daily, cooked together with sea vegetables such as kombu or with onions and carrots. Other beans may be used altogether two to three times a month. For seasoning, a small volume of unrefined sea salt or shoyu or miso can be used. Bean products, such as tempeh, natto, and dried or cooked tofu, may be used occasionally, but in moderate volume.

• **Sea Vegetables:** Five percent or less sea vegetable dishes, including wakame and kombu, daily when cooking grain, in soup, etc. A sheet of toasted nori may also be taken daily. A small dish of hijiki or arame should be prepared two times a week. All other sea vegetables are optional.

• **Condiments:** Condiments to be available on the table are gomashio (sesame salt), on the average made with 1 part salt to 18 parts sesame seeds (reduced to 1:16 after two months); kelp or wakame powder; umeboshi plum; and tekka, though all other regular macrobiotic condiments may be used if desired. These condiments may be used daily on grains and vegetables, but the volume should be moderate to suit individual appetite and taste.

• **Pickles:** Pickles, made at home in a variety of ways, are to be eaten daily, one tablespoon in all, though salty pickles are to be minimized.

• **Animal Food:** Meat, poultry, eggs, and other strong animal food is to be avoided. For melanoma, fish and seafood are also to be avoided, though a small volume of white-meat fish may be eaten once every ten to fourteen days if craved. The fish should be prepared steamed, boiled, or poached and garnished with grated daikon or ginger. Strictly avoid blue-meat and red-meat fish and all shellfish. For skin cancer, depending on the case, a small volume of white-meat fish may be eaten once a week or more frequently after the first month.

• **Fruit:** None the best, the less the better, including both tropical and temperate-climate fruit, until the condition improves. If cravings develop, a small volume of cooked fruit with a pinch of sea salt or dried fruit (also preferably cooked) may be taken. Avoid all fruit juices and cider.

• **Sweets and Snacks:** Avoid all sweets and desserts, including good-quality macrobiotic desserts, until the condition improves. To satisfy a sweet tooth, use sweet vegetables every day in cooking, drink sweet vegetable drink (see special drinks below), and use sweet vegetable jam. Mochi, rice balls, vegetable sushi, and other grain-based snacks may be eaten frequently. Limit rice cakes, popcorn, and other dry or baked snacks, as they may harden the tumor. In the event of cravings, a small volume of amasake, barley malt, or rice syrup may be taken.

• **Nuts and Seeds:** Nuts and nut butters are to avoided due to their high amount of fat and protein, except for chestnuts. Unsalted, roasted seeds such as squash seeds and pumpkin seeds may be consumed as a snack, up to one cup altogether per week.

• **Seasonings:** Seasonings, such as unrefined sea salt, shoyu, and miso, are to be used moderately in order to avoid unnecessary thirst. Avoid mirin and garlic. If you become particularly thirsty after a meal or between meals, you should cut back on these seasonings until the normal level of thirst returns.

• **Beverages:** Beverages and other dietary practices can follow the general recommendations in Part I, with bancha twig tea as the main beverage. Strictly avoid the beverages on the "infrequent" and "avoid" list and don't take grain coffee for the first two to three months after starting this new way of eating.

The most important thing in connection with dietary practice is chewing very well, until all food becomes liquid in the mouth and well mixed with saliva. Chew very, very well, at least 50 times, preferably 100 times, per mouthful. It is also important to avoid overeating and eating within three hours of sleeping.

As noted in the introduction to Part II, persons who have received or who are currently undergoing medical treatment may need to make further dietary modifications.

SPECIAL DRINKS AND PREPARATIONS

Persons with skin cancer and melanoma may also consume some special drinks and dishes, which, taken in small volume, can strengthen blood quality. These dishes include:

• **Sweet Vegetable Drink:** Take one small cup every day for the first month, then two to three times a week the second moth.

• **Carrot-Daikon Drink:** Take one small cup every two days for ten to fourteen days and then once every three days for one month.

• **Kombu-Lotus-Shiitake Drink:** Combine chopped kombu (20 percent), lotus root (40 percent), and shiitake (40 percent). Add four to five times as much water, cook twenty minutes or longer, and add three to four drops of shoyu at the end of cooking and grated ginger and let simmer for several more minutes. Take one small cup daily for three weeks, then twice a week for one month. This is especially good for melanoma.

• **Buckwheat Noodles or Paste:** Buckwheat noodles or buckwheat paste, made with buckwheat flour cooked with chopped scallions, is helpful for skin cancer and melanoma if consumed two to three times per week.

• **Ume-Sho-Kuzu Drink:** A cup of kuzu drink can be helpful if drunk every other day for a two-week period and occasionally thereafter.

• **Miso-Scallion Condiment:** One teaspoon of miso sautéed with sesame oil together with the same volume of scallions and a small volume of grated ginger or garlic added while cooking may be used as a condiment for the meal.

• **Grated Daikon:** Grate about one-half a small cup of fresh daikon, add a few drops of shoyu, and take two to three times a week.

HOME CARES

• **Body Scrub:** Vigorous daily brushing of the skin with a squeezed wet towel will help unblock pores and release excess fat and protein through the skin. When washing, avoid the use of soaps. Skin and scalp normally have a slightly acid pH, and this is upset by most commercial soaps, which are alkaline. Soaps do not really cleanse the skin and can actually prevent excess cholesterol from coming out of pores. Rice bran wrapped in cheesecloth or natural vegetable-quality soaps should be used instead of chemicalized or animal-quality soaps and shampoos.

• **Compress Guidelines:** For a small number of skin cancer or melanoma cases, a compress may be needed to help gradually draw out excess mucus and fat. Please see a qualified macrobiotic teacher for guidance on the proper use and frequency of a compress or plaster. Several types are used, depending on the person's condition. Precede the compress or plaster with application of a towel that has been soaked in hot water and squeezed out over the affected area for about three to five minutes to stimulate circulation.

• **Kombu-Ginger Compress:** Soak a three-inch piece of kombu. Combine with one-half teaspoon of grated ginger and put over the melanoma or other affected area. Cover with a cotton bandage and leave for several hours or overnight. If the ginger is too hot or stimulating, use just 20 percent ginger with cooked rice and barley. Use every day for a maximum of two weeks.

• **Daikon Compress:** A compress made from dried daikon leaves and grated ginger can help speed up the process of discharge. Boil daikon leaves, grate fresh gingerroot, and wrap in cheesecloth. Turn down the flame and place this "ginger sack" (which should contain a lump of grated ginger about the size of a golf ball) in the water. Then, dip a towel into the water, squeeze, and apply to the affected area.

• **Rice Bran Wash:** A rice bran (nuka) skin wash is also beneficial. Wrap nuka in cheesecloth. Place in hot water and shake. The nuka will melt and the water will begin to turn yellow. Then wash the affected area with a towel or cloth that has been dipped in this water.

• **Wood Ash:** The skin may also be washed with wood ash. Place ashes that are left over after burning wood in a fireplace into hot water and stir very well. Let sit until the ashes settle to the bottom, and then use the water to wash the skin. Pat dry with a towel.

• **Fresh Daikon:** In cases where a person with a skin disease suffers from itching, rub a piece of cut fresh daikon directly onto the affected area. If you don't have a daikon, use a scallion or onion.

• **Sesame Oil:** Sesame oil can be applied directly to the affected area in cases where the skin becomes ruptured. Afterward cover the area with cotton cloth to protect from external contact.

• **After Surgery:** In the event the skin cancer and melanoma have been removed in part or whole by surgery, genuine brown rice cream can be used. Two to three bowls may be consumed per day with a small volume of condiments such as scallion-miso, gomashio (sesame salt), tekka, or umeboshi plum for the initial several days. All other regular dishes such as soup, vegetables, beans and bean products, and seaweed should be continued as usual during this time. After that period, regular brown rice and other cereal grains can be introduced gradually. During both times, it is very important to chew the food thoroughly until it assumes a liquid form, up to 100 or more times per mouthful. The removed portion of the skin cancer and melanoma will often restore itself as time passes. Even if the amputated section is not restorable, chewing well can sufficiently serve for digestion.

OTHER CONSIDERATIONS

• Wool and synthetic fabrics are particularly irritating to the skin. Wear cotton and sleep on all-cotton fabrics to allow your skin to breathe naturally.

• Avoid cosmetics or antiperspirants made with synthetic or toxic ingredients. Most commercial deodorants contain aluminum salts that temporarily close the openings of the sweat glands and stop "wetness." They also contain chemical antibacterial agents that are harmful to the body. Body odor is largely caused by consumption of animal food, including all kinds of soft dairy foods, and naturally lessens as the diet becomes more centered on grain and vegetable foods. Even natural deodorants should be minimized, since they may contain ingredients such as beeswax, which can also stop up pores. Among natural cosmetics, one of the safest is clay. Pure clay or clay powder sprinkled on the body can have an antiperspirant effect. Clay also naturally draws wastes and toxins from the skin and can be used as a basis for a facial mask or a compress.

• A sauna, steam bath, or Japanese hot tub can help open clogged skin pores. However, cancer patients should steam or bathe only occasionally, such as a few times a week, and for a short period of time, such as ten minutes. Prepare a thermos of shoyu-bancha tea or miso soup to drink when you come out in order to replace lost fluids and to thicken the blood quality. Unless proper foods have been consumed, this form of inducing sweat is preferable to running, working out in a gym, or other strenuous activity, which may generate more waste products—chiefly urea and lactic acid—than are lost through sweating.

• Do-in or shiatsu massage is beneficial to restoring proper respiration and elimination through the skin. Yoga, martial arts, and other exercises that are grounded in an understanding of the energy meridians can also be used to complement dietary adjustments.

• Avoid direct exposure to the sun as much as possible. Wear a hat or stay in the shade.

• Avoid commercial sunscreen creams that may have chemicals or other harmful ingredients.

PERSONAL EXPERIENCE

Skin Cancer

In early 1975 Roger Randolph, a sixty-one-year-old lawyer from Tulsa, Oklahoma, observed three red spots on his chest and one on his back that did not go away over the course of several weeks. A skin specialist diagnosed his condition as skin cancer and prescribed two types of medicine: one to be applied to these spots twice daily for three weeks, followed by the other medicine for another three weeks. The doctor said the spots on his chest would probably clear up but recommended surgery or radiation therapy to excise the malignancy on his back before it spread.

Randolph discussed his case with his wife and children, and they recommended that he try the macrobiotic approach. Randolph agreed and told his doctor that he would experiment with the Cancer Prevention Diet and report back in three months.

On April 28 Randolph came to see me and I examined him carefully. The spots on his chest had cleared up, but the one on his back was definitely malignant. I recommended the diet described above for three months, with particular emphasis on chewing each mouthful fifty to seventy times. "Mr. Kushi said the cancer would probably continue to grow for a month or two," Randolph recorded, "but that soon thereafter it would definitely disappear. On May 1 I commenced the strict diet, and followed it faithfully for three months."

On August 18 Randolph returned for a medical examination, and his doctor was astonished to find that the tumor on his back had disappeared. "He was flabbergasted and suggested that the cure must have been produced by a delayed reaction to the medicine which I had ceased to apply four and a half months earlier," Randolph wrote. "He urged me to return in three weeks to verify the cancer was gone."

On September 9 Randolph went back and received a clean bill of health. Two months later, in November, he had a final medical check and received a discharge as cured. "In my opinion the macrobiotic diet was the sole cause of the cure," Randolph concluded, "permitting my body to cure itself by providing it with proper nutrition and insulating it from the dreadful food most of us eat." Source: *Case History Report* 1, no. 3 (Boston: East West Foundation, 1976), 1–2.

Malignant Melanoma

In August 1978, Virginia Brown, a fifty-six-year-old mother and registered nurse from Tunbridge, Vermont, noticed a black mole on her arm that kept getting bigger and blacker. She had lost a lot of weight and felt very dull mentally. Doctors at Vermont Medical Center in Burlington performed a biopsy and discovered that she had an advanced case of malignant melanoma (Stage IV). The physicians told her that without surgery she could expect to live only six months. "Even though I had been trained and practiced in the medical profession for years," she later recalled, "I could not go along with surgery. I had professed alternatives for years, but did not really practice them."

At home, her son and daughter-in-law encouraged her to try macrobiotics, and shortly thereafter she attended the EWF's annual cancer conference, meeting that year in Amherst, Massachusetts. At the conference she listened to fifteen cancer patients discuss their experiences on the diet and was impressed with their accounts.

Prior to that time she had followed the standard American way of eating, high in refined foods and fat, especially animal fat from dairy foods, beef, poultry, and fish. At the time she started the diet, she was so sick that she could hardly make it upstairs and slept most of the day. After three weeks eating the new food, which her children prepared for her, she experienced a change in her energy level, attitude, and mental clarity. "I was a new person; I could get up and walk around."

In September she came to Boston to see me, and I made more specific dietary recommendations and advised her to study proper cooking. With the support of her family, she adhered faithfully to the diet, supplemented by Korean yoga exercises, prayer and meditation, and a two-mile walk each morning after breakfast.

She noted afterward:

> I amazed myself at my perseverance, not one of my better qualities. There have been all kind of days—angry, crying, pain, weakness, tension, sadness, and hopelessness, but also thankful times. . . . The most difficult thing has been to see other loved ones go the chemotherapy and radiation route and suffer so.
>
> The most impressive thing was when I first saw Michio. He looked at me and said, "You're doing it. You can get rid of it." He had faith. This was such a contrast to the doctors. The way they look at you is unbelievable.

In October 1979 I met with Virginia again and found that she no longer had any cancer in her body. Medical exams subsequently confirmed this diagnosis. After restoring her health, Virginia went on to study at the Kushi Institute and worked in the macrobiotic health program at the Lemuel Shattuck Hospital in Boston, promoting a more natural way of living among other medical professionals and patients. Sources: "Malignant Melanoma, Stage IV," Cancer and Diet (Brookline, MA: East West Foundation, 1980), 69–70, and interview with Alex Jack, September 30, 1982.

Melanoma

In 1983 Marlene McKenna was diagnosed with malignant melanoma. "As a working mother of four children, radio and TV commentator, and investment broker, I was living a very unbalanced life," she explained in an interview in the Providence Journal.

In August 1985 Marlene began to complain of severe stomach pains, and in January 1986 doctors discovered that five tumors had spread throughout her body. Two feet of her intestines was removed, and Marlene was told she had six months to a year to live.

Declining all treatments, Marlene turned to macrobiotics at the suggestion of her brother and visited me in Boston. In addition to changing her diet, she replaced her electric stove with a gas stove and began to meditate and practice yoga. A devout Catholic, she also did a lot of inspirational reading and praying.

"I promised God that if He walked me through this and helped me live, I would give Him life with life," she recalls.

Within a year Marlene was on the way to recovery, and doctors found no evidence of further cancer. Feeling well enough to return to public life, she ran for state treasurer in Rhode Island. During the campaign, she discovered that she was pregnant. Because of her previous illness and age (forty-two), doctors encouraged her to have an abortion. Marlene refused. "I realized that [having the baby] was part of my promise to give life with life," she explains. Though she lost the election, she gave birth to a healthy baby boy, keeping her promise to God and proving her physicians wrong.

Since then, she has opened Shepherd's, a macrobiotic natural foods restaurant in Providence, and is helping people around the country who have heard of her remarkable recovery.

Source: One Peaceful World Newsletter, Autumn 1989.

22

Bone Cancer

FREQUENCY

This year an estimated 13,550 Americans will die of bone cancer and connective tissue tumors and 20,400 new cases will surface. Bone cancer appears in a variety of forms. The most lethal is multiple myeloma, accounting for about two-thirds of bone cancer deaths. It is one of the fastest-rising cancers in the United States and around the world. Over the last thirty years, death rates from multiple myeloma in this country have soared almost 100 percent.

Multiple myeloma affects both bone tissue and the plasma cells of the blood and usually develops in adults over fifty. This condition is characterized by the spontaneous fracture of the bones, including the vertebrae, ribs, pelvis, and skull, as cancer cells replace normal cells. Other bone cancers include *osteogenic sarcoma*, a tumor affecting children and young adults, which begins in the bone and cartilage and often spreads to the bone marrow, muscles, liver, and lungs; *Ewing's sarcoma*, another cancer of childhood, which appears in the marrow of the longer bones and spread to other bones and organs; *chondrosarcoma*, a slow-growing tumor, which originates in the cartilage of the large bones and affects primarily middle-aged persons; *chordoma*, a rare tumor found at the base of the skull or end of the spine; and *rhabdomyosarcoma*, a soft-tissue tumor in the fat and muscles, which spread rapidly and usually affects children mostly between the ages of two and six. Primary bone cancer is comparatively rare. However, the bones are frequently the site of cancer spreading from other sites.

Amputation is prescribed for many bone cancers, though most myelomas are too advanced for surgery. Radiation therapy and chemotherapy are often used as supplemental treatments. The five-year survival rate for multiple myeloma is 16 to 17 percent. For other bone cancer, it varies with the type and reaches up to 50 percent.

STRUCTURE

The skeletal and muscular system supports the body framework and governs mobility and physical interaction with the environment. The bones also serve to protect vital inner organs and store calcium, phosphorous, and other minerals that are needed for metabolism. Bone is considered both a tissue and an organ and is composed of specialized cells called osteocytes, which are imbedded in a matrix. The matrix includes small fibers and an adhering substance made up of mineral salts. The skeletal structure is also composed of cartilage, which is more flexible than bone; joints, which are junctions between two or more bones; muscles, which control tension and body movement and make up half the body weight; and tendons, which connect muscles and bones.

Bone tissue is made up of thin layers called lamellae. In fully developed bone, these lamellae are classified as either spongy or compact. The skull and ribs, for instance, are more porous or spongelike in structure, while the long bones of the legs and arms consist of a central canal surrounded by concentrically arranged plates of bone tissue. Blood vessels and nerves run through the canals, transporting nutrients and wastes to and from the osteocytes. The bone marrow consists of the soft tissues in the medullary canals of the compact bones and in the interstices of spongy bones.

Bone tissue is constantly changing in order to adapt to stress and varying environmental factors. The bones of infants and children are softer than adults and more subject to malformation or fracture. In the course of aging, the proportion of inorganic mineral salts in the bones increases, slowing their growth. In elderly people, this can cause bones to become brittle and break more easily.

CAUSE OF CANCER

The dense, compact bones are classified as yang in structure, and tumors in this part of the body arise primarily from excess accumulation of refined salt and minerals in combination with excessive animal-quality protein and saturated fat. Foods that can produce this overly contracted condition include meat, eggs, poultry, fish and seafood, and hard, salty cheese.

In addition to these yang influences, strong yin factors are also sometimes involved in bone cancer formation, especially in the case of multiple myeloma. In this disease, the cells of the bone marrow revert to red blood cells, enhancing the susceptibility of the skeletal system to fracture. This condition reflects stagnated intestinal activity caused by excessive consumption of extreme foods in both the yang and yin categories. The latter includes dairy food, refined flour products, sugar and other sweets, coffee and stimulants, soft drinks, tropical fruits and vegetables, drugs and medications, and all kinds of chemicalized or artificially processed foods. The bones and deep inner organs are particularly susceptible to radioactive substances, such as strontium 90, which displace calcium and other minerals in the tissue. Radioactive elements accumulate in the food chain and are consumed principally in animal foods, such as milk and beef. (For a complete description of the relationship between cancer and radiation, see the chapter on leukemia.)

MEDICAL EVIDENCE

• In 1970 Japanese scientists at the National Cancer Center Research Institute reported that shiitake mushrooms had a strong antitumor effect. In experiments with mice, polysaccharide preparations from various natural sources, including the shiitake mushroom commonly available in Tokyo markets, markedly inhibited the growth of induced sarcomas, resulting in "almost complete regression of tumors . . . with no sign of toxicity." Source: G. Chihara et al., "Fractionation and Purification of the Polysaccharides with Marked Antitumor Activity, Especially Lentinan, from *Lentinus edodes* (Berk.) Sing. (an Edible Mushroom)," *Cancer Research* 30:2776–81.

• In 1974 Japanese scientists reported that several varieties of *kombu* and *mojaban*, common sea vegetables eaten in Asia and traditionally used as a decoction for cancer in Chinese herbal medicine, were effective in the treatment of tumors in laboratory experiments. In three of four samples tested, inhibition rates in mice with implanted sarcomas ranged from 89 to 95 percent. The researchers reported that "the tumor underwent complete regression in more than half of the mice of each treated group." Similar experiments on mice with leukemia showed promising results. Source: I. Yamamoto et al., "Antitumor Effect of Seaweeds," *Japanese Journal of Experimental Medicine* 44:543–46.

• Several 1985 studies found a link between pesticide use and increased incidence of multiple myeloma and non-Hodgkin's lymphoma. Source: N. E. Pearce et al., "Malignant Lymphoma and Multiple Myeloma Linked with Agricultural Occupations in a New Zealand Cancer Registry–based Study," *American Journal of Epidemiology* 121:225–37, and D. D. Weisenburger, "Lymphoid Malignancies in Nebraska: A Hypothesis," *Nebraska Medical Journal* 70:300–305.

DIAGNOSIS

Modern medicine commonly tests for bone cancer by a variety of methods, including chest and skeletal surveys, acid and alkaline phosphatase tests, serum calcium tests, and a bone biopsy. For multiple myeloma, detection usually includes a myelogram. In this procedure, a dye is injected into the spinal fluid and X rayed for possible malignancies.

Traditional Oriental diagnosis avoids technological methods of detection that can be harmful to health in favor of simple visual observations, acupressure techniques involving touching certain spots on the body, and other safe but accurate procedures. In this way, development of serious illness, including cancer, can be diagnosed long before it reaches a critical stage and corrective dietary adjustments taken.

In general, the quality of a person's native constitution can be seen in the bone structure, while the quality of the individual's year-to-year, month-to-month, or day-to-day condition appears more in the muscles, skin, and other peripheral areas of the body. The constitution can be judged by feeling the bones, especially in the area of the shoulders, arms, and legs. Stronger and bolder bones indicate a stronger, more yang constitution, while thinner and weaker bones indicate a more yin, weak, and fragile condition. The former type of person has a tendency to be more active in physical and social life, while the latter tends to be more active in mental and artistic life.

Softer muscles show a more yin constitution, nourished by fluid, vegetables, and fruits, while tighter muscles show a more yang constitution, nourished by grains, beans, and animal food, with more minerals. The condition of the skin is also an indication. However, in comparison with the bones, the condition of the muscles and skin is more changeable through diet and exercise, since they are composed of more protein and fat, while the bones are composed of more minerals. Accordingly, while the muscles and skin show the constitution developed during the periods of pregnancy and growth, they also show the present physical and mental conditions. Softer muscles and fine skin indicate a more adaptable and mentally oriented nature, while tighter and harder muscles and skin show a nature that is more physically oriented and active.

These are general tendencies and differ depending upon the individual. In visual diagnosis, both constitution and condition are taken into account in determining relative health or sickness and are examined in assessing the digestive, circulatory, nervous, and excretory systems as well as the skeletal and musculature system.

Bone cancer is a yang disorder and especially affects those who are sturdy in build or lean with very strong constitutions. The development of this form of malignancy can be determined by a variety of observations. Facial color is either red-brown or milky white, and in both cases facial and body skin appears oily.

In bone cancer cases, a green coloration often appears along the spleen meridian, especially from the inside of the big toe up the outside of the leg. Also, in some cases, fatty spots with a green shade appear on the outside of the foot below the ankle. The inside of the wrist may also show a dark green or dark blue color. The outer edge of the palm may become red-white, while the edge on the back of the hand may be green.

In many cases of bone cancer, the toenails may become white or cracked, and often calluses appear on the tips of or between the toes. Hard mucus accumulation and calcification also arise on the forehead and are a possible indication of this condition. A yellow-white color, also showing mucous buildup, often appears on the lower white of the eye. The fingertips, especially the second section, often become white, and the second and third set of knuckles tend to be hard. From these and other signs, developing bone cancer can be detected and protected against naturally.

DIETARY RECOMMENDATIONS

Bone cancer is caused primarily by longtime overconsumption of animal food, especially beef, pork, poultry, eggs, cheese and other dairy food, fish and seafood, and salted and baked foods. Consumption of these and other foods high in fat, protein, and salt should be discontinued. At the same time contributing to bone cancer is the overconsumption of all fatty and oily foods, both of animal and vegetable quality, including sugar, honey, chocolate, carob, and other sweeteners, spices, stimulants, and aromatic foods and drinks, as well as foods that form fat and mucus, such as flour products. These should be limited or avoided completely. Soft drinks, chemical additives, alcohol, and all artificially processed food and beverages are to be avoided, as they are considered possible contributing factors. The following are general dietary guidelines for the relief and prevention of bone cancer:

• **Whole Grains:** Fifty to 60 percent of daily consumption, by volume, should be whole-cereal grains. The first day prepare plain pressure-cooked short-grain brown rice. The following days, prepare brown rice pressure-cooked with 20 to 30 percent millet, then rice with 20 to 30 percent barley, then rice with 20 to 30 percent aduki beans or lentils, and then plain rice again. A delicious morning porridge can be made by taking leftover rice, adding a little more water to soften, and seasoning with a little miso at the end and simmering for two to three minutes more. In daily pressure cooking, the ratio of grain to water should be about 1:2. For seasoning, cook with a postage stamp–sized piece of kombu instead of salt. Other grains can be used occasionally, including whole wheat berries, rye, corn, and whole oats, though oats should be avoided for the first month. However, buckwheat should be avoided for about six months because it is very contractive and may harden the tumor. Seitan is also very yang and should be minimized. Flour products, even unrefined whole wheat bread, chapatis, pancakes, and cookies, should be totally avoided or limited in volume for a period of a few months. Whole-grain pasta and noodles may be eaten a couple times a week. Once or twice a week, fried rice or noodles may be consumed.

• **Soup:** Five to 10 percent soup, consisting of one or two cups or bowls per day of soup cooked with wakame sea vegetable and various vegetables and seasoned lightly with miso or shoyu. To help relieve this condition, pieces of fresh daikon, turnip, or radish can be added almost daily. Occasionally a small volume of shiitake mushroom may be added to the soup. The miso may be barely miso, brown rice miso, or soybean (hatcho) miso and should be naturally aged two to three years. The taste of the soup should be milder than usual. Grain soups, bean soups, and other soups may be taken from time to time.

• **Vegetables:** Twenty to 30 percent vegetables, cooked in a variety of forms, mainly steamed and boiled. While oil is not usually recommended for most cancer patients, for bone cancer one dish of sautéed vegetables cooked with unrefined sesame oil should be eaten daily or every other day. Sweet vegetables such as cabbage, onions, pumpkin, and winter squash can be used most often, though root and leafy vegetables are also to be used regularly. Vegetables may be seasoned during cooking with sea salt, miso, or shoyu, and the taste should be milder than usual. As a rule of thumb, the following dishes may be prepared, though the frequency may differ from person to person: nishime-style vegetables, three times a week; squash-aduki-kombu dish, three times a week; dried daikon, one cup, three times a week; carrots and carrot tops or daikon and daikon tops, three times a week; blanched vegetables, five to seven times a week; pressed salad, five to seven times a week; raw salad, avoid; steamed greens, five to seven times a week; sautéed vegetables, prepared with water the first month, then with sesame oil lightly brushed on the pan once or twice a week after that, kinpira, two-thirds of a cup, two times a week; dried tofu, tofu, tempeh, or seitan with vegetables, two times a week.

• **Beans:** Five percent small beans, such as aduki beans, lentils, chickpeas, or black soybeans, may be used daily, cooked together with sea vegetables such as kombu or with onions and carrots. Black soybeans are highly recommended for regular use for this form of cancer. Beans can be cooked with 10 to 20 percent kombu or other sea vegetable, 30 to 50 percent fall-season squash, or

10 to 30 percent onions and carrots. Season lightly with sea salt, miso, or shoyu. Other beans may be used altogether two to three times a month. For seasoning, a small volume of unrefined sea salt or shoyu or miso can be used. Bean products such as tempeh, natto, and dried or cooked tofu may be used occasionally, but in moderate volume.

• **Sea Vegetables:** Five percent or less sea vegetable dishes, including wakame and kombu, daily when cooking grain, in soup, etc. A sheet of toasted nori may also be taken daily. A small dish of hijiki or arame should be prepared two times a week. All other sea vegetables are optional.

• **Condiments:** Condiments to be available on the table are gomashio (sesame salt), on the average made with 1 part salt to 18 to 20 parts sesame seeds; kelp or wakame powder; umeboshi plum; and tekka, though all other regular macrobiotic condiments may be used if desired. These condiments may be used daily on grains and vegetables, but the volume should be moderate to suit individual appetite and taste.

• **Pickles:** Pickles, made at home in a variety of ways, are to be eaten daily, one tablespoon in all, though salty pickles are to be minimized. Rice bran (nuka) pickles are the most suitable.

• **Animal Food:** Fish and other animal food is to be avoided. However, in the event that animal food is craved, a small volume of white-meat fish may be eaten once every ten days to two weeks. The fish should be prepared steamed, boiled, or poached and garnished with grated daikon or ginger. Strictly avoid blue-meat and red-meat fish and all shellfish.

• **Fruit:** The less the better until the condition improves. If cravings develop, a small volume of cooked fruit with a pinch of sea salt or dried fruit (also preferably cooked) may be taken. Avoid all fruit juices and cider.

• **Sweets and Snacks:** Overuse of sweets is connected with bone disorders, so it is very important to avoid all sweets and desserts, including good-quality macrobiotic desserts, until the condition improves. To satisfy a sweet tooth, use sweet vegetables every day in cooking, drink sweet vegetable drink, or prepare sweet vegetable jam. If cravings arise, a small volume of amasake, barley malt, or rice syrup may be taken. If cravings persist, a little cider, apple juice, or chestnut may be prepared. Mochi, rice balls, vegetable sushi, and other grain-based snacks may be eaten frequently. Limit rice cakes, popcorn, and other dry or baked snacks, as they may harden the tumor.

• **Nuts and Seeds:** Nuts and nut butters are to be avoided due to their high amount of fat and protein, except for chestnuts. Unsalted, roasted seeds such as sunflower seeds and pumpkin seeds may be consumed as a snack, up to one cup altogether per week.

• **Seasonings:** Seasonings, such as unrefined sea salt, shoyu, and miso, are to be used moderately in order to avoid unnecessary thirst. Avoid mirin and garlic. If you become particularly thirsty after a meal or between meals, you should cut back on these seasonings until the normal level of thirst returns.

• **Beverages:** Beverages and other dietary practices can follow the general recommendations in Part I, with bancha twig tea as the principal drink at meals. Carrot juice, one cup, twice a week, is very good for this condition. Strictly avoid the beverages on the "infrequent" and "avoid" list, and don't take grain coffee for the first two to three months after starting this new way of eating.

The most important thing in connection with dietary practice is chewing very well, until all food becomes liquid in the mouth and well mixed with saliva. Chew very, very well, at least 50 times, preferably 100 times, per mouthful. It is also important to avoid overeating and eating within three hours of sleeping.

As noted in the introduction to Part II, persons who have received or who are currently undergoing medical treatment may need to make further dietary modifications.

SPECIAL DRINKS AND DISHES

Several special drinks or side drinks may need to be taken, depending on the individual case. Please see a qualified macrobiotic teacher for guidance. Amounts and frequencies given here are average; these will differ from person to person.

• **Sweet Vegetable Drink:** Take one small cup every day for the first month, then every other day the second month.

• **Carrot-Daikon Drink:** Take one small cup every other day for two weeks, then once every three days for one month.

• **Shiso Powder:** One-half to one teaspoon of shiso powder can be sprinkled daily on grain and vegetable dishes. This is made from roasting and grinding the dried leaves that umeboshi plums usually come prepared with.

• **Kuzu Drink with Grated Daikon:** A cup of kuzu drink is also beneficial for this condition and may be consumed frequently. Prepare by dissolving one teaspoon of kuzu powder in a cup of hot water and cooking briefly with two teaspoons of grated daikon or radish and a little shoyu for taste.

• **Ume-Sho-Bancha:** Ume-sho-bancha tea with half a sheet of crushed, toasted nori sea vegetable can be consumed, up to one cup a day, a few times a week.

• **Carp and Burdock Soup:** For strength, bone cancer patients may prepare occasionally carp soup (koi koku). Mochi or tempeh may also be added to miso soup frequently to restore vitality and generate energy.

HOME CARES

• **Body Scrub:** Scrubbing the whole body, including the abdominal region and the spinal region, with a towel that has been immersed in hot water and squeezed out is very helpful for better circulation of blood, lymph, and other body fluids, as well as for activating physical and mental energies.

• **Compress Guidelines:** For a small number of bone tumors, a compress may be needed to help gradually draw out excess mucus and fat. Please see a qualified macrobiotic teacher for guidance on the proper use and frequency of a compress or plaster. Several types are used, depending on the person's condition. Precede the compress or plaster with application of a towel that has been soaked in hot water and squeezed out over the affected area for about three to five minutes to stimulate circulation.

• **Taro Plaster:** A ginger compress for three to five minutes, followed by a taro potato plaster (mixed 50/50 with grated fresh lotus root) for three to four hours, may be applied on the affected region to help reduce the tumor. Use daily for up to two to four weeks.

• **Vegetable Plaster:** In case of aches and pains, a plaster can be made with cabbage and white potato crushed in a 50/50 mixture. Apply on the affected area until it becomes warm, generally two to three hours, and then repeat.

OTHER CONSIDERATIONS

• Daily physical exercise that does not produce exhaustion is recommended. Ten to fifteen minutes of daily breathing exercises, especially emphasizing long exhalation, is also beneficial. These physical and breathing exercises contribute to relaxing tensions in the body and mind as well as harmonizing physical metabolism.

• Keeping air quality clean and fresh is important for maintenance of general health. For that purpose, green leafy plants can be placed in the house and the windows periodically opened to allow circulation of fresh air. Don't smoke, as this will tighten the bones.

• Avoid wearing wool and synthetic fibers. At the minimum wear cotton underwear and use cotton sheets and pillowcases.

• Avoid watching television for long stretches. Radiation is especially weakening to the bones. Similarly, avoid other artificial sources of electromagnetic energy such as video terminals, smoke detectors, and hand-held electrical appliances, which can weaken the bones and skeletal system.

• Bone cancer patients should particularly avoid damp and humid environments.

PERSONAL EXPERIENCE

Bone Cancer (Metastasized from the Breast)

In November 1980 Bonnie Kramer, a twenty-seven-year-old mother from Torrington, Connecticut, felt discomfort under her arm. She discovered a pea-sized ball that "seemed to float" when touched, but she was not overly concerned about it. She underwent a mammogram the following February, and the results were negative.

During the winter, the lump went through periods of increasing and decreasing in size, and Bonnie started to experience constant pain in her left breast along with fatigue and a milky white discharge from the nipple. Her breasts were enlarged and tender. She also had an unusual number of colds and flu.

A biopsy in February 1982 revealed cancer, and soon afterward Bonnie entered Winsted Memorial Hospital for the removal of her left breast and several lymph nodes under her arm. She also began chemotherapy and was scheduled to undergo six weeks of radiation. The side effects were not severe, although she was irritable at times, lost some hair, and became nauseated after each treatment. Bonnie completed her treatments in March 1983 and was considered by her doctors to be free of cancer. However, periodic bone and liver scans were advised as a precaution. Feeling better, she took a job as a director of social services at a skilled nursing facility and helped raise funds for the American Cancer Society.

Three years later, in April 1986, while playing ball with her son, Bonnie felt a pull in her lower back. The pain continued off and on and by early 1987 had become unbearable. "The pain returned with a vengeance," she recalls. "It just would not go away, and the nurses at work became very concerned. The pain radiated to my face. With each menstrual cycle, I was bloated, suffering with intense cramps." She underwent a bone scan that revealed tumors on her pelvis and upper back. Her doctors advised radiation and aggressive chemotherapy. Bonnie was "numbed to speechlessness" at the news and "couldn't stop crying." As she recalls, "I had to deal with this; that's all I knew. I prayed for strength and guidance in the midst of all the drama. Then, suddenly, out of nowhere, it hit me! Honestly, just like that the answer came. I knew from my readings that more and more was being learned about nutrition and cancer. I remembered my sister telling me about an article she had read several years before, concerning a doctor whose cancer went into remission through a change in diet. It didn't seem relevant to me then, but, suddenly, now it did. 'Oh my God!' I thought. 'That's what I need to do—find out more about this diet—but how?' "

Bonnie's friend went to a local health food store and bought one of my books to read. She found it completely logical but overwhelming. She went to the health food store and bought staple foods and stopped eating meat, sugar, and dairy foods. She also underwent radiation therapy and a hysterectomy. After recovering from surgery, Bonnie decided to attend a seminar presented by the Kushi Institute.

Bonnie supplemented her practice of macrobiotics by taking weekly cooking classes with Sara Lapenta, a Kushi Institute cooking teacher who lived nearby. By May 1987 a blood test revealed that Bonnie's enzyme levels had returned to normal. A bone scan in September showed that the tumors had greatly decreased in size. A friend who worked in the radiation unit at the hospital told Bonnie that she had never seen a report like that before. In September 1988 another bone scan revealed the presence of scar tissue, but no tumors. Bonnie's doctor told her that her remission might have been due to the surgery and radiation, but that macrobiotics may have also helped her. By August 1988 a bone scan produced a totally normal result, with no tumors or scar tissue. Her doctor was now very impressed and fully supportive of her macrobiotic lifestyle.

Bonnie described her experience: "I noticed immediate changes in myself and my son, Ben, who joined in my meals for the first summer. Our allergies seemed to disappear, and Ben no longer got strep throat. We felt stronger, more energetic, more organized, and very well. I had good spirits and stable moods. As my confidence increased, so did the sense of inner peace. I loved feeling at one with nature, at one with God."

Bonnie is now preparing to open a macrobiotic center in her area. Believing that "happiness is real only if it can be shared with others," she would like to help people in her area through classes, food, and guidance. She had dedicated herself to realizing one peaceful world and is grateful to have found a way to "help make this concept a reality."

Source: "A Mother Heals Breast Cancer: Change in Diet Aids Remission of Tumors and Metastases to the Bone," *One Peaceful World Newsletter*, Spring 1990.

23

Leukemia

FREQUENCY

Leukemia, a form of cancer affecting the blood, will claim an estimated 18,200 lives in the United States this year, and 28,200 new cases will arise. Leukemia affects males slightly more than females.

Characterized by the uncontrolled production of white blood cells, leukemia is classified into acute and chronic types. The acute variety tends to grow rapidly, afftects children more commonly, and spreads to the liver, spleen, and lymph nodes. Patients with acute leukemia are very susceptible to anemia, secondary infections, and hemorrhaging and may die from these complications. Chronic leukemia develops more slowly and usually affects those in the middle to older age brackets. The four most common forms of leukemia are: 1) *acute lymphocytic* or *lymphoblastic* (ALL), the most prevalent cancer among children, characterized by diminished granulocytes, the white blood cells that resist infection; 2) *acute myelocytic* (AML), the most prevalent leukemia among adults over forty, characterized by a decrease in platelet production; 3) *chronic myelocytic* or *granulocytic* (CML), an illness accompanied by an abnormal chromosome and affecting young and middle-aged adults; and 4) *chronic lymphocytic* (CLL), a disease that affects primarily the elderly and usually involves malfunction of the spleen.

Modern medicine treats leukemias of all types principally with chemotherapy. Surgery or irradiation by roentgen rays or radioactive phosphorus may also be used if the lymph system is affected or other organs are enlarged. Fresh blood transfusions or bone-marrow transplants are sometimes given in order to provide a fresh source of red blood cells, which scientists believe are produced in the bone marrow. In hospitals, leukemia patients will often be isolated in such devices as the Life Island, a bed enclosed with a plastic canopy designed to provide an environment free of microorganisms. For all forms of leukemia, 35 percent of patients live five years or longer following medical treatment.

STRUCTURE

Our slightly salty bloodstream is a replica of the ancient sea in which biological life developed during most of its evolutionary history. The blood consists of liquid in the form of plasma and formed elements consisting of red blood cells, white blood cells, and platelets. The tighter and more compact red blood cells are yang in structure, while the larger, more expanded white blood cells are yin. The platelets, an important factor in blood clotting, are smaller than red blood cells and because of their contractive ability and size are classified as extremely yang. The plasma comprises about 55 percent of the blood by volume, while the various formed elements, which are suspended in the plasma, constitute the remaining 45 percent.

Our bodies contain about 35 trillion red blood cells. Each of these tiny disc-shaped cells is about 7.7 microns in diameter and about 1.9 microns thick. Men have about 5 million per cubic millimeter and women about 4.5 million per cubic millimeter. The number of red blood cells is dependent on a variety of circumstances, including age, altitude, temperature, and level of activity or rest. For example, as we grow older, the number decreases from the 6 million per cubic millimeter that we had at birth.

Hemoglobin comprises between 60 and 80 percent of the red blood cell and consists of hematin, a more condensed form of protein containing iron, and a simpler, larger protein. Hematin attracts oxygen in the lungs and transports it to the cells of the body. Then, as the oxygen-depleted blood returns through the veins, it attracts and transports carbon dioxide back to the lungs, where it is exhaled. This process is essential for life, and the efficiency with which it is accomplished directly influences our health. In a normal adult, about 20 million red blood cells are destroyed every minute and new red blood cells are continuously formed to replace them. The total volume of hemoglobin in the body is about one kilogram, twenty grams of which are destroyed and rebuilt every day.

The human body contains far fewer white blood cells than red blood cells—about 6,000 per cubic millimeter. They are usually larger than red blood cells, possess a nucleus, and have a power of movement similar to that of an amoeba. White blood cells are attracted to bacteria entering the body, which they envelop and devour. They also gather around inflamed external injuries.

CAUSE OF CANCER

Normal blood is slightly alkaline, with a pH between 7.3 and 7.45, thus giving rise to its mildly salty taste. A pH of less than 7 is acid, while more than 7 is alkaline. If the pH of the blood dips below its normally weak alkaline level and becomes acidic, acidosis arises. Acidity is classified as a yin condition. When the pH factor of the blood moves into the high pH range, the more yang condition of alkalosis occurs. Daily diet is the principal determinant of the blood's relative alkalinity or acidity. More expansive, yin foods and beverages such as sugar, coffee, fruits, juices, milk, and alcohol thin the blood and make it more acid. Contractive foods, including salt, are overly alkaline and construct the circulatory system. The body compensates for poor-quality blood by several mechanisms. For example, when we exhale, excess acids are discharged along with carbon dioxide, and the kidneys continuously filter excess acids from the food and discharge them through urination. Also, our blood contains a variety of buffers, such as sodium bicarbonate, which serve to neutralize acids. In this way the blood can maintain a weak alkaline condition despite regular consumption of extreme foods and beverages.

Under certain circumstances, however, blood equilibrium cannot be maintained, and serious disorders, such as leukemia, result. In blood cancer, the number of red blood cells decreases, while the number of white blood cells increases dramatically. In some cases, leukemia patients may have as many as 1 million white blood cells per cubic millimeter instead of the normal 5,000 to 6,000.

In a normal healthy subject, food reaches the small intestine in the form of chyme, a homogenous liquid that is ready to be absorbed into the bloodstream. The small intestine is akin to a jungle. The villi resemble a forest of hair with millions of bacteria and viruses furthering transmutation by digesting food, changing its quality with their enzymes, and discharging it. Animal foods, strong acids such as sugar and fruits, medications, drugs, and chemicalized food kill these bacteria and cause indigestion, reduce blood production, and create the foundation for serious illness. In properly functioning intestines, molecules of jellified food attach themselves to the ends of the hairs, or villi, become intestinal tissues, and contribute to the production of blood. White blood cells are larger and more flexible than red blood cells and can be classified as yin. They tend to be produced by consumption of expansive foods such as sugar, while red blood cells are created by more yang substances. Leukemia, a condition characterized by too many white blood cells, is caused by overconsumption of yin foods, while scurvy, an excess of red blood cells, is a sign of an overly yang diet.

Scurvy, of course, is no longer a problem because eighteenth-century British sailors learned how to balance their extremely yang diet of salt pork with very yin citrus food. However, leukemia is a modern scourge, and modern medicine has been unable to discover its origin or cure. The rise of leukemia among children and young people has accompanied the explosion of yin foods and beverages manufactured and commonly eaten since World War II. These include snack, party, and dessert foods made with sugar, honey, chocolate, and other sweets; candy and chewing gum; soft drinks, diet colas, and artificial beverages; white bread, rolls, pretzels, and other refined flour products; oranges, bananas, pineapples, and other tropical fruits; french-fried potatoes and potato chips; and milk, cottage cheese, ice cream, milkshakes, and yogurt. Many children today eat a diet with a largely sweet taste that is soft in texture, large in size, and refined or processed in quality. Such a diet will produce an extremely thin quality of blood. Leukemia is also on the rise among Western vegetarians, especially those who eat large amounts of dairy products, fruit, raw foods, curried foods, aromatic herbs, and vitamin pills. Many of these substances are native and natural to tropical or subtropical environments. However, when they become a major part of the diet in temperate climates, serious illnesses will occur.

The increased incidence of leukemia since World War II has often been attributed to nuclear radiation. Estimates of total U.S. cancer deaths from atomic fallout and nuclear power plant emissions over the next generation range from several thousand to a million or more. Epidemiological studies show that residents living near nuclear sites and workers handling nuclear materials have higher cancer rates than other people. While nuclear radiation is dangerous and should be avoided whenever possible, the underlying way of eating governs the degree of susceptibility to cancer in any given instance.

In 1945, for example, there were a small number of people following a macrobiotic diet who lived in Hiroshima and Nagasaki at the time of the first atomic explosions. Among those who survived the initial blast, the individuals who ate macrobiotically were able to function normally and help many other survivors overcome radiation sickness, a form of leukemia, by eating brown rice, well-cooked vegetables, miso soup, sea vegetables, pickled plums, and natural sea salt. From the symptoms of atomic disease they realized that radiation was extremely expansive or yin, and that the blood could be strengthened or yangized with counterbalancing opposite factors such as a salt-rich grain and cooked-vegetable diet.

In traditional Oriental medicine, the hair on the head corresponds with the hairlike villi of the small intestine. When people's hair began to fall out after the bombings, it indicated trouble in the intestine and severely curtailed blood production. In the decades since the first atomic bombings, scientists have confirmed that miso and sea vegetables contain substances in addition to salt that can help protect the body from radiation by binding and discharging radioactive elements.

At the social level, various government agencies have proposed that nuclear waste materials be stored in salt mines or deposits in order to neutralize their deadly emissions. This is an example of how yin and yang are used in the modern world, although scientists do not understand the underlying principle of balance—namely, macrobiotic philosophy—involved.

There are many other sources of artificial radiation in modern society in addition to nuclear energy. Color television, computer and video terminals, photocopier machines, air conditioners, smoke detectors, garage-door openers, supermarket checkout scanners, and numerous other appliances and devices contribute to our rapidly growing electronic environment. Some of this radiation is low-level, such as that emitted by an electric hair dryer. Some radiation is stronger, such as that from microwave ovens. Day by day, all artificial electromagnetic stimuli have a cumulative effect on health and vitality.

A healthy human body has a marvelous capacity to adjust to its environment, even a radioactive or transistorized one. People following the standard macrobiotic way of eating need have no fear of leukemia or other serious illnesses. Of course, in an emergency situation, such as the accident at Three Mile Island, a more limited diet should be followed. However, at current world radiation levels, people still eating the modern refined diet have a much lower tolerance for radioactivity and are at risk of developing leukemia and other cancers. Reversing the biological degeneration of modern society is the key to curing atomic sickness and other forms of cancer. Return to a more natural way of farming, eating, and daily life will make nuclear energy unnecessary and contribute to lasting health and enduring peace.

MEDICAL EVIDENCE

• In 1944 mice on a 60 percent caloric restricted diet registered substantially less induced and spontaneous leukemias than mice fed at pleasure. The incidence of blood cancer in a high leukemia strain of mice fell from 65 to 10 percent and length of life was considerably prolonged. Source: J. A. Saxton, Jr., et al., "Observations on the Inhibition of Development of Spontaneous Leukemias in Mice by Underfeeding," *Cancer Research* 4:401–9.

• In 1947 researchers reported that a high-protein diet enhanced leukemia induced in mice. Source: J. White et al., "Effects of Diets Deficient in Certain Amino Acids on the Induction of Leukemia in DBA Mice," *Journal of the National Cancer Institute* 7:199–202.

• In 1969 medical students linked two common corn-soil pesticides to leukemia in test animals and humans. Tests showed that chlordane and heptachlor were concentrated in the food chain and appeared in the majority of the nation's dairy products, meat, poultry, and fish. The pesticides were phased out of production in the late 1970s by order of the Environmental Protection Agency, but their residues persist. Source: Samuel S. Epstein, M.D., *The Politics of Cancer* (New York: Doubleday, 1979), 271–81.

• In 1972 a Japanese scientist reported that leukemia in chickens could be reversed by feeding them a mixture of whole grains and salt. The experiment was conducted by Keiichi Morishita, M.D., technical chief for the Tokyo Red Cross Blood Center and vice president of the New Blood Association. Source: K. Morishita, M.D., *The Hidden Truth of Cancer* (San Francisco: George Ohsawa Macrobiotic Foundation, 1972).

• Seventh-Day Adventist women in California have 44 percent less leukemia than the general population and men have 30 percent less, according to a 1975 study. The members of this religious group tend to consume whole grains, vegetables, fruit, and nuts and avoid meat, poultry, rich and refined foods, coffee, tea, hot condiments, spices, and alcohol. Source: R. L. Phillips, "Role of Life-style and Dietary Habits in Risk of Cancer among Seventh-Day Adventists," *Cancer Research* 35:3513–22.

• Exposure to high levels of dioxin-laced herbicides substantially increased the rate of cancer deaths among German chemical workers. In a 1991 study, researchers reported male herbicide workers faced a 39 percent greater risk of dying from leukemia, lymphoma, lung cancer, and other malignancies than workers in a control group. In the United States, there has been a controversial debate about whether Vietnam War veterans exposed to Agent Orange, a dioxin-contaminated defoliant, experienced higher risk of cancer. Source: A. Manz et al., "Cancer Mortality among Workers in Chemical Plant Contaminated with Dioxi n," *Lancet* 338:959–64.

• In 1993, researchers reported in the *Archives of Internal Medicine* that smoking cigarettes may increase the risk of leukemia by 30 percent and cause up to 3,600 cases of adult leukemia a year. Source: "Smoking Tied to Leukemia Risk," *New York Times*, February 23, 1993.

DIAGNOSIS

Blood tests and bone-marrow samples are used by doctors to diagnose leukemia. A bone-marrow aspiration and biopsy will also be taken if a malignancy is suspected. Chest X rays, lymphangiogram, liver, spleen, and bone scans, CAT scan of the head, and a lumbar puncture may also be administered.

Oriental medicine diagnoses the quality of the blood by a variety of simple, safe visual techniques. A white color on the lips indicates a deficiency of hemoglobin, abnormal constriction of the blood capillaries, or stagnation and slowness of blood circulation in general. Anemia, leukemia, and similar blood conditions can produce this lip color.

A whitish color in the pink area inside the lower eyelid also indicates a weakened condition caused by excessive intake of either extreme yin or yang foods. This color also often accompanies leukemia.

Whitish fingernails further indicate underactive blood circulation, low hemoglobin, general anemia, and a tendency toward leukemia or other forms of cancer. Normally healthy people do not have this whitish color in the nails except when the fingers are stretched.

DIETARY RECOMMENDATIONS

The major cause of leukemia is the long-time, continuous consumption of foods and beverages in the extreme yin category, including sugar, sugar-treated foods and drinks, ice cream, chocolate, carob, honey, soft drinks and soda, tropical fruits, fruit juices, oily and greasy foods, dairy foods, especially butter, milk, and cream, and many chemicals contained in foods, beverages, and supplements. All of these should be avoided in daily eating. However, the consumption of these items is often accompanied by the intake of foods from the extreme yang category, including meat, poultry, eggs, and cheese, in order to achieve a rough counterbalance. Accordingly, all these animal foods are also to be avoided, with the exception of fish and seafood, which can be consumed occasionally in moderate volume. Although they are not the direct cause, the following enhance leukemic conditions and should also be discontinued: ice-cold food and drinks, hot, stimulant, and aromatic spices, various herbs and herb drinks that have stimulant effects, and vegetables that historically originated in the tropics, including potatoes, tomatoes, and eggplant.

The nutritional recommendations for younger childhood leukemia are included in the chapter on children's cancer. Following are daily dietary guidelines, by volume, for the prevention and relief of leukemia in older children or adults:

• **Whole Grains:** Fifty to 60 percent of daily consumption, by volume, should be whole-cereal grains. The first day prepare plain pressure-cooked short-grain brown rice. On following days, prepare brown rice pressure-cooked with 20 to 30 percent millet, then rice with 20 to 30 percent barley, then rice with 20 to 30 percent aduki beans or lentils, and then plain rice again. A delicious morning porridge can be made by taking leftover rice, adding a little more water to soften, and seasoning with a little miso at the end and simmering for two to three minutes more. In ordinary pressure cooking, the ratio of grain to water should be about 1:2. For seasoning, cook with a postage stamp–sized piece of kombu instead of salt, though in some cases sea salt may be used depending on the person's condition. After the first month, fried rice or fried grain with vegetables can be prepared with a little sesame oil once or twice a week. Other grains can be used occasionally, including whole wheat berries, rye, corn, and whole oats, though oats should be avoided for the first month. Buckwheat and seitan should be minimized. Good-quality sourdough bread may be enjoyed two to three times a week, and noodles, both udon and soba, may also be taken two to three times a week. Avoid all hard baked products until the condition improves, including cookies, cake, pie, crackers, muffins, and the like.

• **Soup:** Five to 10 percent soup, consisting of one or two cups or bowls per day of soup cooked with wakame sea vegetable and various land vegetables such as onions and carrots and seasoned with miso or shoyu. Occasionally a small volume of shiitake mushroom may be added to the soup. The miso may be barley miso, brown rice miso, or soybean (hatcho) miso and should be naturally aged two to three years. To satisfy a sweet tooth, millet soup with sweet vegetables such as squash, cabbage, onions, and carrots may be prepared often. Grain soups, bean soups, and other soups may be taken from time to time. Less frequently, a small portion of white-meat fish or small dried fish can also be cooked into the soup with vegetables, sea vegetables, and/or grains.

• **Vegetables:** Twenty to 30 percent vegetables, cooked in a variety of forms. In general, leafy vegetables, round, hard vegetables grown near the surface of the earth, and root vegetables can be used in about equal volume, i.e., one-third of each type for daily consumption. During cooking, they can be seasoned moderately with sea salt, shoyu, or miso. After the first month, unrefined vegetable oil, especially sesame or corn oil, may be used for sautéeing vegetables several times a week, though oil should not be overconsumed. As a general rule, the following dishes may be prepared, though the frequency may differ from person to person: nishime-style vegetables, four times a week; squash-aduki-kombu dish, three times a week; dried daikon, one cup, three times a week; carrots and carrot tops or daikon and daikon tops, three times a week; blanched vegetables, five to seven times a week; pressed salad, five to seven times a week; raw salad and salad dressing, avoid; steamed greens, five to seven times a week; kinpira, two-thirds of a cup, two times a week, then oil may be used after three weeks; dried tofu, tofu, tempeh, or seitan with vegetables, two times a week.

• **Beans:** Five percent small beans, such as aduki beans, lentils, chickpeas, or black soybeans, may be used daily, cooked together with sea vegetables such as kombu or with onions and carrots. Other beans may be used altogether two to three times a month. For seasoning, a small volume of unrefined sea salt or shoyu or miso can be used. Bean products, such as tempeh, natto, and dried or cooked tofu, may be used occasionally, but in moderate volume.

• **Sea Vegetables:** Five percent or less sea vegetable dishes, including wakame and kombu, daily when cooking grain, in soup, etc. A sheet of toasted nori may also be taken daily. A small dish of hijiki or arame should be prepared two times a week. All other sea vegetables are optional. Sea vegetables can be cooked with other vegetables or sautéed with a small volume of sesame oil after softening them by soaking and boiling lightly in water.

• **Condiments:** Condiments to be available on the table are gomashio (sesame salt), on the average made with 1 part salt to 18 parts sesame seeds (reduced to 1:16 after two months); kelp or wakame powder; umeboshi plum; and tekka, though all other regular macrobiotic condiments may be used if desired. These condiments may be used daily on grains and vegetables, but the volume should be moderate to suit individual appetite and taste.

• **Pickles:** Pickles, made at home in a variety of ways, are to be eaten daily, one tablespoon in all, though salty pickles are to be minimized.

• **Animal Food:** Meat, poultry, eggs, and other strong animal food is to be avoided. A small volume of white-fish may be eaten once a week. The fish should be prepared steamed, boiled, or poached and garnished with grated daikon or ginger. After two months, fish may be eaten twice a week if desired. Strictly avoid blue-meat and red-meat fish and all shellfish.

• **Fruit:** None the best, the less the better, including both tropical and temperate-climate fruit, until the condition improves. If cravings develop, a small volume of cooked fruit with a pinch of sea salt or dried fruit (also preferably cooked) may be taken. Avoid all fruit juices and cider.

• **Sweets and Snacks:** Avoid all sweets and desserts, including good-quality macrobiotic desserts, until the condition improves. To satify a sweet tooth, use sweet vegetables every day in cooking, drink sweet vegetable drink (see special drinks below), and use sweet vegetable jam and a small volume of amasake. Mochi, rice balls, vegetable sushi, and other grain-based snacks may be eaten frequently. Limit rice cakes, popcorn, and other dry or baked snacks, as they may harden the tumor. In the event of cravings, a small volume of barley malt or rice syrup may be taken.

• **Nuts and Seeds:** Nuts and nut butters are to be avoided due to their high amount of fat and protein, except for chestnuts. Unsalted, roasted seeds such as sunflower seeds and pumpkin seeds may be consumed as a snack, up to one cup altogether per week.

• **Seasonings:** Seasonings, such as unrefined sea salt, shoyu, and miso, are to be used moderately in order to avoid unnecessary thirst. Avoid mirin and garlic. If you become particularly thirsty after a meal or between meals, you should cut back on these seasonings until the normal level of thirst returns.

• **Beverages:** Beverages and other dietary practices can follow the general recommendations in Part I, including bancha twig tea as the main beverage. Strictly avoid the beverages on the "infrequent" and "avoid" list and don't take grain coffee for the first two to three months after starting this new way of eating.

The most important thing in connection with dietary practice is chewing very well, until all food becomes liquid in the mouth and well mixed with saliva. Chew very, very well, at least 50 times, preferably 100 times, per mouthful. It is also important to avoid overeating and eating within three hours of sleeping.

As noted in the introduction to Part II, persons who have received or who are currently undergoing medical treatment may need to make further dietary modifications.

SPECIAL DRINKS AND PREPARATIONS

Persons with leukemia may also consume some special drinks and dishes, which, taken in small volume, can strength blood quality. These dishes include:

• **Sweet Vegetable Drink:** Take one small cup every day for the first month, then every third day the second month.

• **Ume-Sho-Kuzu Drink:** Take one small cup every two days for two weeks, then one cup a day for three to four weeks.

- **Aduki Bean Tea:** Take once a day for ten days, then twice a week for two or three more weeks.
- **Shio-Kombu (Salty Kombu):** Sliced sheets of kombu (about one-half-inch square), cooked in a mixture of one-half shoyu and one-half water and boiled down until the liquid becomes completely absorbed by the kombu (usually two to four hours). Consume several pieces daily with cereal grain dishes.
- **Carp and Burdock Soup (Koi Koku):** For energy or to restore vitality, whole carp cooked with shredded burdock roots, seasoned with miso and a little grated ginger. This soup may be used as the soup dish a few times a week for a period of several weeks. See the recipe in Part III.
- **Brown Rice Cream:** In the event of appetite loss, two to three bowls of genuine brown rice cream can be served daily with a condiment of either gomashio (sesame salt), umeboshi plum, or tekka. This rice cream may also be used occasionally as part of the regular whole-grain diet.

HOME CARES

- **Body Scrub:** Scrubbing the whole body, including the abdominal region and the spinal region, with a towel that has been immersed in hot water and squeezed out is very helpful for better circulation of blood, lymph, and other body fluids, as well as for activating physical and mental energies.
- Swelling of the spleen and abdominal regions sometimes accompanies leukemia and is caused by overeating in general, especially protein and fat, and excessive intake of beverages, seasonings, and condiments. In such cases, food consumption should be simplified for a period of several days up to ten days. During this period, daily consumption may consist of pressure-cooked brown rice and barley, one to two cups of miso soup, a small dish of half-dried daikon and daikon leaves pickled for a long period (over two months) with sea salt and rice bran, a dish of vegetables such as onions, carrots, and cabbage sautéed in sesame oil, and several cups of bancha twig tea. However, this simplified diet should not be continued for longer than ten days unless under supervision of an experienced macrobiotic teacher or medical associate.

OTHER CONSIDERATIONS

- General physical exercise and deep breathing exercises are recommended, especially outside in the fresh air. Shiatsu massage and other treatments to relax and loosen any physical and psychological stagnations and hardenings are also very helpful.
- Maintaining clean, fresh air inside the home is important, and for this purpose green plants can be placed in each room. Indoor air circulation can also be maintained by frequently opening the windows.
- Wearing cotton underwear and avoiding synthetic fabrics are helpful for better skin metabolism and facilitate energy flow through the body.
- Avoid exposure to artificial electromagnetic radiation. Keep common hand-held appliances to a minimum. If you have a choice, work and live in areas away from an electronic environment.

PERSONAL EXPERIENCE

Leukemia

Christina Pirello and her mother were very close. When Christina's mother was diagnosed with colon cancer in 1982, Christina thought nothing worse could happen. But following her mother's death two years later, Christina's life was turned upside down. "I watched as conventional methods of treatment hastened her deterioration," Christina recalls. "Watching her suffer more with each treatment strengthened my conviction to seek out alternate treatments should I ever find myself in a similar situation. Interestingly, one of her doctors mentioned macrobiotics to me, but it was too late for her, and I forgot all about it."

Growing up, Christina seemed relatively healthy, though she suffered Mediterranean anemia as a child. She always had a hard time healing cuts and scratches and bruised easily. In her teenage years, her menstrual cycle was irregular and she began hormone treatments that continued for fifteen years.

At age fourteen, Christina became vegetarian. She stopped eating meat but ate lots of dairy foods, sugar, and refined foods. After her mother's death, her fatigue worsened and she felt constantly drained. Meanwhile bruises began to appear everywhere on her body and she felt "as though my insides were on fire."

Seeking a new environment, she moved from Florida north to Philadelphia, but the susceptibility to bruises and infection continued. Finally, a doctor put her through a series of medical tests and diagnosed her condition as CML. The specialists were not helpful. With experimental chemotherapy and a possible bone-marrow transplant, they told her she could live six months to a year. Without treatment, they told her she could expect to survive three months.

Not wanting to repeat her mother's experience, Christina sought an alternative, and a friend introduced her to Robert Pirello, who had been practicing macrobiotics for eight years. Bob helped her clean out her kitchen and gave her a copy of The Cancer Prevention Diet, "telling me to read and cook. I read all night."

Within a few weeks, Christina's energy had returned and gradually her blood tests began to improve. Over the next few months, she experienced several major discharges, as her body began to rid itself of toxins accumulated in past years. "Although the discharge was always unpleasant and almost impossible to bear, I knew I was improving," Christina recounts. "Each blood test revealed an improvement in my white cell count. The doctors were amazed." Thirteen months after she began practicing macrobiotics, her white blood cell count returned to normal, and for the last nine years Christina has been completely free of leukemia.

She and Bob Pirello went on to marry, and today they are leaders of the macrobiotic community in Philadelphia, giving cooking classes, organizing seminars, and pushing MacroNews, one of the nation's major macrobiotic publications.

Source: Christina Pirello, "Macrobiotics: Getting Started," MacroNews, January/February 1990.

24

Lymphatic
Cancer:
Lymphoma and
Hodgkin's
Disease

FREQUENCY

Cancer of the lymphatic system will kill 20,900 Americans this year, while 48,400 new cases will develop. Deaths from Hodgkin's disease have fallen by about two-thirds over the last thirty years, while those from other kinds of lymphoma have risen by almost the same amount.

Lymphoma affects men and women about evenly and is usually divided into two types: *Hodgkin's disease*, which particularly affects people aged fifteen to twenty-four and over fifty, usually involves enlarged lymph nodes in the neck, armpit, or groin. It often spreads to the brain and adjacent lymph nodes. Depending on the case, it is treated with radiation and chemotherapy. A battery of four drugs is commonly given to control Hodgkin's disease, known as MOPP (nitrogen mustard, Oncovin, procarbazine, and prednisone). Between 53 to 57 percent of those with Hodgkin's disease survive five years or longer. *Non-Hodgkin's lymphomas* are divided into eight major types depending on the type of cells affected and their state of differentiation. This form of lymphoma may appear throughout the body and in sites other than the lymph nodes, such as the digestive tract. Non-Hodgkin's lymphomas metastasize in erratic manners. Radiation and chemotherapy are major methods of treatment. Depending on the type, the remission rate for these eight lymphomas is between 18 and 37 percent. There are also several rarer forms of lymphoma such as mycosis fungoides and Burkitt's lymphoma.

STRUCTURE

The lymphatic system consists of lymph capillaries, vessels, ducts, and nodes, as well as such organs as the spleen and tonsils. The lymphatic system is closely related to the blood system. When blood circulates, some of the fluid and other elements in the blood leak out due to the enormous pressure the blood is under. This clear liquid or lymph accumulates between the cells and blood capillaries. The lymph system transports this substance through a network of small, clear tubes and rejoins with the bloodstream near the collarbone. In structure, the bloodstream is generally more yang, since its main function is to transport red blood cells. The lymph stream, consisting primarily of white blood cells, is more yin. Both comprise the circulatory system as a whole and circulate in opposite yet complementary directions. Blood circulation begins in the heart, radiates outward to the more peripheral regions, and then returns. Conversely, the flow of lymph begins in the peripheral body tissues and then enters the central bloodstream.

Unlike the bloodstream, the lymphatic system has no central organ to pump the lymph fluid. The flow of lymph is maintained by several factors such as the activity and contraction of the lungs and diaphragm during breathing and the movements of the villi and the contractions of the small intestine. The spleen is the major organ of the lymphatic system. Located opposite the liver on the left side of the body, the spleen filters substances like bacteria and worn-out red blood cells from the lymph and body fluid. The spleen contributes to the formation of white blood cells, especially lymphocytes; stores blood and minerals, particularly iron; produces antibodies; and contributes to the production of bile. The liver and spleen are complementary. The liver is yang (compact) in comparison and functions in coordination with the bloodstream. The more yin (expanded) spleen serves as the major focus of the lymphatic system.

Also associated with the lymph are the tonsils. The main function of the tonsils is to localize various types of toxic excess for discharging from the body. For example, after consumption of an extreme food, such as an excessive volume of sugar, oil, fats, soft drinks, fruits, juices, refined flour, or chemicals, additional white blood cells are created in the tonsils to neutralize any harmful bacteria that may form in the lymph, while minerals start to gather in this region as a buffer for the discharge of acids. In the meantime the tonsils may become inflamed and the body temperature may rise. If, at this time, the person has the tonsils removed, the fever and inflammation may disappear, but the toxic bodily fluids will continue to circulate throughout the system, and the remaining lymphatic organs will have to work much harder to perform the cleaning and discharge function of the tonsils. The net result is a reduction in the ability of the lymphatic system to efficiently rid the body of toxic excess.

The lymphatic system also contains another major organ, which is located above the heart. Known as the thymus, this organ reaches its largest size at the age of two and then gradually declines until it disappears entirely. The thymus produces white blood cells along with certain types of antibodies.

CAUSE OF CANCER

If the bloodstream is filled with fat and mucus, which are strong in acid, excess will begin to accumulate in the organs. Since the lungs and kidneys are usually affected first, their functions of filtering and cleansing the blood become less efficient. This situation leads to further deterioration of the blood quality and also affects the lymphatic system. General lymphatic troubles can be summarized into two types. The first involves expansion or inflammation of the lymphatic nodes and organs. In extreme cases, this overly yin condition leads to a rupture of the lymphatic vessels. These problems result when the lymph fluid contains too much fatty acid. The other, more yang condition is hardening of the lymph nodes, organs, ducts, and capillaries.

As we have seen, operations such as tonsillectomies contribute to the deterioration of the lymphatic system, since they reduce the ability of this system to cleanse itself. Swollen tonsils and lymph glands result from overconsumption of refined and artificial foods, sugar, soft drinks, tropical fruits and vegetables, milk and dairy products, spices, and other extreme foods from the yin category usually higher in acid. These swellings represent a healthy reaction of the body to localize, neutralize, and discharge this excess. Continued consumption of these foods may produce a chronic deterioration of the quality of the blood and lymph. When the red blood cells begin to lose their capacity to change into normal body cells, the body starts to create a degenerate type of cell that is known as cancerous.

In Hodgkin's disease the lymph nodes and spleen become inflamed, while in lymphomas a malignant tumor develops within the lymphoid tissue and the lymphatic organs become swollen. Both diseases involve an increase in the number of white blood cells. Excessive intake of yin type foods and beverages is the main cause of lymphatic cancers. At the same time a decrease in the number of red blood cells reflects a lack of minerals and other balanced foods centered around natural complex carbohydrate in the diet. Compared to other forms of cancer, especially tumors in the deep, inner organs, lymphatic cancer and leukemia are relatively easy to relieve.

MEDICAL EVIDENCE

• In a 1975 study, French researchers reported that children with chronic radiation enteritis markedly improved on a low-fat diet free of gluten, cow's milk, and milk products. The eleven-year study followed forty-four children, twenty-nine of whom had advanced lymphoma and eleven who had Wilms' tumor. The mean age of the subjects was three years, ten months. Forty-two of the children had received cobalt treatments for cancer resulting in intestinal injury prior to starting the diet. Source: S. S. Donaldson et al., "Radiation Enteritis in Children," *Cancer* 35:1167–78.

• Persons who regularly eat cereal grains, pulses, vegetables, seeds, and nuts are less likely to get lymphoma or Hodgkin's disease than persons who do not usually eat these foods, according to a 1976 epidemiological survey. The sixteen-nation study, based on World Health Organization statistics, found a high correlation between consumption of animal protein, particularly from beef and dairy products, and lymphoma mortality. "Ingestion of cow's milk can produce generalised lymphadenopathy, hepatoslenomegaly, and profound adenoid hypertrophy," the researcher commented on the mechanism of carcinogenesis. "It has been conservatively estimated that more than 100 distinct antigens are released by the normal digestion of cow's milk, which may evoke production of all antibody classes." The studies indicated that beef and dairy food increased the risk of lymphosarcoma and Hodgkin's disease by 70 and 61 percent respectively, while cereal grains lowered the risk by 46 and 38 percent. Source: A. S. Cunningham, "Lymphomas and Animal-Protein Consumption," *Lancet* 2:1184–86.

• The average American eats nine pounds of chemical additives a year, including preservatives, flavoring agents, stabilizers, and artificial colors. Red Dye No. 40, found in imitation fruit drinks, soda pop, hot dogs, jellies, candy, ice cream, and some cosmetics, has been linked to lymphomas in laboratory experiments. Source: Samuel S. Epstein, M.D., *The Politics of Cancer* (New York: Doubleday, 1979), 186–87.

• A California physician reported to a scientific panel on cancer and diet that a high-protein diet reduces the immune mechanism of the body by its action on the T-lymphocyte cell. A diet high in animal products also increases the blood lipids and cholesterol. This, in turn, produces an increased susceptibility to viral infections, a decrease in antibody response, and a decrease in T-cell response, which helps protect against lymphoma. Source: J. A. Scharffenberg, M.D., *Health Consequences of a Good Lifestyle*, American Association for the Advancement of Science, 1981.

• Mice on a low-calorie diet live longer and have a reduced risk of cancer, including lymphoma, than mice on a high-calorie diet. Two UCLA medical researchers reported in 1982 that laboratory animals fed 28 to 43 percent less calories than a control group lived 10 to 20 percent longer and registered fewer tumors of the lymphatic system. Source: R. Weindruch and R. L. Wolford, "Dietary Restriction in Mice Beginning at One Year of Age," *Science* 215:1415–18.

• A 1986 study by the NCI found that farm workers in Kansas who were exposed to herbicides for more than twenty days per year had a six times higher risk of developing non-Hodgkin's lymphoma than nonfarm workers. Source: S. K. Hoar et al., "Agricultural Herbicide Use and the Risk of Lymphomas and Soft-Tissue Sarcoma," *Journal of the American Medical Association* 256:1141–47.

• Exposure to the herbicide (2,4-Dichlorophenoxy) acetic acid (2,4-D) more than twenty days by farm workers in Nebraska increased the risk of developing non-Hodgkin's lymphoma threefold. Source: S. K. Hoar et al., "A Case-Control Study of Non-Hodgkin's Lymphoma and Agricultural Factors in Eastern Nebraska," *American Journal of Epidemiology* 128:901.

DIAGNOSIS

Hodgkin's disease is diagnosed medically by laboratory tests and usually involves surgical removal of a lymph node to be examined under a microscope for malignancy. If the nodes are not involved, a variety of other methods will be used, including a bone-marrow biopsy, lymphangiogram, IVP, liver, spleen, and bone scans, and abdominal or chest CAT scan. In some cases the abdominal wall may be opened surgically for inspection and the spleen will be removed in an operation known as a splenectomy. For non-Hodgkin's lymphomas, an upper and lower GI series is taken, and a spinal tap will be performed to check for metastases to the brain.

Oriental diagnosis focuses primarily on visual features, especially colors, to ascertain the condition of the lymphatic system. A pinkish-white color on the lips indicates weakening lymphatic functions and other disorders, including a tendency toward Hodgkin's disease. This color is caused by excessive consumption of dairy products, fats, sugar, and fruits. A reddish-yellow color inside the lower eyelids shows disorder in the circulatory system, including the spleen function. This color is caused by excessive intake of foods from the extreme yang category, such as poultry, eggs, and dairy products, as well as excess yin type foods, including sugar, fruits, and chemicals.

A white tone to the skin generally indicates contraction of blood capillaries and tissues and inner-organ problems, especially spleen and lymph disorders. This color is caused by excessive yang intake, especially animal food rich in fat, all dairy products, or the overconsumption of salts and minerals. A pale color on the face often arises with a light green shade or tone in the case of lymphoma and Hodgkin's disease due to a lack of balanced minerals and an overall anemic condition.

The temples on the head correspond to the functions of the spleen and other inner organs. Green vessels appearing in this region show abnormal lymph circulation due to an overactive spleen or underactive gallbladder and are caused by excessive fluid and sugar, fats and oils, alcohol and stimulants, and other extreme foods and beverages from the yin category.

The outer layer of the ear shows circulatory and excretory systems. If this area has an abnormally red color, except during vigorous exercise or after being outside in cold weather, it indicates lymphatic and spleen disorders. If the whole nose, not only the tip area, is reddish in color from expansion of the blood capillaries, disorders are indicated also in the spleen and lymph system.

By observing a combination of these and other signs, potential lymph diseases, including cancer, can be detected long before they reach the chronic or degenerative stages and appropriate dietary adjustments be made.

DIETARY RECOMMENDATIONS

The major cause of lymphoma and Hodgkin's disease is the long-time, continuous consumption of foods and beverages in the extreme yin category, including dairy food of all kinds, sweets, including sugar, sugar-treated foods and drinks. All of these should be avoided in daily eating. However, the consumption of these items is often accompanied by the intake of foods from the extreme yang category, including chicken and eggs, meat, poultry, and cheese, in order to achieve a rough counterbalance. Accordingly, all these animal foods are also to be avoided, with the exception of fish and seafood, which can be consumed occasionally in small volume. Although they are not the direct cause, the following enhance lymphomic conditions and should also be discontinued: ice-cold food and drinks, hot, stimulant, and aromatic spices, various herbs and herb drinks that have stimulant effects, and vegetables that historically originated in the tropics, including potatoes, tomatoes, and eggplant. These nightshade plants especially enhance Hodgkin's disease. In preparing food, beware of using an excessive volume of oil. However, after the first month, during which no oil should be used, a reasonable amount of unrefined vegetable oil may frequently be used in sautéeing vegetables. No raw, uncooked foods should be eaten. For lymphatic cancer, it is extremely important to avoid overconsumption of food. Eat less and chew very, very well.

The dietary recommendations for younger children with lymphatic cancer are included in the chapter on children's cancer and those with AIDS-related lymphoma in the chapter on AIDS. Following are daily dietary guidelines, by volume, for the prevention and relief of lymphoma in older children or adults:

• **Whole Grains:** Fifty to 60 percent of daily consumption, by volume, should be whole-cereal grains. The first day prepare plain pressure-cooked short-grain brown rice. On following days, prepare brown rice pressure-cooked with 20 to 30 percent millet, then rice with 20 to 30 percent barley, then rice with 20 to 30 percent aduki beans or lentils, and then plain rice again. A delicious morning porridge can be made by taking leftover rice, adding a little more water to soften, and seasoning with a little miso at the end and simmering for two to three minutes more. In ordinary pressure cooking, the ratio of grain to water should be about 1:2. For seasoning, cook with a postage stamp–sized piece of kombu or a pinch of sea salt, depending on the person's condition. After the first month, once or twice a week these grains can be prepared in the form of fried grains with vegetables. Other grains can be used occasionally, including whole wheat berries, rye, corn, and whole oats, though oats should be avoided for the first month. Buckwheat and seitan should be minimized. Good-quality sourdough bread may be enjoyed two to three times a week, and noodles, both udon and soba, may also be taken two to three times a week. Avoid all hard baked products until the condition improves, including cookies, cake, pie, crackers, muffins, and the like.

• **Soup:** Five to 10 percent soup, consisting of one or two cups or bowls per day of soup cooked with wakame sea vegetable and various land vegetables such as onions and carrots and seasoned with miso or shoyu. Occasionally a small volume of shiitake mushroom may be added to the soup. Lotus root should be used often in soup. The miso may be barley miso, brown rice miso, or soybean (hatcho) miso and should be naturally aged two to three years. To satisfy a sweet tooth, millet soup with sweet vegetables such as squash, cabbage, onions, and carrots may be prepared often.

• **Vegetables:** Twenty to 30 percent vegetables, cooked in a variety of forms. Dishes can be prepared in various ways using round vegetables together with root vegetables, such as carrots, burdock, daikon, and turnip. Unlike in diets for some other cancers, some dishes may be sautéed with a moderate volume of sesame or corn oil, though vegetables should also be cooked frequently using other methods. However, for the first month avoid oil altogether. As a general rule, the following dishes may be prepared, though the frequency may differ from person to person: nishime-style vegetables, four times a week; squash-aduki-kombu dish, three times a week; dried daikon, one cup, three times a week; carrots and carrot tops or daikon and daikon tops, three times a week; blanched vegetables, five to seven times a week; pressed salad, five to seven times a week; raw salad and salad dressing, avoid; steamed greens, five to seven times a week; kinpira, two-thirds of a cup, two times a week; dried tofu, tofu, tempeh, or seitan with vegetables, two times a week.

• **Beans:** Five percent small beans, such as aduki beans, lentils, chickpeas, or black soybeans, may be used daily, cooked together with sea vegetables such as kombu or with onions and carrots. Other beans may be used altogether two to three times a month. For seasoning, a small volume of unrefined sea salt or shoyu or miso can be used. Bean products, such as tempeh, natto, and dried or cooked tofu, may be used occasionally, but in moderate volume.

• **Sea Vegetables:** Five percent or less sea vegetable dishes, including wakame and kombu, daily when cooking grain, in soup, etc. A sheet of toasted nori may also be taken daily. A small dish of hijiki or arame should be prepared two times a week. All other sea vegetables are optional. Sea vegetables can be cooked with other vegetables or sautéed with a small volume of sesame oil after softening them by soaking and boiling lightly in water.

• **Condiments:** Condiments to be available on the table are gomashio (sesame salt), on the average made with 1 part salt to 18 parts sesame seeds (reduced to 1:16 after two months); kelp or wakame powder; umeboshi plum; and tekka, though all other regular macrobiotic condiments may be used if desired. These condiments may be used daily on grains and vegetables, but the volume should be moderate to suit individual appetite and taste.

• **Pickles:** Pickles, made at home in a variety of ways, are to be eaten daily, one tablespoon in all, though salty pickles are to be minimized.

• **Animal Food:** Meat, poultry, eggs, and other strong animal food is to be avoided. A small volume of white-meat fish may be eaten once a week. The fish should be prepared steamed, boiled, or poached and garnished with grated daikon or ginger. After two months, fish may be eaten twice a week if desired. Strictly avoid blue-meat and red-meat fish and all shellfish.

• **Fruit:** None the best, the less the better, including both tropical and temperate-climate fruit, until the condition improves. If cravings develop, a small volume of cooked fruit with a pinch of sea salt or dried fruit (also preferably cooked) may be taken. Avoid all fruit juices and cider.

• **Sweets and Snacks:** Avoid all sweets and desserts, including good-quality macrobiotic desserts, until the condition improves. To satisfy a sweet tooth, use sweet vegetables every day in cooking, drink sweet vegetable drink (see special drinks below), or make sweet vegetable jam. Mochi, rice balls, vegetable sushi, and other grain-based snacks may be eaten frequently. Limit rice cakes, popcorn, and other dry or baked snacks, as they may harden the tumor. In the event of cravings, a small volume of amasake, barley malt, or rice syrup may be taken.

• **Nuts and Seeds:** Nuts and nut butters are to be avoided due to their high amount of fat and protein, except for chestnuts. Unsalted, roasted seeds such as sunflower seeds and pumpkin seeds my be consumed as a snack, up to one cup altogether per week.

• **Seasonings:** Seasonings, such as unrefined sea salt, shoyu, and miso, are to be used moderately in order to avoid unnecessary thirst. Avoid mirin and garlic. If you become particularly thirsty after a meal or between meals, you should cut back on these seasonings until the normal level of thirst returns.

• **Beverages:** Beverages and other dietary practices can follow the general recommendations in Part I, including bancha twig tea as the main beverage. Strictly avoid the beverages on the "infrequent" and "avoid" list and don't take grain coffee for the first two to three months after starting this new way of eating.

The most important thing in connection with dietary practice is chewing very well, until all food becomes liquid in the mouth and well mixed with saliva. Chew very, very well, at least 50 times, preferably 100 times, per mouthful. It is also important to avoid overeating and eating within three hours of sleeping.

As noted in the introduction to Part II, persons who have received or who are currently undergoing medical treatment may need to make further dietary modifications.

SPECIAL DRINKS AND PREPARATIONS

Persons with lymphatic cancer may also consume some special drinks and dishes, which, taken in small volume, can strengthen blood quality. These dishes include:

• **Sweet Vegetable Drink:** Take one small cup every day for the first month, then two to three times a week the second month, and then occasionally as desired.

• **Carrot-Daikon Drink:** Take one small cup two to three times a week for two to four weeks and then once every three days for one month.

• **Lotus-Carrot Drink:** Take one small cup every two or three days for four to six weeks. When soft, you can eat the lotus. Prepare by cooking fresh lotus root that has been chopped with an equal volume of grated carrots, add an equal volume of water, simmer, and use the liquid as tea. Alternatively, you can add kombu to this mixture, about 25 percent by volume, and, toward the end of cooking, season with a few drops of shoyu.

• **Ume-Sho-Kuzu Drink:** For energy or vitality, if needed, make one small cup every two or three days for ten days to two weeks, then two times a week for three to four weeks.

• **Grated Daikon:** Grate about one-half a small cup of fresh daikon, add a few drops of shoyu, and take two to three times a week.

• **Fasting:** Swelling of the spleen and abdominal regions sometimes accompanies lymphatic cancer and is caused by overeating in general, especially protein, and excessive intake of beverages, seasonings, and condiments. In such cases, food consumption should be simplified for a period of several days up to ten days. During this period, daily consumption may consist of pressure-cooked brown rice and barley, one to two cups of miso soup, a small dish of half dried daikon and half daikon leaves pickled for a long period (over two months) with sea salt and rice bran, a dish of vegetables such as onions, carrots, and cabbage sautéed in sesame oil, and several cups of bancha twig tea. However, this simplified diet should not be continued for longer than ten days unless under supervision of an experienced macrobiotic teacher or medical associate.

HOME CARES

• **Body Scrub:** Scrubbing the whole body, including the abdominal region and the spinal region, with a towel that has been immersed in hot water and squeezed out is very helpful for better circulation of blood, lymph, and other body fluids, as well as for activating physical and mental energies.

• **Compress Guidelines:** For a small number of lymphatic tumors, a compress may be needed to gradually help draw out excess mucus and fat. Please see qualified macrobiotic teacher for guidance on the proper use and frequency of a compress or plaster. Several types are used, depending on the person's condition. Precede the compress or plaster with application of a towel that has been soaked in hot water and squeezed out over the affected area for about three to five minutes to stimulate circulation.

• **Tofu–Green Vegetable Plaster:** A plaster of mashed tofu mixed with the same volume of mashed green leafy vegetables is recommended for swollen glands and inflammation of the spleen.

• **Buckwheat Plaster:** A plaster of buckwheat flour kneaded with warm water or green clay may also be applied to inflamed lymph nodes or glands to help reduce the swelling.

• **Sweating:** If sweating occurs at night, relief can be provided by eating a small volume of sliced burdock roots and carrot roots, sautéed with sesame oil and seasoned with shoyu.

• **Bathing:** Hot baths and showers should be taken quickly. Soaking the body for a long time in the tub causes the body to lose important minerals.

OTHER CONSIDERATIONS

• Good exercise is strengthening to the lymph and circulatory systems, but do not exercise to the point of exhaustion. Deep bathing exercises, massage, and tai chi–type movements are generally preferable to strenuous activities. Walking is excellent.

• Maintaining clean, fresh air inside the home is important, and for this purpose green plants can be placed in each room. Indoor air circulation can also be maintained by frequently opening the windows.

• Wearing cotton underwear and avoiding synthetic fabrics are helpful for better skin metabolism and facilitate energy flow through the body.

• Avoid exposure to artificial electromagnetic radiation. Keep common hand-held appliances to a minimum. If you have a choice, work and live in areas away from an electronic environment.

• Avoid frequent exposure to artificial radiation, including medical and dental X rays, smoke detectors, television, and video terminals, which are weakening to the lymph and blood.

• Try to be happy, positive, and outgoing. Singing, dancing, and playing are particularly beneficial for improving overall health and mentality and harmonizing with the rhythms of nature.

PERSONAL EXPERIENCE

Hodgkin's Disease

In January 1973 nineteen-year-old Maureen Duney of Belle Mead, New Jersey, discovered a lump in the right side of her throat. In April a biopsy of the lymph node gland proved malignant, and doctors at Memorial Hospital in New York diagnosed her condition as Hodgkin's disease, stage III B.

In June Maureen began radiation therapy, and by August the tumors were dispersed. However, in March 1975 she noticed a thickening in the intestinal area to the left of the navel, and tests showed that the cancer had come back. There was also a tumor on the last rib on her left side.

In September 1975 Maureen began experimental chemotherapy, but after one month friends persuaded her to try macrobiotics. At the end of the month, Maureen came to see me, and I recommended the Cancer Prevention Diet and an application of a ginger compress to the spleen and rib areas.

"Mr. Kushi projected that I would be cured in four to six months," she recorded. "I took the information back to my parents, family, and doctors. I began cooking and eating macrobiotically immediately. From September following my first treatment of MOPP [chemotherapy], my sediment rate was 42; in November, after eating macrobiotically for two months, it had dropped to a normal count of 14. I felt alive again, was active daily, my strength increased, and my hair stopped falling out."

Prior to this time, Maureen had always been a poor eater. She did not eat as much meat but, in her words, "devoured sweets, ice cream, fruits, liquids, hoagies, and pizza." By early 1976 the Hodgkin's disease was gone, and she no longer suffered from itching or night sweating. "I consume none of the foods that caused my illness at the first," she concluded. "I continue to eat macrobiotically gratefully every day." Source: *Case History Reports*, Vol. 1, no. 3 (Boston: East West Foundation, 1976), 5–7.

Hodgkin's Disease

Emily Bellew, a resident of Columbus, Ohio, was twenty-two and had been married for three years. She was expecting her first child but had a very difficult pregnancy and delivery. She gained 80 pounds, ballooning up to 205 pounds, and craved large amounts of ice cream, red meat, and anything else she could find.

Three days after the birth of her son, Bryan, Emily experienced a swollen and stiff neck. She attributed it to holding him in the wrong position. During her postpartum checkup, a few weeks later, she mentioned the sore neck to her doctor. Medical tests found that she had Hodgkin's disease, stage II B.

For the next several months Emily underwent radiation treatment. But her condition worsened. The cancer spread to the lower portion of the hipbone, and she had to use a wheelchair. Following chemotherapy treatments for the next several months, the cancer in the hip cleared up, but it had spread to the abdomen. This was followed by another round of chemo and discovery of a lump in the groin. After two and half years of treatment, Emily came across a book on macrobiotics and decided that she had nothing to lose. Doctors had now told her that she could expect to live several more months, a year at most.

Emily came to see me where I was giving a seminar. "The next three days changed my life," she recalled. "I heard lectures and attended cooking classes. I also began to eat macrobiotic food for the first time. I took new knowledge and new cookbooks back home and began cooking. I started to feel the difference right away, and it was all so really simple. This was the way our bodies were meant to be nourished."

Within a year, the tumors went away and doctors could find no trace of cancer. Within two more years, her weight stabilized at 113 pounds. It is now nine years since Emily walked away from the hospital to begin the "Great Life."

Source: Ann Fawcett and the East West Foundation, *Cancer-free: 30 Who Triumphed over Cancer Naturally*, (New York and Tokyo: Japan Publications, 1991).

25

Brain Cancer

FREQUENCY

Brain tumors and cancer of the central nervous system will kill an estimated 11,800 Americans this year, and 16,900 new cases will develop. Men between age fifty and sixty are most at risk, but between 1958 and 1988 the death rate increased almost 25 percent for both sexes. Brain tumors are on the rise in children and now account for about 35 percent of all cancer deaths in both males and females under fifteen. Brain cancer is also on the rise among the elderly, with the incidence of brain tumors more than doubling from 1968 to 1985. For people over eighty, the rate of increase was even more dramatic, soaring 300 to 400 percent over this period, or as much as 23 percent a year. This trend appears to be global, with deaths from brain tumors rising 500 percent in Italy, England, and Wales, and up to 200 percent in France, Germany, and Japan.

A majority of brain tumors affect the brain tissue itself and are called gliomas. These are subdivided into four main types: 1) *glioblastoma multiforme*, a malignant tumor affecting both children and adults and one that may spread quickly through the cerebrum, cerebellum, brain stem, and spinal cord; 2) *astrocytoma*, a tumor found mostly in children, affecting the cerebellum and brain stem; 3) *ependymoma*, another childhood tumor, which grows in the ventricles of the brain; 4) *oligodendroglioma*, a slow-growing tumor that affects the white matter in the frontal lobe and is found in both children and adults.

Other brain tumors include *medulloblastoma*, a childhood cancer that spreads from the cerebellum to other regions of the brain and central nervous system; *meningioma*, a tumor affecting the membrane covering the brain and spinal cord; *pituitary adenoma*, a tumor that affects the hypothalamus and optic nerve; *gaulioneuroblastoma*, a malignancy that spreads quickly through the nerve cells; *neurofibrosarcoma*, a cancer affecting the peripheral nervous system; and *neuroblastoma*, a tumor that affects children three years old or younger and spreads through the nervous network in various regions including the chest, neck, abdomen, lower back, eye, and adrenal glands. About 15 percent of brain tumors have metastasized from other organs, especially the lungs, kidney, breast, or the lymph nodes in the case of Hodgkin's disease.

Because of their location within one of the most sensitive parts of the body, many brain tumors are considered untreatable by modern science. However, depending on the type and staging, surgery and radiation therapy are often employed. The operation is called a craniotomy and involves removing part of the skull, removing the malignant tissue, and putting back the excised bone. The risk of damaging the brain during such a procedure is high.

When surgery is ruled out, radiation is commonly used, especially for medulloblastomas and ependymomas. However, X ray treatments may cause permanent damage to the spinal cord, especially in children. Hormone therapy is sometimes used in conjunction with surgery to decrease the swelling or control metastases. Steroids are given and followed up by drugs such as prednisone, which may be administered intravenously or intramuscularly for the rest of the patient's life. Other methods of treating brain tumors include hypothermia (lowering the temperature of the brain or body), cryosurgery (freezing), and implanting radiosensitizers to enhance radiation therapy. The present survival rate for all forms of brain tumors is 25 percent for males and 33 percent for females.

STRUCTURE

The human nervous system has two anatomical divisions: the central nervous system, which includes the brain and spinal cord, and the peripheral nervous system, which includes all of the nervous structures outside of the skull and vertebral canal, such as the craniospinal nerves and the orthosympathetic branch of the autonomic nervous system. The central nervous system acts as a switchboard for incoming impulses from receptors and outgoing impulses to effectors; it regulates all body activities except for chemically controlled ones and is the seat for the higher consciousness processes.

The autonomic nervous system is not considered to be an anatomical division, but a functional unit, which handles the involuntary, unconscious body activities, such as the beating of the heart, breathing, digestive peristalsis, and so on. The autonomic system is, in turn, composed of two antagonistic branches: the parasympathetic (yang) and the orthosympathetic (yin). The parasympathetic nerves have a more central position of origin in the body, beginning in the brain stem and sacral region of the spinal cord and passing outward through four pairs of cranial nerves and three pairs of sacral nerves. The orthosympathetic nerves have a more peripheral position, beginning in the central section of the spine and passing outward through the corresponding spinal nerves. In almost all organs, tissues, and smooth muscles, there are pairs of autonomic nerves, one ortho- and one parasympathetic, which act in opposite ways. When the parasympathetic nerves act on expanded (yin) organs, such as the bronchi of the lungs or the wall of the digestive tract, there is naturally a resultant contraction. Their action on compact organs (yang), such as the iris of the eye or cardiac muscles, brings about expansion or dilation. The orthosympathetic nerves have a complementary, opposite effect. They inhibit hollow organs, such as the bladder, and stimulate compact ones, such as the uterus, during pregnancy.

The two major divisions of the brain are the large forebrain, including the cerebrum, and the more compact hindbrain, including the cerebellum. Since the forebrain is more open and expanded, it is classified as yin, while the smaller, more compact hindbrain is yang. The brain can also be divided into its more central region, known as the midbrain, and more peripheral region, called the cortex. In order for communication to proceed smoothly, incoming and outgoing impulses need to be balanced. Within the brain, the more compact or central regions tend to be areas where images and impulses are received, while outgoing communication originates in the more peripheral or expanded areas. Thus nervous impulses from the eyes, ears, nose, skin, and other sense organs gather in the midbrain, while images, dreams, and thoughts are dispatched outward from the more peripheral cortex regions. Also in terms of receiving and dispatching, the hindbrain receives incoming vibrations and stores them as memory, while outgoing vibrations, including our images of the future, arise in the forebrain.

CAUSE OF CANCER

In the last several years there has been considerable research concerning the relationship between the right and left hemispheres of the brain. Studies show that the right hemisphere in most people is the origin of more simple or mechanical action and consciousness, while the left hemisphere produces more complex and creative thinking. In terms of language, more simple or basic expressions originate in the right hemisphere, while the left hemisphere creates more refined and original expression. Imagination, which is based mostly on futuristic thinking, develops more in the left hemisphere, while analytical thinking, based more on actual past experiences, arises in the right hemisphere.

Our modern technological civilization has arisen due to the active development of right-hemisphere thinking. This more focused, yang type of thinking and activity has resulted from a way of eating centered around meat, dairy food, and other animal products. Imbalance in one direction produces a corresponding pull in the other. To balance the increasing amounts of food, modern society has witnessed a proliferation of extreme substances in the yin category, including alcohol, spices, coffee and other stimulants, refined sugar, imported tropical fruits and vegetables, chemical additives, and a variety of drugs, including tranquilizers, birth-control pills, and hallucinogens.

Within many modern countries, especially during the last fifteen or twenty years, young people have been exposed to these types of food from birth, and many have experimented and become regular users of marijuana, hashish, cocaine, or LSD. These extremely yin substances have produced a rapid shift in thinking from the right side of the brain, which is predominant in modern society, toward the left side, and also from the back of the brain more toward the front. As a result, many young people started looking more toward the future, while neglecting or forgetting previous traditions, including the relationship with their parents, elders, and ancestors. Similarly, they lost interest in school, business or professional careers, and the political and economic condition of society. Instead they turned to music, the arts, spiritual teachers from the East, and other nonlinear pursuits.

In many cases, the continuous intake of yin-type foods and drugs has led to very unbalanced conditions and expression. By moving to the other extreme, vegetarians who eat primarily fruits, juices, and raw foods, and members of the psychedelic counterculture risk a variety of illnesses. These include mental disease, herpes, multiple sclerosis, leukemia, and brain cancer.

Tumors that affect the outer regions of the brain or the nerve cells of the peripheral nervous system are caused primarily by foods, drinks, and medications or drugs in the yin category. These forms of brain malfunction or nervous disorders are more commonly found in children or young adults who have grown up on sugar-coated breakfast cereals, honey, chocolate, and other sweeteners, orange juice, soda pop, ice cream, and oily and greasy foods, as well as many chemical additives, in conjunction with constant intake of milk, butter, and other dairy foods.

Tumors in the inner region of the brain or spinal cord are more yang in structure and location. They arise primarily from consumption of excess animal food, including meat, poultry, eggs, and cheese, and refined salt and thus tend to affect older persons. As a whole, the brain and central nervous system are extremely compact (yang) and therefore a magnet to attract drugs, medications, synthetic vitamins, food and mineral supplements, and other extremely expansive (yin) substances. By avoiding these things and centering the diet, the brain and nervous system can maintain their normal functions.

MEDICAL EVIDENCE

• A 1974 study reported an increase in brain tumors and other cancers in men who had been occupationally exposed to vinyl chloride for at least one year. Vinyl chloride is widely used in plastic wrapping for packaging and storing foods. The FDA classifies it as an indirect food additive, and its residues are found in many foods. Source: I. R. Tabershaw and W. R. Gaffey, "Mortality Study of Workers in the Manufacture of Vinyl Chloride and Its Polymers," *Journal of Occupational Medicine* 16:509–18.

• In 1978 researchers reported fourteen cases of neuroblastoma, a brain tumor, over a sixteen-month period in people exposed to chemical pesticides. Five cases were children who were unintentionally exposed before or after birth to chlordane formulations. These pesticide residues tend to accumulate in high-fat foods such as meat, poultry, dairy products, and fish. Source: P. F. Infante et al., "Blood Dyscrasias and Childhood Tumors and Exposure to Chlordane and Heptachlor," *Scandinavian Journal of Work and Environmental Health* 4:137–50.

• In 1981 medical doctors reported a unique approach to brain tumor therapy regulating plasma levels of an essential amino acid and putting the terminal brain cancer patients on a natural foods diet. Developed at the University of Tennessee Center for Health Sciences, the experiment was conducted on three patients with glioblastomas beginning in 1975. Two of the three showed marked improvement. The first lived fifteen months and the tumor initially disappeared before reappearing. The second lived twenty-three months. The third survived eight months. In contrast, the mean survival for patients with this disease is four to six months. Source: C. R. Greer et al., "Surgery, Irradiation, and Metabolic Control of Brain Tumors" (letter), *American Journal of Clinical Nutrition* 34:600–601.

• In a follow-up to the above study, researchers at the University of Tennessee reported on the safety and feasibility of dietary management for brain cancer. Six patients with glioblastomas who had been treated with surgery and irradiation were put on a natural foods diet high in foods such as oatmeal, corn, carrots, and zucchini and a dietary supplement that restricted an essential amino acid. The regime was low in meat, dairy products, and other high-protein foods. "Amino acid restriction resulted in no additional patient morbidity," the researchers concluded. "There were no alterations in laboratory values to indicate the need for [medical] intervention. Quality of life for the patients did not diminish." Source : J. B. Burgess et al., *Nutrition and Cancer* 1, no. 4:16–21.

• In 1993 scientists reported that diets rich in soyfoods, especially miso soup, produced genistein, a natural substance that blocked the growth of new blood vessels that feed a tumor. Researchers from Children's University Hospital in Heidelberg, Germany, reported that genistein also deterred cancer cells from multiplying and could have significant implications for the prevention and treatment of solid malignancies, including those of the brain, breast, and prostate. Source: "Chemists Learn Why Vegetables Are Good for You," *New York Times*, April 13, 1993.

DIAGNOSIS

Brain tumors are commonly detected by X rays or CAT scans to the skull, spinal cord, and chest. Other medical techniques may include an electroencephalogram, cerebral angiogram, brain scan, spinal puncture, and myelogram.

Oriental medicine uses a variety of simple observations to ascertain the condition of the nervous system. A purplish-red color around the eyes shows an overworked nervous system caused mainly by consumption of drugs, chemicals, medications, refined simple sugars, and other extreme foods and drinks from the yin category. The parasympathetic system is especially affected by these substances. However, the orthosympathetic system will also be weakened, making all body reflexes and functions less sharp. The immediate effect can often be seen in the eyes, where the pupils contract, and in the vascular system, where the blood vessels dilate. After continued drug use, however, the parasympathetic nerves become worn out, expanding more and more. The pupils then dilate and the vessels contract.

The middle region of the forehead also shows the condition of the nervous system. A red color here shows nervousness, oversensitivity, excitability, and instability due to the overconsumption of yin-type foods, drinks, stimulants, and drugs. A white color is caused by excess intake of dairy products, especially milk, cream, and yogurt, together with excessive liquid. Nervous functions are generally slow and dull, and mental activities are cloudy and unclear. A yellow color indicates alertness but a tendency toward narrow-mindedness and inflexibility. The major cause is excessive intake of eggs, poultry, and dairy food. Dark spots or patches on the forehead indicate elimination of excessive sugars, fruits, honey, milk sugar, and other sweets as well as chemicals and drugs. Red pimples or spots on the middle forehead show the elimination of sugar and fruits combined with refined white flour products or dairy products.

The middle layer or ridge of the ear reflects the condition of the entire nervous system. A red color here indicates nervous disorders. The earlobe corresponds to the brain, and pimples, discolorations, or other abnormalities in this region may show developing cysts or tumors.

A loose mouth shows a variety of disorders, including nervous-system malfunctions. This condition usually also reflects trouble in the small intestine, the brain's complementary opposite organ.

The color on the back of the hand may also indicate nervous problems. If marijuana, hashish, or other hallucinogenic substances, as well as medications, are used repeatedly for some time, the body will begin to discharge these toxins and the color of the hands and fingers will change to red or purple.

Rough skin also shows nervous disorders caused by extreme yin-type foods or drugs. This condition may be accompanied by an irregular pulse, excessive sweating, frequent urination, diarrhea, vertigo, excessive sensitivity, and emotional instability.

The sensitively trained hand can also locate the approximate region of brain tumors and cancer by detecting vibrations produced and discharged from each part of the brain. In some cases, brain tumors may cause paralysis, seizure, loss of sight, and loss of physical and mental coordination. By examining the paralyzed parts and functions of the body, indirect detection of the area of the brain affected can be done.

Generally, brain tumors are comparatively easier than other cancers to relieve through proper eating. This is because they tend to grow slowly in this very compact region, and the abundance of blood supply to the brain means that a change in blood quality from an altered diet will quickly affect the condition of the brain and nervous system.

DIETARY RECOMMENDATIONS

There are two basic types of brain tumors. The harder carcinoma type, usually occurring deep inside the brain, is caused by the gathering of excess protein and fat, especially of animal quality. Animal products, including eggs, meat, poultry, dairy food, and oily, fatty fish, and other strong yang foods should be strictly avoided. Sugar and other strong yin foods may enhance this type of tumor. The second type of brain tumor, sarcoma, is softer and usually occurs more on the surface of the brain. It is caused primarily by the consumption of extreme yin foods and beverages, especially milk, butter, cream, yogurt, sugar and sweets, and excessive fruit and juice. The growth of brain tumors is promoted by chemicals in artificially processed food as well as exposure to industrial pollutants, though these are usually not the primary cause. It is therefore advisable to avoid the continued use of all synthetic food products and for patients with this condition to restore their health in a relatively fresh and clean atmospheric environment. Although they are not direct causes of brain tumors, spices, stimulants, alcohol, and aromatic beverages and substances are to be avoided because they tend to accelerate tumor growth. Because of their potential for contributing to cancer creation and growth, flour products, especially refined flour treated with oil, fat, and sweets, as well as overconsumption of liquid, are also to be avoided. Nutritional advice for infants and young children, including those with brain tumors, is given in the chapter on children's cancer. Following are general dietary guidelines for older children and adults.

• **Whole Grains:** Fifty to 60 percent of daily consumption, by volume, should be whole-cereal grains. The first day prepare plain pressure-cooked short-grain brown rice. On following days, prepare brown rice pressure-cooked with 20 to 30 percent millet, then rice with 20 to 30 percent barley, then rice with 20 to 30 percent aduki beans or lentils, and then plain rice again. A delicious morning porridge can be made by taking leftover rice, adding a little more water to soften, and seasoning with a little miso at the end and simmering for two to three minutes more. In ordinary pressure cooking, the ratio of grain to water should be about 1:2. For seasoning, cook with a postage stamp–sized piece of kombu or a pinch of sea salt, depending on the person's condition. After the first month, once or twice a week these grains can be prepared in the form of fried grains with vegetables. Other grains can be used occasionally, including whole wheat berries, rye, corn, and whole oats, though oats should be avoided for the first month. For more yang tumors deep inside the brain or in the back of the head, avoid buckwheat and seitan for several months. For tumors on the periphery or surface of the head and toward the front, buckwheat and seitan may be taken occasionally. Good-quality sourdough bread may be enjoyed two to three times a week, and noodles (udon for more yang cancers and both udon and soba for more yin cancers) may also be taken two to three times a week. Avoid all hard baked products until the condition improves, including cookies, cake, pie, crackers, muffins, and the like.

• **Soup:** Five to 10 percent soup, consisting of one or two cups or bowls per day of soup cooked with wakame sea vegetable and various land vegetables such as onions and carrots seasoned with miso or shoyu. Occasionally a small volume of shiitake mushroom may be added to the soup. Lotus root should be used often in soup. The miso may be barley miso, brown rice miso, or soybean (hatcho) miso and should be naturally aged two to three years. To satisfy a sweet tooth, millet soup with sweet vegetables such as squash, cabbage, onions, and carrots may be prepared often. Frequently these vegetables can be sautéed with a little sesame oil before cooking in the soup. Among vegetables, more round vegetables are preferred, such as onions, pumpkin, and winter squash, though other root and green leafy vegetables may also occasionally be used in soup. Grain soups, bean soups, and other soups may be taken from time to time. Less frequently, a small portion of white-meat fish or small dried fish can also be cooked into the soup with vegetables, sea vegetables, and/or grains. After the first month, when no oil should be consumed, two to three times a week vegetables may be lightly sautéed with a small volume of sesame oil or corn oil before cooking them in the soup.

• **Vegetables:** Twenty to 30 percent vegetables, cooked in a variety of forms. Dishes can be prepared in various ways using round vegetables, together with root vegetables such as carrots, burdock, daikon, and turnip. Avoid oil for the first one to two months, after which some dishes may be sautéed with a moderate volume of sesame or corn oil. As a general rule, the following dishes may be prepared, though the frequency may differ from person to person: nishime-style vegetables, three times a week for those with more yang tumors and four times for those with more yin tumors; squash-aduki-kombu dish, three times a week; dried daikon, one cup, three times a week; carrots and carrot tops or daikon and daikon tops, three times a week; blanched vegetables, five to seven times a week; pressed salad, five to seven times a week; raw salad and salad dressing, avoid; steamed greens, five to seven times a week; sautéed vegetables, twice a week, using water the first month and then a volume of sesame oil; kinpira, two-thirds of a cup, two times a week, using water the first month and then sautéing in oil (this dish is particularly beneficial for brain tumors); tofu, dried tofu, tempeh, or seitan with vegetables, two times a week.

• **Beans:** Five percent small beans, such as aduki beans, lentils, chickpeas, or black soybeans, may be used daily, cooked together with sea vegetables such as kombu or with onions and carrots. Other beans may be used altogether two to three times a month. For seasoning, a small volume of unrefined sea salt or shoyu or miso can be used. Bean products, such as tempeh, natto, and dried or cooked tofu, may be used occasionally, but in moderate volume.

• **Sea Vegetables:** Five percent or less sea vegetable dishes, including wakame and kombu, daily when cooking grain, in soup, etc. A sheet of toasted nori may also be taken daily. A small dish of hijiki or arame should be prepared two times a week. All other sea vegetables are optional. Sea vegetables can be cooked with other vegetables or sautéed with a small volume of sesame oil after softening them by soaking and boiling lightly in water.

• **Condiments:** Condiments to be available on the table are gomashio (sesame salt), on the average made with 1 part salt to 18 parts sesame seeds (reduced to 1:16 after two months); kelp or wakame powder; umeboshi plum; and tekka, though all other regular macrobiotic condiments may be used if desired. These condiments may be used daily on grains and vegetables, but the volume should be moderate to suit individual appetite and taste. One to two teaspoons a day of sliced lotus root cooked together with kombu and a bit of grated ginger, seasoned with shoyu, is especially good for this condition. Several small pieces of kombu cooked with shoyu can also be helpful if consumed daily with any meal. This is called shio kombu or salty kombu.

• **Pickles:** Pickles, made at home in a variety of ways, are to be eaten daily, one tablespoon in all, though salty pickles are to be minimized.

• **Animal Food:** Meat, poultry, eggs, and other strong animal food is to be avoided. A small volume of white-meat fish may be eaten once every two weeks by those with more yang cancers and once a week by those with more yin tumors. The fish should be prepared steamed, boiled, or poached and garnished with grated daikon or ginger. After two months, fish may be eaten twice a week if desired. Strictly avoid blue-meat and red-meat fish and all shellfish.

• **Fruit:** None the best, the less the better, including both tropical and temperate-climate fruit, until the condition improves. If cravings develop, a small volume of cooked fruit with a pinch of sea salt or dried fruit (also preferably cooked) may be taken. Avoid all fruit juices and cider.

• **Sweets and Snacks:** Avoid all sweets and desserts, including good-quality macrobiotic desserts, until the condition improves. To satisfy a sweet tooth, use sweet vegetables every day in cooking, drink sweet vegetable drink (see special drinks below), and use sweet vegetable jam and a small volume of amasake. Mochi, rice balls, vegetable sushi, and other grain-based snacks may be eaten frequently. Limit rice cakes, popcorn, and other dry or baked snacks, as they may harden the tumor. In the event of cravings, a small volume of barley malt or rice syrup may be taken.

• **Nuts and Seeds:** Nuts and nut butters are to be avoided due to their high amount of fat and protein, except for chestnuts. Unsalted, roasted seeds such as squash seeds and pumpkin seeds may be consumed as a snack, up to one cup altogether per week. Avoid sunflower seeds.

• **Seasonings:** Seasonings, such as unrefined sea salt, shoyu, and miso, are to be used moderately in order to avoid unnecessary thirst. Avoid mirin and garlic. If you become particularly thirsty after the meal or between meals, you should cut back on these seasonings until the normal level of thirst returns.

• **Beverages:** Beverages and other dietary practices can follow the general recommendations in Part I, including bancha twig tea as the main beverage. Strictly avoid the beverages on the "infrequent" and "avoid" list and don't take grain coffee for the first two to three months after starting this new way of eating.

The most important thing in connection with dietary practice is chewing very well, until all food becomes liquid in the mouth and well mixed with saliva. Chew very, very well, at least 50 times, preferably 100 times, per mouthful. It is also important to avoid overeating and eating within three hours of sleeping.

As noted in the introduction to Part II, persons who have received or who are currently undergoing medical treatment may need to make further dietary modifications.

SPECIAL DRINKS AND PREPARATIONS

Persons with brain tumors may also consume some special drinks and dishes, which, taken in small volume, can strengthen blood quality. These dishes include:

• **Sweet Vegetable Drink:** Take one small cup every day or every other day for the first month, then two to three times a week in the second month.

• **Carrot-Daikon Drink:** Take one small cup every day for seven to ten days for more yang cancers, then every other day for the next month. For more yin tumors, take one small cup two to three times a week for two to four weeks, and then once every three days for one month.

• **Lotus-Kombu Drink:** Soak one-half dried lotus root and chop finely. Combine with a little kombu that has been soaked and chopped. Add one and one-half cups spring water, cook, and simmer fifteen to twenty minutes. Take one small cup of the liquid for one month, then two or three times a week for the second month. (The lotus and kombu may also be eaten when soft.)

• **Umeboshi Plums:** Take one-half to one plum daily for two to four weeks, then two to three times a week thereafter.

• **Ume-Sho-Kuzu Drink:** Those with more yin brain tumors may take this drink for energy and vitality. Take one small cup every two or three days for ten days to two weeks, then two times a week for three to four weeks.

• **Grated Carrots:** For more yang tumors, one-half cup of raw grated carrots with a few drops of shoyu may be taken twice a week at mealtime, for two to three months, to help discharge accumulated fat and oil.

• **Grated Daikon:** Taken occasionally, one-half small cup of grated daikon with a few drops of shoyu is beneficial for this condition.

HOME CARES

• **Body Scrub:** Scrubbing the whole body, including the abdominal region and the spinal region, with a towel that has been immersed in hot water and squeezed out is very helpful for better circulation of blood, lymph, and other body fluids, as well as for activating physical and mental energies.

• **Soaking the Feet:** Soak the feet in salty cold water three to five minutes before going to bed. This will help bring the energy from the head to the lower part of the body.

• **Lotus-Root Plaster:** Heavy pressures and pains in the head or brain can be relieved by reducing the consumption of fruit, juices, and beverages or temporary avoidance of salty food. A lotus-root plaster, consisting of a 50/50 mixture of grated fresh lotus root and mashed cabbage leaves or other greens, with 10 to 20 percent white flour and 5 percent granted ginger, is also helpful if applied directly on the region and kept there about three hours.

OTHER CONSIDERATIONS

• Good exercise is always helpful, but do not exercise to the point of exhaustion. Deep breathing exercises, massage, and tai chi–type movements are generally preferable to strenuous activities. Walking is excellent.

• Maintaining clean, fresh air inside the home is important, and for this purpose green plants can be placed in each room. Indoor air circulation can also be maintained by frequently opening the windows.

• Avoid frequent exposure to artificial radiation, including medical and dental X rays, smoke detectors, television, and video terminals, which often emit radiation toward the face or head.

• Brain tumors and cancer can be accelerated if the intestinal functions are stagnated, for example, from constipation or menstrual difficulties. Accordingly, keeping the bowels smooth and the menstrual function regular is very helpful and can also help relieve pressure and pain in the head regions. An enema for inducing elimination may be needed as well as a massage or ginger compress applied on the abdomen. Douching to eliminate stagnated fat and mucus in the uterine region may also be necessary.

• Avoid wearing shoes or socks while indoors. Walk barefoot or on the grass or soil outside, when possible, to stimulate the flow of electromagnetic energy from the earth to the nervous system.

• Avoid synthetic clothing, especially underwear, stockings, socks, hats, and scarves. Wigs and hairpieces should also be avoided. Synthetic rugs, curtains, furniture, blankets, and other home furnishings should gradually be replaced with more natural materials.

• Long hot baths or showers should be avoided in order to prevent depletion of minerals from the body. Limit bathing to a few times a week.

• Brain and nervous disorders are often accompanied by excitability, hypersensitivity, despondency, or lowered will to live. Short but regular periods of meditation—including visualization, prayer, chanting, yoga, or other exercises—can help to calm the mind and center the thoughts.

• Mental nourishment is as important to self-development as physical sustenance. Avoid loud and frenzied music, chaotic art, brutal and violent films, and depressing magazines and literature. Within moderation, select strong, meaningful mental outlets. Reading, music, and arts that help to create a positive attitude should be selected.

PERSONAL EXPERIENCE

Brain Tumor

In August 1986 Mona Sanders had just turned thirty-seven and was enjoying life. However, after a grand mal seizure that sent her sprawling onto a tennis court, hospital tests, and two surgeries showed that she had an anaplastic astrocytoma, grade 3. The brain tumor, the size of a small grapefruit, was fast-growing and, according to physicians, inoperable.

The diagnosis devastated Mona and she began to experience nausea, vomiting, and numbness in her right leg. "I had always enjoyed life, living by my own decisions—until now," she recalled. "The doctors' prognosis rang through my mind: 'It was bad,' 'It would never go away,' 'Chemo might be able to slow its growth,' 'It was close to a motor area and I would eventually lose control,' 'Wheelchair in the future,' 'Six to eighteen months to live.' "

An aunt from New Orleans recommended macrobiotics, and Mona began reading *Recovery,* by Elaine Nussbaum (see personal account in the chapter on female cancer). Mona reasoned that if Elaine, also a housewife, could heal herself, she could, too, even though she lived in a small town in northeast Mississippi where no one had ever heard of macrobiotics.

Checking with the American Cancer Society hotline to see if there was anything else she could do, Mona was told "Nothing. Good luck." The line went dead. "We'll see about that!" Mona said to herself.

Several days later, in January 1987, Mona came to Boston to begin macrobiotics. Although she was on many pills and her thinking was cloudy, she videotaped the seminar and reviewed the tapes when she returned home. In February, Mona returned to Boston and came to see me for personal guidance and instruction.

With the help of several macrobiotic cooks, Mona began to experience the benefits of the diet. In addition, she used imaging and visualization to help shrink the tumor, imaging it decreasing in size from the size of a grapefruit to a golfball, to a pinhead, and then to nothing.

Medical tests confirmed the steady remission of her malignancy, and a CAT scan in April, just four months after she started macrobiotics, showed no evidence of cancer. Since then, five years ago, she has remained cancer-free.

"Today with God's help and the love and support of my husband, children, family, and friends, I am alive with the chance to work, play, and love," Mona reports. "I want to share my experiences with others to spare them the anguish I went through and to offer a practical alternative to degenerative disease."

Source: Mona Sanders, "Healing a Terminal Brain Tumor," *One Peaceful World Newsletter*, Autumn/Winter, 1990.

Brain Tumor

Brian Bonaventura worked in the automotive industry in Columbus, Ohio. He had been suffering flulike symptoms for several months when, in September 1983, he suffered from a seizure at work. Doctors found a benign brain tumor the size of a small orange in the right frontal lobe of his brain.

Following surgery, Brian decided to forego chemotherapy and radiation treatments. However, personal and marital problems caused him anxiety, and after panic attacks he started taking tranquilizers. A CAT scan in autumn 1984 proved normal, but the new doctor advised him to avoid fried foods and decrease his meat consumption. "This was the first advice I had received from a doctor about changing my diet," Brian recalled.

His emotional life continued to be stressful, and soon his diet returned to the former pattern of high amounts of fat and sugar. In 1988 Brian's marriage ended, and later that year MRI tests revealed a new tumor in the brain, this one malignant.

While recovering from his second surgery, Brian read a book on macrobiotics that his sister-in-law gave him and decided to give it a try. "I couldn't put the book down and felt it made complete sense, reviewing my past. As soon as I got out of the hospital, I located the nearest health food co-op and began eating as close to the macrobiotic diet as I knew how, while reading all I could. After a meeting with Michio, I followed his suggestions very closely for many months."

Over the next three years, Brian's health improved dramatically. Emotionally, he says he feels more stable than he ever did, and he hasn't had a panic attack in years. He rarely gets depressed and has become an active snow and water-skier. Active in the macrobiotic community in Columbus, Brian is attending the Kushi Institute Extension Program in Cleveland and hopes someday to become a teacher and counselor.

Source: Ann Fawcett and the East West Foundation, *Cancer-free: 30 Who Triumphed over Cancer Naturally*, (New York and Tokyo: Japan Publications, 1991).

26

Children's Cancer

FREQUENCY

Cancer is the number one cause of death by disease in this country in children between the ages of one and fourteen. This year, an estimated 7,800 American children will be diagnosed with cancer and another 1,500 will die, about a third of them from leukemia. Childhood leukemia in the United States has climbed 11 percent from 1973 to 1988. Brain tumors are also on the rise in children and now account for about 35 percent of all cancer deaths in both males and females under fifteen. Other common sites include the bone, bone marrow, lymph nodes, kidneys, and soft tissues. Overall, the incidence of childhood cancer increased 28 percent from 1950 to 1987.

The principal malignancies are: 1) ALL, the most prevalent cancer among children, characterized by diminished granulocytes, the white blood cells that resist infection; 2) *osteogenic sarcoma* and *Ewing's sarcoma*, bone cancers; 3) *neuroblastoma*, which can appear anywhere but mostly appears in the abdomen, where swelling results; 4) *rhabdomyosarcoma*, the most common soft tissue sarcoma, which can occur in the head, neck, genito-urinary tract, trunk, or extremities; 5) *brain cancers*, characterized in the early stages by headaches, blurred or double vision, dizziness, difficulty in walking or handling objects, and nausea; 6) *lymphomas* and *Hodgkin's disease*, which involves swelling of lymph nodes in the neck, armpit, or groin, general weakness and fever, and other possible symptoms; 7) *retinoblastoma*, an eye cancer that affects children under the age of four; and 8) *Wilms' tumor*, a kidney cancer that appears as a swelling or lump in the abdomen.

Medical treatment usually involves radiation or chemotherapy. Survival rates vary from about 25 to 85 percent, depending on the type of cancer and staging. In the last thirty years, there has been a dramatic increase in survival among children with leukemia from 4 percent to 73 percent.

CAUSE OF CANCER

During the embryonic period, energy and nutrients that support the formation of the body, the mind, and associated functions are supplied through the placenta and the embryonic cord. During pregnancy, from the time of conception to the time of birth, the human embryo increases in weight approximately 3 billion times. The food we eat as human beings recapitulates the entire course of biological evolution.

In the womb, we eat the essence of animal food in mother's blood. Until about one year of age, we eat the more diluted essence of animal food in mother's milk. After that, whole grains, which co-evolved with human beings in the most recent 25 million year period, become our principal food, initially in soft, easily digestible form. If we don't eat grains during the entire course of our life, we begin to lose our unique human status. Grains are customarily cooked with a pinch of salt or seaweed and taken with salt- or mineral-rich soup or broth, representing the primordial ocean in which life began and the slightly saline quality of our blood. Plant foods—the major supplement to grains—include ancient and modern vegetables and beans, representing the continuing course of biological evolution on land. Since grains and beans are already fruits, consumption of tree and ground fruits (which co-evolved with and gave rise to monkeys and apes), as well as nuts and seeds, is not essential for our development, but these foods may be eaten in moderation for enjoyment and variety. Animal foods, which share a similar quality with human beings, should generally be avoided or limited and, if consumed, eaten in the forms further away from us on the spiral of evolution. Fish and seafood, representing more primitive forms of animal life, are more suitable than birds and mammals. Daily food is the essence of biological life, and the kind, amount, frequency, and way of preparing food we take largely shape and determine our human destiny on this planet.

If a mother's eating habits are imbalanced and her diet consists largely of acid-producing foods—including excessive consumption of animal protein and fat, dairy foods, simple sugars, fruits and fruits juices, soft drinks, chemicalized food and beverages, and others—a baby developed in her womb may be born with deformities, congenital heart disease, or a tendency toward natural immune deficiency that could lead to cancer, AIDS, or other serious disorders. This orientation may manifest during childhood, especially if improper foods continue to be consumed after birth throughout the growing period.

The modern way of life tends to produce a child that is weaker physically and mentally than children in the past. Children today tend to be larger and heavier than necessary. Physical and mental response tends to be duller. On the average, a smaller, thinner, and shorter child is stronger than a larger, fatter, and taller one. Compared with children from a few generations ago, modern children are weaker in their physical and mental resistance, endurance, and response in general. This means that modern newborns are also weaker in natural immunity than in the past.

Because increasing numbers of newborns are physically larger and heavier and many mothers have weak contracting power during delivery, cesarean surgery has tripled in modern society, accounting for about one in every four births. In addition, the use of forceps, drugs, and other emergency measures to assist in delivery has become more widespread. If the newborn does not experience passing through the natural birth canal with strong repeated contractions, the child tends to be weaker in physical endurance and resistance in general.

At the same time, nursing is often intentionally stopped, and artificially produced formula is substituted for mother's milk. During the first few days after delivery, the mother's breast secretes a yellow fluid called colostrum, which has ample immune factors. Throughout the next period of breast-feeding, as regular mother's milk is produced, the newborn continues to receive essential natural immune factors. These include antibodies that resist the growth of undesirable viruses and bacteria, provide immunity against infectious disease (especially against rickettsia, salmonella, polio, influenza, strep, and staph), promote strong white blood cells, and produce *B. bifidum,* a unique type of healthy bacteria found in the intestines of babies that creates resistance to large variety of microorganisms. These immune factors decrease as time passes. It is more difficult for the newborn to develop natural immunity, including a strong blood and lymphatic system, if it has not been breast-fed.

The rise of childhood cancer and other degenerative and immune diseases began in the 1950s. At that time, dietary habits began to change dramatically when a high-protein, high-fat diet became standardized in the United States and most of the industrialized world. Chemical agriculture replaced organic farming, and grain and flour products were increasingly refined. Commercially prepared fast foods replaced home cooking, and modern advertising elevated sensory appeal and satisfaction, along with packaging, especially through the new medium of television, which was often directed at children. In the 1960s and early 1970s, fast foods, including hamburgers, french fries, pizza, and fried chicken, became popular, further weakening the younger generation. Finally, in the 1980s and early 1990s, microwave cooking, food irradiation, and other highly artificial methods of preparing and preserving foods became widespread, contributing to further decline. This vast fundamental change in the modern way of eating naturally altered the biological, mental, and spiritual status of human beings, contributing to degenerative disease. The lack of whole grains and natural minerals in fresh vegetables and sea vegetables has particularly contributed to the decline.

In addition, the last half-century has seen an abuse of medication and pills, the overuse of antibiotics and medical treatment, the rise of recreational drugs, exposure to X rays and other potentially harmful medical and dental procedures, exposure to electrical generators, television, computers, and other appliances and devices that emit artificial electromagnetic energy, and environmental pollution. Out of a misunderstanding of the nature and function of the human body, millions of children (and adults) have had their tonsils removed. The tonsils are one of several important immune glands that serve to cleanse toxins, excess mucus, and other substances from the lymph system. Chronic swelling and inflammation show that they are doing their job of localizing and neutralizing dietary excess. The way to relieve tonsillitis is not to take out the tonsils, but to stop the intake of improper foods and drinks that are overburdening the lymphatic system. If the tonsils are removed, diseases can spread more rapidly.

Together these factors have resulted in the biological decline of modern children. In extreme cases, this can result in childhood cancer, especially leukemia, lymphoma, cancer on the surface or in the front of the brain, bone cancer, and central nervous system cancer, which are all classified as more yin.

From the macrobiotic view, the primary dietary causes of childhood malignancies are: 1) dairy food of all kind, including whole milk, low-fat or skim milk (high in protein), yogurt, butter, cheese, and ice cream; 2) sugar, sweets, chocolate, honey, carob, and foods and candy containing these simple sugars; 3) soft drinks, cold drinks, and drinks served with ice cubes; 4) white flour, white bread, and other refined flour products, including pizza, crackers, muffins, cookies, cakes, and pies; 4) excessive oily and fatty foods of all kinds, including animal and vegetable quality, including meat, poultry, eggs, salad dressings, mayonnaise, and others; 5) tropical fruits and vegetables, including bananas, mangoes, pineapple, tomatoes, potatoes, eggplant, and others; 6) too much temperate-climate fruit and especially juice; 7) too much chemically grown food and foods containing artificial additives, preservatives, and stabilizers; 8) too many canned, frozen, precooked, and other prepared foods; 9) food that is cooked on an electric range or microwave oven, which gives a chaotic energy and vibration.

MEDICAL EVIDENCE

• In an analysis of seventeen pesticides, toxins, and other chemical substances in the breast milk of vegetarian and nonvegetarian mothers, scientists found that except for PCBs (which were about equal), "the highest vegetarian value was lower than the lowest value obtained in the [nonvegetarian] sample. . . . [T]he mean vegetarian levels were only one or two percent as high as the average levels in the United States." Source: J. Hergenrather et al., "Pollutants in Breast Milk of Vegetarians," (letter), *New England Journal of Medicine* 304 (1976):792.

• In a review of the medical evidence linking dairy food with disease, two doctors reported that milk "may contribute to the formation of kidney stones, may cause intestinal malabsorption and diarrhea, and may even cause malnourishment of the older infants, especially leading to iron deficiency anemia. Good evidence has been presented that milk products are associated with the development of cancer, skin lesions, musculoskeletal abnormalities, pulmonary obstruction, immunological disorders, and liver function abnormalities." Source: Agatha and Calvin Thrash, M.D., *The Animal Connection* (Seale, AL: Yuchi Pines Institute, 1983), 69.

• In 1985 the American Heart Association issued revised dietary guidelines stating that fat intake could be reduced even lower than 30 percent, as usually recommended. The list of recommended daily foods for children and adults included a wide range of vegetables and fruits, including broccoli, cabbage, mustard greens, kale, collards, carrots, pumpkin, and winter squash; whole grains and their products, including brown rice and whole-grain bread, cereals, and pasta; dried beans, peas, and other meatless main entrées, including tofu; fish and seafood; nuts, and vegetable-quality fats and oils. The list of foods for everyone to avoid, including children and adults in good health, included whole milk, most cheese, ice cream, and other high-fat dairy products; eggs (maximum two per week) and foods prepared with eggs; red meat (except for lean cuts), cured meat, and organ meats; butter and other animal fats and hydrogenated fats and oils; sugary desserts, store-bought desserts and mixes, and highly processed snacks. Source: *The American Heart Association Handbook* (New York: Dutton, 1980), and "The American Heart Association Diet" (Dallas: American Heart Association, 1985).

• In 1986, in a small pilot study, eight of ten AIDS patients reported having had a tonsillectomy in childhood. "The possibility of an observed relationship between AIDS and tonsillectomies is due to the fact that individuals who have undergone chronic infections reflect an underlying immunological abnormality that puts them at increased risk for AIDS. . . . A better understanding of the intricate relationship of the immune system to the development of viral malignancies may result from the study of the effect of lymphoid tissue removal on susceptibility to leukemia, lymphoma, and AIDS." Source: S. McCombie, "Tonsillectomy as a Co-Factor in the Development of AIDS," *Medical Hypotheses* 19:291.

• In a symposium on nutrition, infection, and the immune system, a researcher reported that casein and bovine gammaglobulin, two antigenic proteins found in milk, may be absorbed directly into the bloodstream, especially in people with IgA deficiency, and contribute to the development of a variety of auto immune disorders, including rheumatoid arthritis, lupus erythematosus, Hodgkins' disease, brain tumors, and various other cancers. IgA is an antibody normally found in children who are breast-fed. Source: C. Cunningham-Rundles, "Failure of the G.I. Tract Barrier in Patients with a Suppressed Immune System," Lecture at the College of Physicians and Surgeons, Columbia University, December 4–5, 1986.

• Breast-feeding can reduce the risk of certain cancers for both mother and child. In 1988 researchers from the National Institute of Child Health and Human Development in Bethesda, Maryland, found that infants breast-fed more than six months had a lower risk of developing cancer in childhood, especially lymphomas. In this study, children who were formula-fed or breast-fed for less than six months had approximately twice the risk of getting some childhood cancers by age fifteen as those breast-fed for longer than six months. They also had five times the risk of getting lymphoma. "Mother's milk contains substantial antimicrobial benefits for infants, increasing their resistance to many infections and possibly protecting them from many diseases, including lymphomas," researchers reported. Source: "Breast-feeding Linked to Decreased Cancer Risk for Mother, Child," *Journal of the National Cancer Institute* 80:1362–63.

• In 1983 the U.S. Department of Agriculture approved the use of soy products and other vegetable protein products as partial substitutes for meats, poultry, and seafoods in school lunch and some other feeding programs. In a review of the health benefits of soy, medical researchers in 1989 noted that soy products were comparable with milk in protein quality for preschool and older children; except for premature infants, soy protein can serve as a sole protein source in the human diet; soyfoods are high in protease inhibitors that inhibit the action of various enzymes that have been associated with causing cancer; soy formulas are lactose-free and may benefit infants and small children who are sensitive to cow-milk protein, which can cause diarrhea, emesis, vomiting, and weight loss; soy products can reduce cholesterol and triglycerides in subjects with high lipid levels and protect against heart disease; and soy foods are useful in decreasing blood glucose responses compared with other high-fiber foods and may prevent diabetes. "One desirable way to alter typical American diet patterns to meet the above [U.S. Department of Agriculture] dietary recommendations involves partial replacement of foods of animal origin with cereals and legumes," the scientists concluded. Source: John Erdman and Elizabeth Fordyce, "Soy Products and the Human Diet," *American Journal of Clinical Nutrition* 49:725–37.

• In tests of the acceptability of tofu in the lunch menus of preschoolers in 1990, analysis showed that the nutritional quality of the nine tofu recipes adhered more closely to national dietary guidelines than the beef, chicken, eggs, and cheese originally served. The children accepted tofu well, preferring it to dairy and meat in several dishes, including macaroni and cheese, lasagna, tuna casserole, and quiche. Source: H. L. Ashraf et al., "Use of Tofu in Preschool Meals," *Journal of the American Dietetic Association* 90:114–16.

• In a survey of sixty AIDS patients, a medical researcher reported that all had been formula-fed as babies with the exception of one person, who had been breast-fed for less than three months. Source: Michio Kushi and Martha Cottrell, M.D., *AIDS, Macrobiotics, and Natural Immunity* (New York and Tokyo: Japan Publications, 1990), 158.

• Recent studies show a clear association between childhood cancers and exposure to carcinogenic chemicals. The three most common—kidney, brain, and acute leukemia—are often related to occupational exposure of fathers and mothers to such products as organic solvents, hydrocarbons, paints, dyes, and pigments. Children of mechanics and mining and aircraft workers are also at risk. "Clusters of acute leukemia are found in agricultural countries with heavy pesticide use, particularly for cotton production. Additionally, brain tumors have been associated with home termite treatment. Of 34 pesticides repeatedly applied commercially to lawns, at up to five times agricultural rates, 10 are well recognized carcinogens." Source: Samuel S. Epstein, M.D., and Ralph W. Moss, authors of *The Cancer Industry*, letter to the *New York Times*, July 16, 1991.

• The risk of childhood leukemia correlates with the location of power lines, according to researchers at the University of Southern California in Los Angeles. In a study of 219 children with leukemia and 207 healthy children, they found that the children with the highest estimated exposure had double the leukemia incidence seen in children with the lowest estimated exposures. The researchers also found a relationship between childhood leukemia and exposure to electric hair dryers and televisions. Source: *American Journal of Epidemiology*, November 1, 1991, and "Fickle Fields: EMFs and Epidemiology," *Science News*, November 30, 1991.

• Children treated for leukemia, the most common childhood cancer, are at an extremely high risk for developing a second tumor. In 1991 researchers reported that children with leukemia receiving radiation treatments contracted a second malignancy seven times more often than expected and a brain tumor twenty-two times more often. The second cancer came an average of six years after treatment. Though radiation treatment was singled out, smaller studies have found that chemotherapy also raises the odds of subsequent tumors. Source: Joseph Neglia, *New England Journal of Medicine*, November 7, 1991, and "A Special Risk for Leukemia Patients," *New York Times*, November 7, 1991.

DIAGNOSIS

Civilized life as a whole is making people more yin. They are more passive and sedentary. Their thinking is more yin. They are dropping out from discipline at all levels—family life, schools, religions, work. Today people don't want to do hard work or help others. Parents don't want to make the effort to bring up children, so they take birth-control pills (yin) and have abortions (which is also weakening and makes the woman very yin).

Children today are weaker, more yin, than children used to be. This is shown not just by declining SAT test scores over the last generation, but by physiological signs. These include smaller ears and ears lacking in detached earlobes, weaker bones and teeth, and bodies that are taller and heavier. Children today are becoming lazier. They can't stand cold weather, hardships, or difficulties as their grandparents used to. Many lack self-discipline due to a lack of good-quality yang in their diet—whole grains, vegetables, good-quality salt and mineral-rich seaweed.

While everyone's condition is unique, those susceptible to cancer in childhood often share some of the following characteristics: 1) general fatigue, physically and mentally, with a tendency to become inactive and seek more comfortable situations and surroundings; 2) development of frequent colds and infections accompanied by light fever; 3) skin rashes, similar to allergic reactions; 4) intestinal disorders including gas, constipation, and frequent diarrhea; 5) feeling of nausea; 6) irregular appetite, fluctuating from insatiable to almost no appetite, and frequent cravings for sweets, fruit, pastries, and similar foods; 7) hypoglycemia, including a tendency to be more depressed, irritable, and sad, particularly in the late afternoon; 8) difficulty sleeping at night; 9) peripheral parts of the body are often colder than normal; 10) susceptibility to bruises and cuts and slower than normal healing; 11) swelling of lymph glands; and 12) inability to focus or concentrate on what they are doing.

DIETARY RECOMMENDATIONS

The major cause of cancer in children, including leukemia, lymphoma, brain tumors, and kidney cancer, is the consumption of foods and beverages in the extreme yin category, including sugar, sugar-treated foods and drinks, ice cream, chocolate, carob, honey, soft drinks and soda, tropical fruits, fruit juices, oily and greasy foods, dairy foods, especially butter, milk, and cream, and many chemicals contained in foods, beverages, and supplements. All of these should be avoided in daily eating. However, the consumption of these items is often accompanied by the intake of foods from the extreme yang category, including meat, poultry, eggs, and cheese, in order to achieve a rough counterbalance. Accordingly, all these animal foods are also to be avoided, with the exception of fish and seafood, which can be consumed in small volume after one month on a stricter diet. Although they are not the direct cause, the following enhance malignant conditions and should also be discontinued: ice-cold food and drinks, hot, stimulant, and aromatic spices, various herbs and herb drinks that have stimulant effects, and vegetables that historically originated in the tropics, including potatoes, tomatoes, and eggplant.

Compared to adults, children are smaller and more compact—more yang— and therefore require less salt, miso, shoyu, and other salty seasonings and slightly more oil, fruit, sweets, and desserts. When cooking for a family, it is advisable to season according to the children's needs and for adults to add slightly more condiments at the table.

First we give the dietary guidelines for babies and infants and then for children. For older children with cancer (those over fifteen), follow the guidelines under the specific cancers in this section of the book.

Guidelines for Babies and Infants

Our diet should change in accordance with the development of our teeth. The ideal food for the human infant is mother's milk, and all of the baby's nourishment should come from this source for the first six months. At about that age, the quantity of breast milk can gradually be decreased over the next six months while soft foods, containing practically no salt, are introduced and proportionately increased. Mother's milk should be usually be stopped around the time the first molars appear (twelve to fourteen months) and the baby's diet by then consist entirely of soft mashed foods.

Harder foods should be introduced around the time the first molars appear and gradually increase in percentage over the next year. By the age of twenty to twenty-four months, softly mashed foods should be replaced entirely by harder foods, which will comprise the mainstay of the diet.

At the beginning of the third year, a child can receive one-third to one-fourth the amount of salt used by an adult, depending upon its health. A child's intake of salt should continue to be less than an adult's until about the seventh or eighth year.

At age four, the standard diet may be introduced, along with mild sea salt, miso, and other seasonings, including ginger. Until this age, infants ideally should not have any animal food, including fish, except in special cases where the child is weak, slightly anemic, or lacks energy. Then give about one tablespoon of white-meat fish or seafood that has been well boiled with vegetables and mashed. At age four, if desired, a small amount white-meat fish or seafood may be included from time to time for enjoyment. Different tastes appeal to us at different periods of our development. A natural sweet taste particularly nourishes babies and children.

The following dietary recommendations may be followed for healthy infants as well as those with serious sicknesses, including childhood leukemia, lymphoma, or brain or kidney tumors.

Whole Grains. These can be introduced after eight months to one year as the baby's main food. The cereal should be in the form of a soft whole-grain porridge consisting of 4 parts brown rice (short-grain), 3 parts sweet brown rice, and 1 part barley. The porridge is preferably cooked with a piece of kombu, although this sea vegetable does not always have to be eaten. Millet and oats can be included in this cereal from time to time. However, buckwheat, wheat, and rye are usually not given.

The porridge may be prepared by pressure cooking or boiling. To pressure-cook, soak cereals for two to three hours and pressure-cook with five times more water for one hour or longer, until soft and creamy in consistency. To boil, soak cereals for two to three hours and boil with ten times more water until one-half the original volume of water is left. Use a slow flame after the rice comes to a boil. If rice boils over, turn off flame and start it again when rice stops boiling over.

If the cereal is introduced to a baby less than five months old, the porridge is best digested if mashed well, preferably in a *suribachi* or with a mortar and pestle. If the baby is less than one year old, rice syrup or barley malt may be added to maintain a sweet taste similar to the mother's milk.

The proportion of water to grains depends upon the age of the baby and usually ranges from 10 to 1, to 7 to 1, to 3 to 1. Younger babies require a softer cereal and thus more water.

The porridge can also be given the baby as a replacement for mother's milk if the mother cannot breast-feed.

Be careful to avoid giving babies porridges or ready-to-eat creamy grain cereals made from flour products.

Soup can be introduced after five months, especially broth. The contents may include vegetables that have been well mashed until creamy in form. No salt, miso, or shoyu should be added before the baby is ten months old. Thereafter, a slightly salty taste may be used for flavoring. However, in such special cases as a baby with green stools or a baby experiencing digestive troubles, a salty taste may need to be used, only in small volume and for a short period.

Vegetables can be introduced after five to seven months, usually when teeth come in and grains have been given for one month. When introducing vegetables to children, start by giving sweet vegetables such as carrots, cabbage, squash, onions, daikon, and Chinese cabbage. These may be boiled or steamed and should be well cooked and thoroughly mashed. Because it is usually difficult for children to eat greens, parents should make a special effort to see that they are eaten. Sweet greens such as kale and broccoli are generally preferred over slightly bitter-tasting ones such as watercress and mustard greens. Very mild seasoning may be added to vegetables after ten months to encourage the appetite.

Beans can be introduced after eight months, but only small amounts of adzuki beans, lentils, or chickpeas, cooked well with kombu and mashed thoroughly, are recommended. Other beans such as kidney beans, soybeans, and navy beans can also be used occasionally, provided they are well cooked until very soft and mashed thoroughly. Beans may be seasoned with a tiny amount of sea salt or shoyu or sweetened with squash, barley malt, or rice syrup.

Sea vegetables can be introduced as a separate side dish after the child is from one and one-half to two years old, although grains are preferably cooked with kombu, and vegetables and beans may also be cooked with sea vegetables even if they are not always eaten.

Fruit should be given to babies or infants occasionally. Temperate-climate fruit, in season, can be introduced in small volume, about one tablespoon, in cooked and mashed form, after one and one-half and two years of age. However, in some special cases, cooked apples or apple juice may be used temporarily as an adjustment for some conditions.

Pickles that are traditionally made, quick and light in aging and seasoning, can be introduced after the child is two to three years old.

Beverages may include spring or well water, boiled or cooled, bancha twig tea, cereal grain tea, apple juice (warmed or hot), and amasake (which has been boiled with two times as much water and cooled).

For further information on infant and childhood nutrition or health, please refer to my book *Macrobiotic Pregnancy and Care of the Newborn* (New York and Tokyo: Japan Publications, 1984) or contact a qualified macrobiotic teacher or medical professional.

Guidelines for Younger Children

• **Whole Grains:** Fifty to 60 percent of daily consumption, by volume, should be whole-cereal grains. The first day prepare plain pressure-cooked short-grain brown rice. On following days, prepare brown rice pressure-cooked with 20 to 30 percent millet, then rice with 20 to 30 percent barley, then rice with 20 to 30 percent aduki beans or lentils, and then plain rice again. A delicious morning porridge can be made by taking leftover rice, adding a little more water to soften, and seasoning with a little miso at the end and simmering for two to three minutes more. In ordinary pressure cooking, the ratio of grain to water should be about 1:2. For seasoning, cook with a postage stamp–sized piece of kombu instead of salt, though in some cases sea salt may be used, depending on the child's condition. Other grains can be used occasionally, including whole wheat berries, rye, corn, and whole oats, though oats should be avoided for the first month. Buckwheat and seitan should be minimized, since they are usually too energizing for children. Good-quality sourdough bread may be enjoyed two to three times a week, and noodles, both udon and soba, may also be taken two to three times a week. Avoid all hard baked products until the condition improves, including cookies, cake, pie, crackers, muffins, and the like.

• **Soup:** Five to 10 percent soup, consisting of one or two cups or bowls per day of soup cooked with wakame sea vegetable and various land vegetables such as onions and carrots and seasoned with miso or shoyu. Occasionally a small volume of shiitake mushroom may be added to the soup. The miso may be barley miso, brown rice miso, or soybean (hatcho) miso and should be naturally aged two to three years. To satisfy a sweet tooth, millet soup with sweet vegetables such as squash, cabbage, onions, and carrots may be prepared often. Grain soups, bean soups, and other soups may be taken from time to time.

• **Vegetables:** Twenty to 30 percent vegetables, cooked in a variety of forms. In general, leafy vegetables, round, hard vegetables grown near the surface of the earth, and root vegetables can be used in about equal volume, i.e., one-third of each type for daily consumption. During cooking, they can be seasoned moderately with sea salt, shoyu, or miso. After the first month, unrefined vegetable oil, especially sesame or corn oil, may be used for sautéing vegetables several times a week, though oil should not be overconsumed. As a general rule, the following dishes may be prepared, though the frequency may differ from person to person: nishime-style vegetables, four times a week; squash-aduki-kombu dish, three times a week; dried daikon, one cup, three times a week; carrots and carrot tops or daikon and daikon tops, three times a week; blanched vegetables, five to seven times a week; pressed salad, five to seven times a week; raw salad and salad dressing, avoid; steamed greens, five to seven times a week; sautéed vegetables, two to three times a week, using a small volume of sesame oil; kinpira, two-thirds of a cup, two times a week; dried tofu, tofu, or tempeh with vegetables, two times a week. Limit seitan.

• **Beans:** Five percent small beans, such as aduki beans, lentils, chickpeas, or black soybeans, may be used daily, cooked together with sea vegetables such as kombu or with onions and carrots. Other beans may be used altogether two to three times a month. For seasoning, a small volume of unrefined sea salt or shoyu or miso can be used. Bean products, such as tempeh, natto, and dried or cooked tofu, may be used occasionally, but in moderate volume.

• **Sea Vegetables:** Five percent or less sea vegetable dishes, including wakame and kombu, daily when cooking grain, in soup, etc. A sheet of toasted nori may also be taken daily. A small dish of hijiki or arame should be prepared two times a week. All other sea vegetables are optional. Sea vegetables can be cooked with other vegetables or sautéed with a small volume of sesame oil after softening them by soaking and boiling lightly in water.

• **Condiments:** Condiments to be available on the table are gomashio (sesame salt), on the average made with 1 part salt to 18 parts sesame seeds (reduced to 1:16 after two months); kelp or wakame powder; umeboshi plum; and tekka, though all other regular macrobiotic condiments may be used if desired. These condiments may be used daily on grains and vegetables, but the volume should be moderate to suit individual appetite and taste.

• **Pickles:** Pickles, made at home in a variety of ways, are to be eaten daily, one tablespoon in all, though salty pickles are to be minimized.

• **Animal Food:** Meat, poultry, eggs, and other strong animal food is to be avoided. A small volume of white-meat fish may be eaten once or twice a week. The fish should be prepared steamed, boiled, or poached and garnished with grated daikon or ginger. After two months, fish may be eaten twice a week if desired. Strictly avoid blue-meat and red-meat fish and all shellfish.

• **Fruit:** The less the better, including both tropical and temperate-climate fruit, until the condition improves. If cravings develop, a moderate volume of cooked fruit with a pinch of sea salt or dried fruit (also preferably cooked) may be taken. Juice, such as apple cider, may be taken in moderation.

• **Sweets and Snacks:** Avoid all sweets and desserts made with sugar, chocolate, honey, carob, maple syrup, and other simple sugars. To satisfy a sweet taste, use sweet vegetables every day in cooking, drink sweet vegetable drink (see special drinks below), or eat sweet vegetable jam. Mochi, rice balls, vegetable sushi, and other grain-based snacks may be eaten frequently. Limit rice cakes, popcorn, and other dry or baked snacks, as they may harden the tumor. Macrobiotic desserts made with good-quality grain-based sweeteners such as amasake, barley malt, or rice syrup may be enjoyed in moderation.

• **Nuts and Seeds:** Nuts and nut butters are to be limited. Unsalted, roasted seeds such as sunflower seeds and pumpkin seeds may be consumed as a snack, up to one cup altogether per week.

• **Seasonings:** Seasonings, such as unrefined sea salt, shoyu, and miso, are to be used moderately in order to avoid unnecessary thirst. Avoid mirin and garlic. If the child become particularly thirsty after the meal or between meals, you should cut back on these seasonings until the normal level of thirst returns.

• **Beverages:** Good spring or well water of natural quality may be used as a daily beverage. Bancha tea may also be taken frequently. Strictly avoid the beverages on the "infrequent" and "avoid" list and don't take grain coffee for the first two to three months after starting this new way of eating.

The most important thing in connection with dietary practice is chewing very well, until all food becomes liquid in the mouth and well mixed with saliva. Chew very, very well, at least 50 times, preferably 100 times, per mouthful. It is also important to avoid overeating and eating within three hours of sleeping.

As noted in the introduction to Part II, children who have received or who are currently undergoing medical treatment may need to make further dietary modifications.

SPECIAL DRINKS AND PREPARATIONS

Children with cancer may also consume some special drinks and dishes, which, taken in small volume, can strengthen blood and lymph quality. These dishes include:

• **Sweet Vegetable Drink:** Take one small cup every day for the first month, then every third day the second month.

• **Ume-Sho-Kuzu Drink:** Take one small cup every two days for two weeks, then one cup a week for three to four weeks. This will help energize and restore vitality.

• **Grated Daikon:** Grate one-half small cup of fresh daikon and add a few crops of shoyu. Taken occasionally, two or three times a week, this will help digestion and discharge old fat and oil from the body.

• **Carp and Burdock Soup (Koi Koku):** Cook whole carp with shredded roots, seasoned with miso and a little grated ginger. This soup may be used as the soup dish a few times a week for a period of several weeks. It is very, very energizing and to be used only medicinally. See the recipe in Part III.

• **Brown Rice Cream:** In the event of appetite loss, two to three bowls of genuine brown rice cream can be served daily with a condiment of either gomashio (sesame salt), umeboshi plum, or tekka. This rice cream may also be used occasionally as part of the regular whole-grain diet. If the child requires a sweet taste, add sweet vegetable jam, amasake, barley malt, or rice syrup or a small amount of cooked fruits to the cereal.

HOME CARES

• **Body Scrub:** Scrubbing the whole body, including the abdominal region and the spinal region, with a towel that has been immersed in hot water and squeezed out is very helpful for better circulation of blood, lymph, and other body fluids, as well as for activating physical and mental energies.

• **Swelling:** Swelling of the spleen and abdominal regions sometimes accompanies children's cancers and is caused by overeating in general, especially protein, and excessive intake of beverages, seasonings, and condiments. In such cases, food consumption should be simplified for a period of several days up to ten days. During this period, daily consumption may consist of pressure-cooked brown rice and barley, one to two cups of miso soup, a small dish of half dried daikon and half daikon leaves pickled for a long period (over two months) with sea salt and rice bran, a dish of vegetables such as onions, carrots, and cabbage sautéed in sesame oil, and several cups of bancha twig tea. However, this simplified diet should not be continued for longer than ten days unless under supervision of an experienced macrobiotic teacher, nutritionist, or medical associate or professional.

OTHER CONSIDERATIONS

• General physical exercise and deep breathing exercises are recommended, especially outside in the fresh air. Shiatsu massage and other treatments to relax and loosen any physical and psychological stagnations and hardenings are also very helpful.

• Maintaining clean, fresh air inside the home is important, and for this purpose green plants can be placed in each room. Indoor air circulation can also be maintained by frequently opening the windows.

• Wearing cotton underwear and avoiding synthetic fabrics are helpful for better skin metabolism and facilitate energy flow through the body.

• Avoid exposure to electromagnetic fields. Keep common hand-held appliances to a minimum. If you have a choice, have the child live, play, and go to school in areas away from an artificial electronic environment.

27

Radiation- and Environmentally- Related Cancer

FREQUENCY

Nuclear radiation has been associated with various cancers, including leukemia, lymphoma, bone cancer, brain cancer, and thyroid cancer, since the 1940s. Survivors of the bombing of Hiroshima and Nagasaki, workers in atomic weapons and nuclear power plants, persons exposed to atomic fallout, residents near Three Mile Island and Chernobyl (sites of two major nuclear accidents), and other individuals contaminated by radioactive particles have been most affected. Tens of millions of people are believed to have been directly exposed to high levels of nuclear radiation from these sources, while nearly everyone living on the planet since 1945 has been affected to some extent. Estimates of total deaths from cancer related to atomic fallout and nuclear power plant emissions over the last generation range from several thousand to a million or more. In the last decade, nonionizing, as well as ionizing, radiation has come under increasing review, and studies are beginning to associate leukemia, lymphoma, brain tumors, bone cancer, and other malignancies with exposure to power lines, computer terminals, and other sources of artificial electromagnetic radiation. Over the next few years, we can expect the magnitude of this problem to be more clearly defined. Presently, 3 percent of cancers in the United States are related to radiation.

CAUSE OF CANCER

Radioactive particles emitted by nuclear reactions can ionize, or alter, the electrical charge of the atoms and molecules that comprise body cells and tissues. Such particles can also accumulate in different parts of the body, leading to destruction and deterioration of surrounding organs and tissues. Radiation can also damage the genetic structure of cells, such as those involved in reproductive functions, leading to genetic abnormality, sterility, and other disorders in future generations. The accumulation of radioactive particles in the environment may result in long-term imbalances in the food supply and in plant and animal life. The effects of radiation are cumulative, and even small doses may lead to leukemia or other cancer within several years, though often malignancy does not show up for ten, twenty, thirty years, or more.

The symptoms of radiation sickness include nausea, vomiting, loss of appetite, diarrhea, hair falling out, internal bleeding, sores on the skin, convulsions, and premature aging. According to traditional Far Eastern medicine, these are signs of yin, dispersing energy. Also, susceptibility to infection and anemia are common signs of radiation sickness due to abnormally low levels of red blood cells and high levels of white blood cells. Diagnostically, the hair on the head corresponds with the hairlike villi of the small intestine. When people's hair began to fall out after the bombings, it indicated trouble in the intestine and severely curtailed blood production. In addition to the blood and lymphatic system, the bones and deep inner organs are particularly susceptible to radioactive substances, such as strontium 90, which displace calcium and other minerals in the tissue and bone. From the macrobiotic view, radiation sickness and related cancers are caused primarily by overall weakening of the intestines, which are connected with the transformation of metabolized foodstuffs into healthy red blood cells. Weakening of the intestines would also produce vomiting, diarrhea, loss of appetite, nausea, and other common symptoms. Because the brain receives the greatest flow of blood, and because blood is stored in the bone marrow, these organs are often the site of malignancy following exposure to radiation.

The Earth is constantly being bathed by natural electromagnetic radiation from the sun, moon, stars, and distant galaxies. These light waves, sound waves, radio waves, and other rays and vibrations ordinarily represent no danger to human beings or other life on the planet. However, during the last century, modern civilization has developed communications and industrial technologies that produce large amounts of artificial electromagnetic energy that vibrate at the more extreme octaves of the radiation spectrum. This development has paralleled the increasing production of highly unnatural and artificial food. With the Industrial Revolution, we have moved from wood and coal to oil, gas, electricity, and most recently nuclear energy, as a source of energy. Characterized by accelerating speed, energy, heat, and density, modern civilization has sought for ever more increasingly extreme materials to fuel its unchecked expansion. Extreme technologies characterize the modern food system, from chemical agriculture and highly refined processing to irradiation, genetically altered foods, and microwave cooking.

While nuclear radiation and other forms of artificial energy are dangerous and should be avoided whenever possible, returning to a natural way of eating may help eliminate the toxic effects of exposure and enable us to maintain general good health. In 1945, for example, there were a small number of people following a macrobiotic diet who lived in Hiroshima and Nagasaki at the time of the world's first atomic explosions. Among those who survived the initial blast, the individuals who ate macrobiotically were able to function normally and help many other survivors overcome radiation sickness by eating brown rice, well-cooked vegetables, miso soup, sea vegetables, pickled salt plums, and natural sea salt. From the symptoms of atomic disease they realized that radiation was extremely expansive, or yin, and that the blood could be strengthened, or yangized, with counterbalancing opposite factors such as a salt-rich grain and cooked-vegetable diet.

In the decades since the first atomic bombings, as a result of these macrobiotic experiences scientists in Canada and Japan have confirmed that miso and sea vegetables contain substances in addition to salt that can help protect the body from radiation by binding and discharging radioactive elements. In 1986, within two weeks after the nuclear accident at Chernobyl, all the macrobiotic food disappeared from stores in Europe. People knew its power.

At the social level, various government agencies have proposed that nuclear waste materials be stored in salt mines or deposits in order to neutralize their deadly emissions. This is an example of how yin and yang are used in the modern world, although scientists do not understand the underlying principle of balance—namely, macrobiotic philosophy—involved.

In addition to nuclear radioactivity, which is a form of ionizing radiation, nonionizing radiation such as that given off by conventional power generators, common household and office equipment, and hand-held appliances has come under increasing scrutiny in the last ten years. In the past, it was believed that nonionizing radiation was safe. However, research has begun to emerge showing that leukemia, lymphoma, brain cancer, and other tumors, as well as many other serious illnesses, are more frequent among those who live in close proximity to power lines, transformers, and electrical stations, those whose work exposes them to artificial electromagnetic fields, and possibly users of computers, electric hair dryers, and other equipment and devices (see Table 19).

In the laboratory, medical tests recently have associated exposure to artificial electromagnetic fields with affecting the flow of chemicals across membranes, interfering with the synthesis of genetic materials, altering the activity of hormones and other chemicals, and enhancing the growth of cancer cells. From the macrobiotic view, again these are all yin effects—expansive, weakening, disintegrating, decomposing.

The spread of computers, television, copy machines, air conditioners, smoke detectors, garage-door openers, supermarket scanners, and numerous other appliances and devices has contributed to our rapidly growing electronic environment. Some of this radiation is low-level, such as that of a quartz watch or a TV remote, while others are stronger, such as that of a microwave oven or a hospital X ray. Day by day, however, all artificial electromagnetic stimuli have a cumulative effect on health and vitality.

A healthy human body has a marvelous capacity to adjust to its environment, even one with radioactivity and artificial electromagnetic fields. People eating macrobiotically retain greater resistance but should minimize their exposure or counterbalance the potentially harmful effects with special foods, green plants, and other methods noted below. People eating the modern diet have a much lower tolerance for radioactivity and electromagnetic fields (EMFs) and are at a higher risk of developing leukemia and other cancers.

Once, about twenty-five years ago, at Erewhon, the pioneer natural foods store in Boston, we had a rat problem. Not wanting to use harmful chemicals or kill the rats, the staff decided to use an ultra-high-frequency sound to disperse them. When the device was sounded, the rats all started to eat brown rice and seaweed. They stopped eating everything else. They instinctively knew that it was survival food. In the future, I hope that we humans are as smart as rats and mice.

TABLE 19.   THE ELECTROMAGNETIC SPECTRUM, AND HEALTH AND DISEASE

Wave	Frequency (in hertz)	Applications	Associated Conditions
(Ionizing)			
Gamma	10^{20-21}	Nuclear energy	Leukemia, brain tumors, lymphonoma, birth defects, genetic damage
X rays	10^{17-20}	Medical exams	Leukemia, breast cancer, reproductive disorders, genetic damage
Ultraviolet	10^{15-17}	Ozone-depleted sunlight, sunlamps	Skin cancer
(Nonionizing)			
Visible	10^{14-15}	Natural light, wood, gas, coal, charcoal energy	Good health
Infrared	10^{12-14}		
Microwave	10^{10-12}	Radar, satellites, microwave ovens, computers	Heat damage, eye disorders, certain cancers, birth defects
UHF	10^{8}	Communications, computers	Various disorders
VHF	10^{7}	Communications, computers	Various disorders
HF	10^{6}	Communications, computers	Various disorders
LF	10^{5}	Communications, computers	Various disorders
VLF	10^{4}	Communications, computers	Various disorders

TABLE 19. (*Con't.*)

Wave	Frequency (in hertz)	Applications	Associated Conditions
(Nonionizing)			
ULF	10^3	Communications, computers	Various disorders
ELF	10^2	Ordinary electricity, high power lines, home wiring, appliances, computers	Reproductive and birth defects, cancer promotion, central nervous system disorders

MEDICAL EVIDENCE

Related to Nuclear Radiation

• In 1964 scientists at the Gastrointestinal Research Laboratory at McGill University in Montreal reported that a substance derived from the sea vegetable kelp could reduce by 50 to 80 percent the amount of radioactive strontium absorbed through the intestine. Stanley Skoryna, M.D., said that in animal experiments sodium alginate obtained from brown algae permitted calcium to be normally absorbed through the intestinal wall while binding most of the strontium. The sodium alginate and strontium were subsequently excreted from the body. The experiments were designed to devise a method to counteract the effects of nuclear fallout and radiation. Source: S. C. Skoryna et al., "Studies on Inhibition of Intestinal Absorption of Radioactive Strontium," *Canadian Medical Association Journal* 91:285–88.

• In a follow-up experiment in 1968, Canadian researchers reported that sea vegetables contained a polysaccharide substance that selectively bound radioactive strontium and helped eliminate it from the body. In laboratory experiments, sodium alginate prepared from kelp, kombu, and other brown seaweeds off the Atlantic and Pacific coasts was introduced along with strontium and calcium into rats. The reduction of radioactive particles in bone uptake, measured in the femur, reached as high as 80 percent, with little interference with calcium absorption. "The evaluation of biological activity of different marine algae is important because of their practical significance in preventing absorption of radioactive products of atomic fission as well as in their use as possible natural decontaminators." Source: Y. Tanaka et al., "Studies on Inhibition of Intestinal Absorption of Radio-active Strontium," *Canadian Medical Association Journal* 99:169–75.

• In 1979, 64 veterans or widows of U.S. soldiers stationed in Hiroshima and Nagaski in 1945 to help clean up the A-bombed cities filed claims asserting that their exposure to radiation had contributed to serious or fatal illness, including bone cancer, leukemia, and blood-related diseases. Source: Harvey

Wasserman and Norman Soloman, *Killing Our Own* (New York: Delta, 1982), 14–15.

• A team studying atomic bomb radioactivity has found miso is effective in helping to remove radioactive elements from the body and controlling inflammation of organs caused by radioactivity. In experiments conducted on male and female rats four weeks after birth, radioisotopes of iodine 131 and cesium 134 were injected into the animals' stomachs. Both isotopes are secondary elements produced in nuclear reactor accidents. The iodine 131 isotope is absorbed in the thyroid gland, while the cesium 134 accumulates in muscles and in the intestines.

Researchers at Hiroshima University Medical Center found that there was only half the amount of iodine 131 in the blood of the group fed with miso in contrast to the control group three and six hours after the injections. Lower amounts of radioactive particles were also measured in the kidneys, liver, and spleen. Although there was no difference in the amount of radioactive cesium in the blood, a high amount of cesium was eliminated from the muscles of the group eating miso.

In other tests of exposure to a half-lethal dose of radiation to test the effect of miso on victims of a nuclear explosion, more than 80 percent of the rats from each group died within one week. However, the inflammation of organs commonly seen after exposure to radiation was less for the rats eating miso. Akihiro Ito, head of the Hiroshima University medical team, said that this showed that miso stimulated the body's circulation and metabolic system. Source: "Miso Shows Promise as Treatment for Radiation," *Japan Times*, September 27, 1988.

• People who eat miso regularly may be up to five times more resistant to radiation than people who do not eat miso. This is the conclusion of scientific studies conducted by Kazumitsu Watanabe, professor of cancer and radiation at Hiroshima University's atomic bomb radiation research center.

In laboratory experiments, he tested the cells in the small intestine of mice. These cells absorb nutrients and are particularly sensitive to radiation. They are easily destroyed by radiation. The victims of Hiroshima and Nagasaki suffered from severe cases of diarrhea after the atomic bomb because of massive destruction of these cells.

Forty-nine-week-old mice were given miso as 10 percent of their food for seven days prior to exposure to radiation. Mice were exposed to full-body X rays 1,400 to 2,400 times stronger than a regular medical X ray (seven to ten curies). Three days later their cells were examined. The loss of cells was less severe in the miso-eating mice than in regular mice. When nine curies were administered, the gap between miso-eating and regular mice's loss of cells became greater. Ten curies is a lethal dose for humans. When ten curies were given to miso-eating mice, 60 percent survived, compared to only 9 percent of the mice that did not eat miso.

"I don't know specifically what element in miso is effective," Professor Watanabe told the South Western Japan Conference on the Effects of Radiation. "The small intestines of mice and humans are quite similar. Therefore this study indicates that miso is a preventive measure against radiation."

In other tests at Hiroshima University, it has already been shown that miso has the property of eliminating radiation from the body and can help relieve liver cancer. Plans for further studies include how miso affects cancer of the large intestine and stomach as well as the effect of radiation on blood pressure. Sources: "Miso Protects against Radiation," *Yomiuri Shinbun*, July 16, 1990, and "People Who Consume Miso Regularly Are More Resistant to Radiation," *Nikan Kogyo Shinbun*, July 25, 1990.

• In 1977 researchers found that workers at the Hanford Reservation in Washington State, which manufactured plutonium for atomic weapons, had high death rates for multiple myeloma. Federal standards for maximum exposure in the workplace are currently 5 rems (radiation equivalent in man, a unit indicating biological effect of radiation) a year, equivalent to 100 to 125 bone X rays. The study found unexpectedly high cancer rates in workers whose total exposure not just yearly, but over an entire career, was 4 rems. Four rems is equivalent to the natural background radiation received by the average person in modern society in forty years.

In 1991 scientists reported that workers exposed to low levels of radiation at the Oak Ridge National Laboratory in Tennessee, site of nuclear weapons production since the 1940s, had higher death rates from leukemia, bone cancer, and other cancers than unexposed workers. The study was the first to show a clear association between low levels of radiation and all types of cancer. The Oak Ridge workers were exposed to an average of 1.7 rems over their careers, about a third of the annual limit. Source: *Journal of the American Medical Association* 265 (1991):1397–1402, and "Study Links Cancer Deaths and Low Levels of Radiation," *New York Times*, March 20, 1991.

Related to Electromagnetic Fields

• In the late 1970s, seven unusual clusters of birth defects and miscarriages were reported in Canada and the United States among women who operated video display terminals (VDTs). A 1979 study showed that children in the Denver area who lived in homes near electric distribution wires carrying high current had died of cancer at twice the expected rate. Source: *Science News*, April 21, 1979.

• In 1982 researchers reported a slightly elevated incidence of breast cancer in women living near high-current power lines. Source: *Science News*, September 28, 1991.

• In Britain, researchers found that exposure to fluorescent lights was associated with a two to two and a half times higher risk of malignant melanoma. Source: J. A. Treichel, *Science News* 122 (August 28, 1982).

• In 1986 researchers found that children living within fifteen meters of lines carrying electricity from the power company's substation to the neighborhood transformer faced five times the risk of all forms of cancer compared with children who lived farther away. Source: *Science News*, February 14, 1987.

• The average annual exposure to radiation for a person in the United States is about .1 rem. One chest X ray gives about .02 rem. In 1989 the NRC issued a study predicting that the risk of getting cancer from low levels of radiation appeared to be four times as high as previously estimated. Warren Sinclair, president of the National Council on Radiation Protection and Measurements, said that current limits for nuclear workers may have to be dropped from 5 rems a year to 1 or 2. The recommended maximum exposure for the public is .1 rem. Source: "Higher Cancer Risk Found in Radiation," *New York Times*, December 20, 1989.

• In 1989 researchers reported that exposure to medical X rays during infancy can significantly increase women's chances of breast cancer in their thirties. Source: Nancy Hildreth, "The Risk of Breast Cancer after Irradiation of the Thymus in Infancy," *New England Journal of Medicine* 321:1281–84.

• A 1984 study found that men who had died from brain cancer frequently had been employed in electrical occupations. In 1986 investigators for the New York State Department of Health reported that "prolonged exposure to low-level magnetic fields may increase the risk of developing cancer in children." The incidence of cancer in this study, and in another study in Sweden, was associated with magnetic field strengths of two to three milligauss, which was considered relatively low to begin with. A 1988 study of men who had died of brain cancer in East Texas found that the risk for electric-utility workers was thirteen times greater than for other workers. In 1989 epidemiologists at Johns Hopkins University reported that an elevated risk of all cancers was greater among cable splicers working for the New York Telephone Company. Their rate of leukemia was seven times higher than that for other workers in the company. The mean level of field to which they had been exposed was 4.3 milligrauss. A pulsed extremely low frequency (ELF) magnetic field of between 4 to 4 milligrauss has been measured at a distance of twelve inches from most common types of personal computers.

In the 1980s scientists found that low-level electromagnetic fields can interfere with the ability of T-lymphocyte cells to kill cancer cells, suggesting that the fields may be acting as cancer promoters by suppressing the immune system.

In 1988 researchers demonstrated that weak 60Hz electric fields similar in strength to those encountered while standing beneath a typical overhead high-voltage power line or close to a computer monitor could increase the activity of an enzyme called ornithine decarboxylase, which is associated with cancer promotion.

In the early 1980s, Spanish researchers found that when chicken eggs were exposed to weak pulsed ELF magnetic fields nearly 80 percent developed abnormally, with malformations of the cephalic nervous system.

In 1988 researchers found that women who worked with VDTs for more than twenty hours a week experienced a risk of both early and late miscarriages that was 80 percent higher than normal. Sources: "The Risk of Miscarriage and Birth Defects among Women Who Use Visual Display Terminals during Pregnancy," *American Journal of Industrial Medicine*, June 1988, and Paul Brodeur, "The Magnetic-Field Menage," *MacWorld*, July 1990, 136–47.

• In 1991 researchers reported that men whose occupations involve frequent exposure to EMFs, such as power-line installers and workers involved in power-plant operations, have a six times higher rate of breast cancer than other men. The investigators concluded that "studies of exposure to electromagnetic fields and the risk of breast cancer in women are warranted." Source: P. A. Demers et al., "Occupational Exposure to Electromagnetic Fields and Breast Cancer in Men," *American Journal of Epidemiology* 134;340–47.

• In a 1991 study, researchers found that childhood leukemia is linked with proximity to power lines and the use of certain appliances, like hair dryers and black-and-white television sets. Source: "Electric Currents and Leukemia Show Puzzling Links in New Study," *New York Times*, February 8, 1991.

• A 1990 study found a weak risk between childhood leukemia and brain cancer and prenatal exposure to electric blankets. Source: D. A. Savitz et al., "Magnetic Field Exposure from Electric Appliances and Childhood Cancer," *American Journal of Epidemiology* 131: 763–73.

• In Connecticut, police officers have filed lawsuits claiming that their work with radar guns caused thyroid or testicular cancer. Around the country, other police officers with cancer have also begun to associate their condition with use of radar equipment. Source: NBC News, June 19, 1992.

• In 1992 Sweden's National Board for Industrial and Technical Development announced that from now on it "will act on the assumption that there is a connection between exposure to power frequency magnetic fields and cancer, in particular childhood cancer."

Marking the first time that a national government has recognized the EMF-cancer link, Sweden is expected to establish safety standards for new power lines and evacuate families with children away from existing lines.

Swedish researchers reported a fourfold increase in the risk of leukemia among children who live near power lines. Scientists also showed that cancer risk goes up with increasing exposure.

Source: Thomas H. Maugh II, "Swedish Research Finds EMF-Cancer Link," *Los Angeles Times*, November 9, 1992.

• In 1993, public concern focused on cellular telephones and their possible association with cancer, especially brain cancer, following a highly publicized lawsuit by a Florida man who asserted that his wife died of brain cancer following chronic use of a cellular telephone. Meanwhile, the death of the chairman of TLC Beatrice Co. from brain cancer and the diagnosis of brain cancer in another nationally known executive, both of whom may have been heavy users of cellular phones, fueled the controversy. Several other people with brain tumors came forward and reported that they had used cellular phones several hours a day and their tumors arose in the part of the brain nearest to where their telephone antennaes pressed against their skulls when they talked.

While comprehensive studies have not been done on cellular phones, which have been available only for the last ten years, some preliminary findings are suggestive. Dr. Stephen Cleary at the Medical College of Virginia reported that when he exposed human brain tumor cells and normal human blood cells to two hours of radio waves, the cells grew 30 percent faster than unexposed cells and maintained that brisk pace for days. He performed the experiment at two frequencies, the high frequency of a microwave oven and a low frequency used in factories to seal plastics. The cellular phone frequency—840 to 880 megahertz—fell in between.

In Sweden, a medical study sponsored by a cellular phone maker found that laboratory animals exposed to continuous and pulsed waves at slightly higher frequencies than cellular phones showed some biological effects as radiation penetrated the blood-brain barrier. Source: *New York Times*, February 2, 1993 and *Boston Globe*, February 8, 1993.

DIAGNOSIS

The symptoms of radiation sickness are noted above. Exposure to artificial electromagnetic fields usually results in less severe symptoms. For example, among computer users, eye disorders, including eye strain, blurred vision, and cataracts, are commonly reported. In traditional Oriental medicine, eye problems are related to the liver, which has the overall responsibility of protecting the body from toxins and harmful influences. Eye troubles show that the liver is also affected. Other signs include general weakness, fatigue, and moist or dry lips. These indicate intestinal weakness and possible disturbances in blood and lymph production.

DIETARY RECOMMENDATIONS

The foods and beverages that primarily enhance radiation-related cancers are those in the extreme yin category, including sugar, sugar-treated foods and drinks, ice cream, chocolate, carob, honey, soft drinks and soda, tropical fruits, fruit juices, oily and greasy foods, dairy foods, especially butter, milk, and cream, stimulants and aromatic foods and drinks, and many chemicals contained in foods, beverages, and supplements. All of these should be avoided in daily eating. However, the consumption of these items is often accompanied by the intake of foods from the extreme yang category, including meat, poultry, eggs, and cheese, in order to achieve a rough counterbalance. All these foods create a more acidic environment within the body and, accordingly, are also to be avoided, with the exception of white-meat fish, which can be consumed occasionally in moderate volume. The following also enhance leukemic and malignant conditions and should be discontinued: ice-cold foods and drinks, hot spices, various herbs and herb drinks that have stimulant effects, and vegetables that historically originated in the tropics, including potatoes, tomatoes, and eggplant.

Conversely, brown rice and other whole grains that contain a certain acid that can chemically unite with and discharge radioactive factors such as strontium 90 should be taken daily. Minerals contained in miso soup and sea vegetables have the same kind of effect. In general, a slightly saltier—more yang— way of eating can be observed, emphasizing slightly stronger foods, stronger cooking methods, stronger seasonings, and other more contractive qualities.

In the event of a nuclear accident or explosion, observe the following general dietary guidelines for several days to several weeks or longer, depending on the magnitude of the event. The more detailed dietary guidelines that follow should be implemented depending on the severity of the symptoms. Of course, if the explosion is serious, you may need to evacuate the area (see "Other Considerations" below for advice on this procedure). Pregnant women and children within 100 miles of the accident should leave the area.

Within a radius of 30 miles of the reactor or explosion:
Whole grains—60 to 70 percent
Miso soup with vegetables and sea vegetables—3 to 5 percent (1 or 2 cups or bowls)
Vegetables—20 percent (cooked, no raw food)
Beans and sea vegetables—5 to 10 percent
No animal food, fruit, sweets, desserts

Within a radius of from 30 to 150 miles:
Whole grains—60 percent
Miso soup with vegetables and sea vegetables—3 to 5 percent (1 or 2 cups or bowls); occasionally grain or bean soup
Vegetables—20 to 25 percent (cooked, no raw food)
Beans and sea vegetables—5 to 10 percent
Limit animal food (fish once a week); limit fruit (cooked or dried cooked fruit once a week); avoid sweets and desserts

Within a radius of 150 to 300 miles:
Whole grains—50 percent or more
Miso soup with vegetables and sea vegetables—3 to 5 percent (1 or 2 cups or bowls); occasionally grain or bean soup
Vegetables—25 to 30 percent (cooked, no raw food)
Beans and sea vegetables—5 to 10 percent
Occasional fish or fruit (cooked); limit sweets and desserts

Following are daily dietary guidelines, by volume, for the prevention and relief of radiation-related cancers in general or exposure to extreme radioactivity:

• **Whole Grains:** Fifty to 60 percent of daily consumption, by volume, should be whole-cereal grains. The first day prepare plain pressure-cooked short-grain brown rice. On following days, prepare brown rice pressure-cooked with 20 to 30 percent millet, then rice with 20 to 30 percent barley, then rice with 20 to 30 percent aduki beans or lentils, and then plain rice again. A delicious morning porridge can be made by taking leftover rice, adding a little more water to soften, and seasoning with a little miso at the end and simmering for two to three minutes more. In ordinary pressure cooking, the ratio of grain to water should be about 1:2. For seasoning, cook with a pinch of sea salt. Other grains can be used occasionally, including whole wheat berries, rye, corn, and whole oats, though oats should be avoided for the first month. Buckwheat and seitan may be eaten in moderation. Good-quality sourdough bread may be enjoyed two to three times a week, and noodles, both udon and soba, may also be taken two to three times a week. Avoid all hard baked products until the condition improves, including cookies, cake, pie, crackers, muffins, and the like.
• **Soup:** Five to 10 percent soup, consisting of one or two cups or bowls per day of soup cooked with wakame sea vegetable and various land vegetables such as onions and carrots and seasoned with miso or shoyu. (Use about one quarter

to one half teaspoon of miso per cup.) Occasionally a small volume of shiitake mushroom may be added to the soup. The miso may be barley miso, brown rice miso, or soybean (hatcho) miso and should be naturally aged two to three years. Grain soups, bean soups, and other soups may be taken from time to time. Less frequently, a small portion of white-meat fish or small dried fish can also be cooked into the soup with vegetables, sea vegetables, and/or grains.

• **Vegetables:** Twenty to 30 percent vegetables, cooked in a variety of forms. In general, leafy vegetables, round, hard vegetables grown near the surface of the earth, and root vegetables can be used in about equal volume, i.e., one-third of each type for daily consumption. During cooking, they can be seasoned moderately with sea salt, shoyu, or miso. After the first month, unrefined vegetable oil, especially sesame or corn oil, may be used for sautéing vegetables several times a week, though oil should not be overconsumed. As a general rule, the following dishes may be prepared, though the frequency may differ from person to person: nishime-style vegetables, four times a week; squash-aduki-kombu dish, three times a week; dried daikon, one cup, three times a week; carrots and carrot tops or daikon and daikon tops, three times a week; blanched vegetables, five to seven times a week; pressed salad, five to seven times a week; raw salad and salad dressing, avoid; steamed greens, five to seven times a week; sautéed vegetables, two to three times a week (with water the first month and sesame oil thereafter); kinpira, two-thirds of a cup, two times a week, then oil may be used after three weeks; dried tofu, tofu, tempeh, or seitan with vegetables, two times a week.

• **Beans:** Five percent small beans, such as aduki beans, lentils, chickpeas, or black soybeans, may be used daily, cooked together with sea vegetables such as kombu or with onions and carrots. Other beans may be used altogether two to three times a month. For seasoning, a small volume of unrefined sea salt or shoyu or miso can be used. Bean products, such as tempeh, natto, and dried or cooked tofu, may be used occasionally, but in moderate volume.

• **Sea Vegetables:** Five percent or less sea vegetable dishes, including wakame and kombu, daily when cooking grain, in soup, etc. A sheet of toasted nori may also be taken daily. A small dish of hijiki or arame should be prepared two times a week. All other sea vegetables are optional. Sea vegetables are excellent for this condition, but be careful not to take too much volume or cook too strongly, as tightness may develop.

• **Condiments:** Condiments to be available on the table are gomashio (sesame salt), on the average made with 1 part salt to 16 parts sesame seeds; kelp or wakame powder; umeboshi plum (which is very good for this condition); and tekka, though all other regular macrobiotic condiments may be used if desired. These condiments may be used daily on grains and vegetables, but the volume should be moderate to suit individual appetite and taste.

• **Pickles:** Pickles, made at home in a variety of ways, are to be eaten daily, one tablespoon in all, though salty pickles are to be minimized.

• **Animal Food:** Meat, poultry, eggs, and other strong animal food are to be avoided. A small volume of white-meat fish may be eaten once a week. The fish should be prepared steamed, boiled, or poached and garnished with grated daikon or ginger. After two months, fish may be eaten twice a week if desired. Strictly avoid blue-meat and red-meat fish and all shellfish.

• **Fruit:** None the best, the less the better, including both tropical and temperate-climate fruit, until the condition improves. If cravings develop, a small volume of cooked fruit with a pinch of sea salt or dried fruit (also preferably cooked) may be taken. Avoid all fruit juices and cider.

• **Sweets and Snacks:** Avoid all sweets and deserts, including good-quality macrobiotic desserts, until the condition improves. To satisfy a sweet tooth, use sweet vegetables every day in cooking, drink sweet vegetable drink (see special drinks below), and use sweet vegetable jam. Mochi, rice balls, vegetable sushi, and other grain-based snacks may be eaten frequently. Limit rice cakes, popcorn, and other dry or baked snacks, as they may harden the tumor. In the event of cravings, a small volume of amasake, barley malt, or rice syrup may be taken.

• **Nuts and Seeds:** Nuts and nut butters are to be limited due to their high amount of fat and protein, except for chestnuts. Unsalted, roasted seeds such as sunflower seeds and pumpkin seeds may be consumed as a snack, up to one cup altogether per week.

• **Seasonings:** Seasonings, such as unrefined sea salt, shoyu, and miso, are to be used moderately in order to avoid unnecessary thirst. Avoid mirin and garlic. If you become particularly thirsty after a meal or between meals, you should cut back on these seasonings until the normal level of thirst returns.

• **Beverages:** Beverages and other dietary practices can follow the general recommendations in Part I, including bancha twig tea as the main beverage. Strictly avoid the beverages on the "infrequent" and "avoid" list and don't take grain coffee for the first two to three months, after starting this new way of eating.

The most important thing in connection with dietary practice is chewing very well, until all food becomes liquid in the mouth and well mixed with saliva. Chew very, very well, at least 50 times, preferably 100 times, per mouthful. It is also important to avoid overeating and eating within three hours of sleeping.

As noted in the introduction to Part II, persons who have received or who are currently undergoing medical treatment may need to make further dietary modifications.

SPECIAL DRINKS AND PREPARATIONS

Persons with radiation-related cancers may also consume some special drinks and dishes, which, taken in small volume, can strengthen blood quality. These dishes include:

• **Sweet Vegetable Drink:** Take one small cup every day for the first month, then every third day the second month.

• **Ume-Sho-Kuzu Drink:** Take one small cup every two days for two weeks, then one cup a day for three to four weeks. This will give energy and vitality.

• **Grated Daikon:** Grate ½ cup of fresh daikon, add several drops of shoyu, and take two to three times a week.

• **Shio Kombu (Salty Kombu):** Sliced sheets of kombu (about one-half-inch square), cooked in a mixture of one-half shoyu and one-half water, and boiled down until the liquid becomes completely absorbed by the kombu (usually two to four hours). Consume several pieces daily with cereal grain dishes.

• **Carp and Burdock Soup (Koi Koku):** This soup is very energizing. Cooked whole carp with shredded burdock roots, seasoned with miso and a little grated ginger. This soup may be used as the soup dish a few times a week for a period of several weeks. See the recipe in Part III.

• **Brown Rice Cream:** In the event of appetite loss, two to three bowls of genuine brown rice cream can be served daily with a condiment of either gomashio (sesame salt), umeboshi plum, or tekka. This rice cream may also be used occasionally as part of the regular whole-grain diet.

HOME CARES

• **Body Scrub:** Scrubbing the whole body, including the abdominal region and the spinal region, with a towel that has been immersed in hot water and squeezed out is very helpful for better circulation of blood, lymph, and other body fluids, as well as for activating physical and mental energies.

• **Swelling:** Swelling of the spleen and abdominal regions sometimes accompanies radiation-related cancers and is caused by overeating in general, especially protein, and excessive intake of beverages, seasonings, and condiments. In such cases, food consumption should be simplified for a period of several days up to ten days. During this period, daily consumption may consist of pressure-cooked brown rice and barley, one to two cups of miso soup, a small dish of half-dried daikon and daikon leaves pickled for a long period (over two months) with sea salt and rice bran, a dish of vegetables such as onions, carrots, and cabbage sautéed in sesame oil, and several cups of bancha twig tea. However, this simplified diet should not be continued for longer than ten days unless under supervision of an experienced macrobiotic teacher, nutritionist, or medical associate or professional.

OTHER CONSIDERATIONS

• General physical exercise and deep breathing exercises are recommended, especially outside in the fresh air. Shiatsu massage and other treatments to relax and loosen any physical and psychological stagnation and hardening are also very helpful.

• Maintaining clean, fresh air inside the home is important, and for this purpose green plants can be placed in each room. Indoor air circulation can also be maintained by frequently opening the windows.

• Wearing cotton underwear and avoiding synthetic fabrics are helpful for better skin metabolism and facilitate energy flow through the body.

• Avoid exposure to artificial electromagnetic radiation. Keep common hand-held appliances to a minimum. If you have a choice, work and live in areas away from an electronic environment.

Nuclear Radiation

If it becomes necessary to evacuate an area because of an accident, explosion, war, or other exposure to nuclear radiation, observe the following guidelines:

• Seek a location 250 to 300 miles from the site, toward a more rural area.
• Seek a more northern or colder location.
• Seek an area away from major industrial and population centers, including nuclear plants and military installations.
• If available, seek a high mountainous area, with access to spring or stream water. Ideally, an open valley high on a mountain range where air currents can pass through but not collect, as in a closed valley, is recommended.
• If a mountain is not available, seek an unpopulated seacoast or a cave.
• Check prevailing winds beforehand. Winds from major areas of radioactivity should be avoided; ocean winds may be helpful. The leeward slope of a mountain may offer some protection.
• Foods to take for emergency evacuation include: sea salt (at least one to two pounds per person), roasted short-grain brown rice or other whole grains; hatcho miso or other natural miso fermented over at last two summers; sea vegetables especially kombu and wakame; umeboshi plums with shiso leaves; aduki beans; sesame seeds; drinking and cooking water for several days; and grains, beans, and vegetable seeds for planting.
• Materials to take in case of an emergency include: flint and waterproof matches, hatchet or small ax, pressure cooker, woolen blanket roll, twenty-five to thirty-five feet of one-quarter-inch nylon cord, compass and map of area, scissors, and knife.
• Apparel and storage materials should include: warm clothing, sturdy trousers and shirt, double pair warm socks, heavy boots, gloves, head protection (leather or woolen), and heavy-duty-thickness plastic sheets to wrap food items and for general use in protecting supplies from moisture at site.
• Books and writing materials to take include: several key books or documents, such as texts on cosmology, history, and health, along with myths, poetry, and songs. Paper and writing implements to keep a personal or community journal.

Computers

In case of serious illness, including cancer, we strongly advise that computer use be avoided or, if that is not possible, limited to thirty minutes a day until usual good health is restored. To minimize harmful radiation from computers:

• Use LCD (liquid crystal displays) screens, which are generally safer than CRTs (cathode ray tubes), i.e., ordinary monitors.
• Use black-and-white monitors, which emit less radiation than color monitors.
• Obtain a radiation shield that fits over the front of CRTs and another one that goes around the sides and top of the computer. These can reduce exposure to ELF fields.
• Keep back at least two feet from the front of the computer and laser printer and four feet from the sides or back. This substantially reduces the strength of the electromagnetic field you are exposed to.
• Take regular exercise breaks.

• Keep green plants in the room to provide oxygen and to help absorb harmful vibrations.

• Be sure to eat mineral-rich seaweed every day, which has been shown to help eliminate radiation from the body. If you feel tired or other effects at the computer, try snacking on some toasted nori squares, shio kombu, roasted dulse, or other sea vegetable snacks. The protein in beans and bean products such as tempeh is also good to help neutralize radioactivity.

Television

For cancer patients, we advise that TV be avoided or limited to one half hour a day and that you sit at least ten feet from the screen.

PERSONAL EXPERIENCES

Radiation Sickness in Nagasaki

At the time of the world's first plutonium atomic bombing, on August 9, 1945, Tatsuichiro Akizuki, M.D., was director of the Department of Internal Medicine at St. Francis's Hospital in Nagasaki, Japan. In his book, Dr. Akizuki explained how he was able to save numerous survivors of the blast from radiation sickness and cancer of the blood:

On August 9, 1945, the atomic bomb was dropped on Nagasaki. Lethal atomic radiation spread over the razed city. For many it was an agonizing death. For a few it was a miracle. Not one co-worker in the hospital suffered or died from radiation. The hospital was located only one mile from the center of the blast. My assistant and I helped many victims who suffered the effects of the bomb. In the hospital there was a large stock of miso and shoyu. We also kept plenty of rice and wakame (seaweed used for soup stock or in miso soup). I had fed my co-workers brown rice and miso soup for some time before the bombing. None of them suffered from atomic radiation. I believe this is because they had been eating miso soup. . . .

On the tenth of August at 8 A.M., the Uragami Hospital was still burning. It was truly a miracle that there was not a single death in the hospital. I took up again the treatments of the maladies at 9 A.M., praying to God as I could not believe what happened. The supply of medicine was low. The hospital attendants prepared as usual a meal consisting of brown rice, miso soup with Hokkaido pumpkin and wakame, two times per day, at 11 A.M. and 5 P.M. They distributed the trays of brown rice to our grim neighbors and to the wounded.

At this period the scientific Americans declared that the center of the explosion area would be uninhabitable for the next seventy-five years. We disregarded this horrible declaration and continued, in straw sandals, to go around the city of Nagasaki the next day after the explosions to visit the sick in their homes.

The third day: at the clinic the number of injured grew; they were affected with bleeding gums, diarrhea, hemorrhages with no signs of any considerable wounds. The patients usually said: "It is because I have breathed a toxic gas that I bleed." One notices these violet bloody spots under the skin and in the membranes. Is it dysentery or purpura? The fact is very curious that the persons affected by these symptoms are not burned. It happened in the shade at the moment of the explosion. Now we know the symptoms were in reality those of the first stage of radioactive contamination. . . .

I resolved to try my method—using miso soup, unpolished brown rice, and salt. Sugar is poison to the blood. Obstinately I persuaded the people around me, again and again. I myself was more or less eccentric. I had no knowledge of the new biophysics or atom-biology; no books, no treatise, on atomic disease yet . . . I had no idea what kind of ray the atomic detonation might produce. I made a diagnosis and reasoned thus far: it may be radium, Roentgen ray, or gamma ray, which probably destroys hematogenic tissue, and marrow tissue of the human body. . . .

I gave the cooks and staff strict orders that they should make unpolished whole-grain rice balls, adding some salt to them, make salty thick miso soup at each meal, and never use sugar. When they didn't follow my order, I scolded them without mercy: "Never take sugar, no sweets, sugar will destroy blood."

My mineral method made it possible for me to remain alive and go on working vigorously as a doctor. The radioactivity may not have been a fatal dose but ever since, Brother Iwanaga, Reverend Noguchi, Chief Nurse Miss Murai, I, and other staff members and in-patients kept on living on the lethal ashes of the bombed ruins. It was thanks to this salt mineral method that all of us could work away for people day after day, overcoming fatigue or symptoms of atomic disease, and survived the disaster free from severe symptoms of radioactivity.

In addition to the testimony of Dr. Akizuki, there are additional accounts by survivors of Nagasaki and Hiroshima who healed themselves of radiation sickness, keloid tumors, and other serious effects of the bombing. Source: T. Akizuki, M.D., *Documentary of A-bombed Nagasaki* (Nagasaki: Nagasaki Printing Company, 1977), Ida Honoroff, "A Report to the Consumer," May 1978, and Hideo Ohmori, "Report from Japan," *A Nutritional Approach to Cancer* (Boston: East West Foundation, 1977), 28–32.

Radiation Sickness in Hiroshima

In 1945 Sawako Hirago was a ten-year-old schoolgirl in Hiroshima. In the atomic bombing on August 6, she was exposed to severe radiation that burned her face, head, and legs. The burned parts swelled up to nearly three times their normal size. In the hospital, doctors feared for her recovery because one-third of her body was burned. Her mother gave her palm healing therapy over the abdomen every night, and Sawako ate the only food available, two rice balls and two daikon radish pickles each day. Inside the rice balls was umeboshi (pickled salted plums).

Although the medical doctors gave up on her, Sawako survived: "My mother didn't show me a mirror until I was cured. However, I was able to see my hands and leg, which were very dirty and had a bad, rotten smell. On the rotten spots there were always flies. When the skin healed, I broke it because it was itchy; finally it became a keloidal condition. I didn't see my face until it was finally cured. However, sores remained on my nose and pus remained on my chest. My hands and chest had masses of skin which remained until I was twenty."

Because of her disfiguration, Sawako was ridiculed, nicknamed "Hormone Short," and told she could never marry or have children. After completing school, she became a high school physics teacher and met a young chemistry teacher who ate very simply. The couple married and attended lectures by George Ohsawa, the founder of modern macrobiotics in Japan, and he said that only people practicing macrobiotics would survive future nuclear war.

After talking with Mr. Ohsawa, Sawako gave up the modern, refined food that she had been eating since her survival and started eating brown rice and other foods. To her surprise, her problems including anemia, leukemia, low blood pressure, falling hair, and bleeding from the nose, started to clear up. Within two months, she was elated: "My face became beautiful."

Sawako went on to have seven healthy children and raised all of them on brown rice, miso soup, vegetables, seaweed, and other healthy food. Source: Sawako Hiraga, "How I Survived the Atomic Bomb," *Macrobiotic,* November/December 1979.

Diet and Radiation-related Cancers in Russia

In 1985 Lidia Yamchuk and Hanif Shaimardanov, medical doctors in Chelyabinsk, organized Longevity, the first macrobiotic association in the Soviet Union. At their hospital, they have used dietary methods and acupuncture to treat many patients, especially those suffering from leukemia, lymphoma, and other disorders associated with exposure to nuclear radiation. Since the early 1950s, wastes from Soviet weapons production had been dumped into Karachay Lake in Chelyabinsk, an industrial city about nine hundred miles east of Moscow. In particular they began incorporating miso soup into the diets of patients suffering from radiation symptoms and cancer. "Miso is helping some of our patients with terminal cancer to survive," Yamchuk and Shaimardanov reported. "Their blood (and blood analysis) became better after they began to use miso in their daily food."

Meanwhile, in Leningrad, Yuri Stavitsky, a young pathologist and medical instructor, volunteered as a radiologist in Chernobyl after the nuclear accident on April 26, 1986. Since then, like many disaster workers, he suffered symptoms associated with radiation disease, including tumors of the thyroid. "Since beginning macrobiotics," he reported, "my condition has greatly improved."

In Leningrad, in 1990, a visiting delegation of macrobiotic teachers from the United States, Japan, Germany, and Yugoslavia gave macrobiotic lectures at the Cardiology Center, the Institute of Cytology (the main cancer research center), and the State Institute for the Continuing Education of Doctors. Zoya Tchoueva, a Leningrad psychiatrist and medical researcher, is translating *The Cancer Prevention Diet* into Russian.

In Pushkin, the former country estate of the Russian emperors and a children's convalescent center, town officials and the Agricultural Institute of Leningrad invited the macrobiotic association to set up an Ecological Village and donated 100 acres of land for organic production of grains and vegetables. Soviet medical and environmental groups such as Union Chernobyl and Peace to the Children of the World hope to begin distributing miso, sea vegetables, and other macrobiotic-quality foods that may help protect against the effects of harmful nuclear radiation.

In 1992 Galina Sanderson, a filmmaker from Belarus, and her husband, Cliff Sanderson, a natural medical practitioner from the United States, announced plans to establish an international rehabilitation center near Lake Baikal, in eastern Siberia, for children from Chernobyl and other sites affected by radiation sickness. Michio Kushi was asked to be on the board of directors and provide macrobiotic dietary recommendations for children and their parents. About 3 million children in the former Soviet Union are estimated to have been exposed to high levels of nuclear radiation as a result of the Chernobyl explosion. Sources: Alex Jack, "Soviets Embrace Macrobiotics," *One Peaceful World Newsletter,* Autumn/Winter 1990, personal communication to Alex Jack, April 1991, and personal communication to Michio Kushi, May 4, 1992.

28

AIDS-related Cancer

FREQUENCY

AIDS is spreading rapidly around the world, with the number of deaths from AIDS doubling in many countries about every two years. Tens of millions of people are presently infected with the AIDS virus, and unless a remedy is found, the disease threatens to affect a majority of the earth's inhabitants by the early decades of the next century. By the year 2000, an estimated 120 million persons around the world will be infected with the AIDS virus.

Kaposi's sarcoma, or KS, was the first cancer associated with AIDS. A form of skin cancer characterized by brown or purple spots on the skin, usually the legs, it may initially appear as a simple dark spot of small size. Gradually the number of spots may cover various body surfaces. The lymph nodes of the neck often become extremely swollen. KS may also manifest in the body, such as in the cavity of the mouth or around the anus. Until the AIDS epidemic, KS was a rare disease that affected primarily men of Mediterranean origin over the age of fifty. It was limited to the skin and could be controlled medically, rarely proving fatal. Over 24,000 cases of KS have been reported in connection with AIDS. The incidence is decreasing, with 35 to 40 percent of AIDS cases having KS in the early 1980s and 14 percent in 1992. The average age of someone with AIDS-KS is thirty-four, and median life expectancy ranges from fourteen to thirty-two months, depending on symptoms and T-cell counts. Standard treatment is surgery to remove localized lesions, radiation treatment for lesions in the mouth, and chemotherapy for widespread KS.

A variety of other malignancies may occur with AIDS. Non-Hodgkin's lymphoma (NHL) is the next most frequent cancer, affecting about 3 percent of AIDS cases. The risk of NHL in single men has reached epidemic proportions in some cities, such as San Francisco, where it has risen more than tenfold and is associated with those with HIV infection 104 times as much as in the general population. Females are at less risk to develop lymphoma than males. Primary central nervous system lymphoma (PCL) accounts for 0.6 percent of all AIDS cases, though it may eventually affect up to 2 percent of all individuals with the disease. Hodgkin's disease is associated with AIDS in a small number of cases, and disorders with possible links to HIV include T-cell NHL, cervical dysplasia, and pediatric smooth muscle tumors. Prognosis for these other malignancies is also low, ranging from several months to a year or more. Noncancerous AIDS-related symptoms include nervous system dysfunctions and various forms of encephalitis, meningitis, viral myelitis, Candida albicans, CMV, toxoplasmosis, herpes, and others.

STRUCTURE

The purpose of the immune system is to maintain personal existence and to develop an individual's biological and spiritual quality under ever-changing environmental conditions. Human natural immunity includes: 1) intuition and instinct, which are constantly at work helping us avoid danger and reacting to new factors and influences; 2) consciousness, including different levels of awareness that operate through the processes of discrimination, selection, and attraction or repulsion to avoid extremes and protect us from danger; 3) autonomic response, including the sympathetic and parasympathetic nervous system, which provides corrective balance and harmony to new stimuli; 4) body surface protection and reaction, including the skin, sweat glands, pores, and white blood cell and lymphatic reactions, which serve to protect the body and expel toxins and unnecessary energies from the inside of the body to the surface; 5) internal liquid protection, including saliva, digestive enzymes and acids, immunoglobulin A (IGA), and other secretions that are active in neutralizing and minimizing the undesirable activities of viruses, bacteria, and other microorganisms; 6) blood and intercellular fluid protection and reaction, including B cells, T cells, and other lymphocytes, which neutralize or harmonize the adverse effects of viruses or their microorganisms; 7) lymphatic protection, including lymph nodes, which help cleanse the body of undesirable wastes; and 8) cellular protection, including cell membranes and intercellular fluids, which act to protect the nucleus of the cell from undesirable physical stimuli and harmful chemicals.

CAUSE

The decline of natural immunity, or AIDS, is not the result of a sudden failure, defect, or ineffectiveness in one or more of these immune functions. It is the result of partial or total failure or decay of all of them, usually over a period of time. The primary origin of natural immune deficiency is cloudiness of intuition and instinct. The decline of intuitive and instinctive judgment causes us to observe abnormal lifestyles and dietary practices that exceed the natural limitations of our environment, climate, constitution, or condition. Adopting imbalanced ways of life and eating, in turn, results in the further decay and weakening of other levels of the natural immune system.

While this is the primary origin of immune deficiency, the biological cause of natural immunity is improper dietary habits. Through longtime dietary abuse we create a weakened internal environment in which harmful viruses and bacteria can easily take hold, grow, and multiply. The energy and nutrients of the food we eat day to day create, nourish, and govern the quality and volume of blood and intercellular fluids, the quality of lymphatic fluids, and the quality of organs, tissues, and cells as well as their functions. Daily food largely shapes and determines our destiny in life and whether our natural immunity remains strong or weakens and decays.

A daily diet composed of rich animal meat, poultry, dairy food, sugar, refined products, and oily, greasy food, together with frequent consumption of tropical fruits, soft drinks, and aromatic, stimulant beverages—in other words, the modern way of eating—produces a more acidic condition within the body. Harmful viruses such as HIV thrive in this kind of environment. In contrast, a traditional diet centered on whole grains and vegetables, beans and sea vegetables, and other natural foods tends to produce a more alkaline condition in the blood and body as a whole.

According to our careful observations since the beginning of the AIDS epidemic, people who have weakened their natural immunity and are susceptible to infection by the AIDS virus tend to consume the following foods: 1) a great amount of sweets, including foods containing chocolate, sugar, carob, honey, and chemical sweeteners; 2) a great amount of fruits and fruit juices, including such tropical fruits as bananas, papayas, mangoes, avocado, kiwis, and others; 3) a great amount of dairy products, especially milk, yogurt, cream, butter, ice cream, and foods containing dairy; 4) refined flour products, including refined white flour, yeasted bread, and other baked products; 5) nightshade plants such as tomatoes, potatoes, eggplant, and peppers, as well as plants that originated in a tropical climate; 6) a great deal of oily and fatty food products, including salad dressing, spreads, sauces, and deep-fried foods; and 7) soft drinks, carbonated waters, and wine and other sweet alcoholic beverages.

The items in these seven categories all fall more within the category of extreme yin foods and beverages. They produce expanding, decomposing, and loosening, and weakening results in various organs and glands and their functions. At the same time, they generate overwhelming acid-producing conditions in the body. The following disorders commonly arise as a result of their consumption: 1) intestinal weakness, including a deterioration in food absorption and production of fresh, healthy blood; 2) liver infection, hepatitis, and mononucleosis as fat and mucus burden the liver and cause overeating and cravings for foods rich in sweets and easily digested foods; 3) lymphatic disorders, including swollen lymph nodes overworked from trying to cleanse poisonous waste from the body; an imbalance in white blood cells, including T-4 and T-8 cells; 4) weakening of respiratory function as fat and mucus gather in the lungs and carbon dioxide builds up in the blood; 5) pancreatic disorders, especially hypoglycemia, or chronic low blood sugar, as fat gathers around this organ and hinders the secretion of anti-insulin; 6) weakness of bones as alkaline minerals stored in these areas are mobilized to neutralize acidosis; 7) skin disorders as the body attempts to discharge this excess through the skin; 8) KS or skin cancer, which represents the body's attempt to eliminate excess fat and protein, combined with excessive simple sugar and often animal-quality protein, to the surface of the body; 9) reproductive disorders; 10) nervous sensitivity; 11) mental indecision; and 12) receptivity toward infectious viruses and bacteria, including HIV.

Essentially, we can say that the body—including blood, lymph, body cells, and immune cells—becomes more yin from poor eating, and, as in other autoimmune disorders, the body begins to attack itself. Ordinarily, the immune system creates balance through attraction/repulsion. At all levels, it operates according to yin and yang (see chart). At the cellular level, T cells "read" a virus and signal the B cells to produce a complement to the virus, or an antibody, which perfectly matches the virus. This antibody coats the virus, attaches itself, and changes the virus from yin to yang. The neutralized virus no longer attacks cells but repels them. A yin enzyme is secreted that decomposes or melts the coated virus, allowing it to be discharged naturally from the body, e.g., through the filtering system of the kidneys into the urine. With AIDS, there is a deficiency of T-4 cells, which activate this immune function and which are classified as more yang. As a consequence, the virus continues to multiply, invading, devouring, and eventually killing the host.

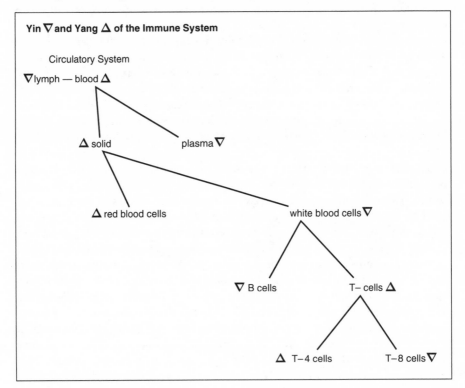

Kaposi's Sarcoma (KS), the most common cancer associated with AIDS, appears in the form of dark, brownish-black marks and may spread all over the skin. They continuously appear and spread as long as excessive fat, protein, and simple sugar remain within the system beyond the capacity of normal elimi-natory functions, especially respiratory and urinary elimination. KS can also appear in the inner lining of the oral cavity and gums, as well as inside the respiratory tract, the digestive tract, the rectum, and the anal region.

Following a change in dietary practice, KS may still continue for some period until the accumulation of fats caused by longtime consumption of oily, greasy food, dairy fats, and sugars is eliminated. Thereafter, the sarcoma usually dries up gradually and the dark discolorings change to a lighter shade. However, it may take several years before the lesions completely disappear, provided physical metabolism and other body functions have been restored to normal healthy conditions.

In the United States, I began working with people with AIDS in the early 1980s. I observed many cases of men with AIDS, KS, and other symptoms declared terminal by the medical profession who recovered as a result of adopting a macrobiotic way of eating. In New York and Boston, medical doctors began to research our approach and reported to their colleagues that the macrobiotic group they studied for several years showed marked improvement and on the average outlived every other control group or experimental group under study.

Though AIDS is now global, affecting practically every culture and nation, it is spreading most rapidly in the tropical regions of the world, including Africa, Latin America, India and Pakistan, and other warmer latitudes. The unifying principle of yin and yang helps us understand the incidence and spread of AIDS. Viral infections, as well as infectious conditions caused by bacteria, parasites, and other organisms, spread more rapidly in warm, hot regions where people are balancing the yang, contracted environment with proportionately more yin, expansive food and beverages. In many tropical countries, people are no longer eating a diet centered around whole grains and vegetables like their ancestors. Instead, they are eating large amounts of sugar, spices, oil, stimulant beverages, nightshade plants, and other items with strong yin energy, as well as animal food, dairy food, refined flour, highly processed foods, and other foods imported from the West. Uprooted from their traditional farmland to make way for cattle ranching, sugar plantations, and other aspects of modern agriculture and food production, they have flocked to cities and urban slums, where they are subject to malnutrition, unemployment, and destitution. Well-meaning relief agencies then compound the problem by distributing evaporated milk and infant formula, canned goods, refined grains, sugar, and other high-caloric items. AIDS, as well as many other infectious conditions, breeds in such an environment.

Several years ago, I was invited to give a seminar to medical doctors and World Health Organization officials in West Africa, where AIDS has reached epidemic proportions. I observed that AIDS was frequent in big cities and among people eating in the modern way, but in the rural areas, where grains, vegetables, and other more natural foods were still eaten, AIDS was much less common.

In my seminars, I meet many young men with AIDS or borderline AIDS who go to the Caribbean or other warm, tropical climates for vacation. There tropical fruits, including bananas, mangoes, guava, pineapple, and papayas, are plentiful, along with rum and alcohol, marijuana and cocaine, and other extreme yin substances. For AIDS, these are suicide zones. In addition to the food quality, the hot weather allows the virus to spread more quickly. If you want to vacation in the tropics, eat a lot of meat and chicken beforehand and develop heart disease (more yang). The hot climate and relaxing food will help cool you out. For recovering from AIDS, a colder, more temperate climate is advisable.

Fewer women than men get AIDS. The reason for this is that women are more yang in structure and condition and therefore are better able to take in yin than men. Conversely, men are more yin and can handle yang better. Traditionally, women ate proportionately more vegetables, especially salad, fruit, sweets, desserts, and other yin foods and beverages, while men ate more animal food, more salt, more baked food, and other more yang items. Females have a very hard time with yang—salty, baked food, meat, fish, etc.—and the intake of these kinds of foods in modern society by women and girls underlies the spread of ovarian cancer, lung cancer, and other yang disorders. Conversely, men have a hard time handling strong yin, and taking too much fruit, salad, ice cream, dairy food, and other items predisposes them to leukemia, lymphoma, AIDS, and other yin disorders. Overall, women are healthier than men and live longer because they are able to exchange energy more harmoniously with the environment through menstruation and lactation. Breast-feeding contributes to the health of the mother, as well as the child, and strengthens her natural immunity to disease.

In addition to improper diet, many aspects of modern life promote and encourage the development of natural immune deficiency. In our experience, the following factors enhance or contribute to immune deficiency: 1) the mother's way of life and eating during pregnancy, which largely shapes and determines her child's physical, mental, and spiritual constitution; 2) weakening of natural immunity at birth through Cesarean section and/or the substitution of infant formula for mother's milk; and 3) weakening of natural immunity during the growing period, including abuse of medication, removal of tonsils and other glands, exposure to X rays, exposure to other artificial electromagnetic radiation, drug abuse, abuse of medical treatment, overuse of antibiotics, environmental pollution, and promiscuous sexual behavior.

According to modern medicine, becoming infected with the HIV virus amounts practically to a death sentence. There is no cure. From the macrobiotic view, this is not necessarily true. First, the aim is to keep the virus dormant. If the virus is dormant, a person can live ten, twenty, thirty years, or more, and there is no need to worry. For those newly infected, the standard macrobiotic diet will usually keep the virus inactive and the person symptom-free, so there is no need to worry. For cases that have already begun to symptomatize, it will generally take about two years eating in a macrobiotic way to become normal, and then five to seven years in total for the virus to disappear completely from the body.

MEDICAL EVIDENCE

• In 1983 a small group of men in New York City with AIDS began macrobiotics under the inspiration of Michio Kushi and Lawrence H. Kushi, D.Sc. They hoped to change their blood quality, recover their natural immunity, and survive this otherwise always fatal illness. In May 1984 a research team led by Elinor N. Levy, Ph.D., and John C. Beldekas, Ph.D., of the Department of Immunology and Microbiology at Boston University's School of Medicine, and Martha C. Cottrell, M.D., director of student health at the Fashion Institute of Technology in New York, began to monitor the blood samples and immune functions of ten men with KS (a usual symptom of AIDS). Preliminary results indicated that most of the men were stabilizing on the diet. "Survival in these men who have received little or no medical treatment appears to compare very favorably with that of KS patients in general. We suggest that physicians and scientists can feel comfortable in allowing patients, particularly those with minimal disease, to go untreated as part of a larger [dietary] study or because non-treatment is the patient's choice." Source: "Patients with Kaposi Sarcoma Who Opt for No Treatment" (letter), *Lancet*, July 1985.

• At the International AIDS Conference in Paris in June 1986, Elinor Levy and associates presented further findings concerning the men with KS who had been practicing macrobiotics. In their conclusion, the researchers noted:

1. Lymphocyte number increases over the first two years from diagnosis with KS in men who are following a macrobiotic diet. A linear regression analysis model predicts that lymphocyte number becomes normal within this two-year period.

2. During this time period the percentage of T-4 cells does not change. The percentage of T-8 cells possibly decreases.

3. These results compare favorably with those from any of the medical treatments reported.

4. There are several possible explanations for these positive findings, including: a) the macrobiotic diet and/or lifestyle is of benefit to men with KS; and b) the decision to become and remain macrobiotic selects for men with a better prognosis.

Source: Elinor Levy, J. C. Beldekas, P. H. Black, and L. H. Kushi, "Patients with Kaposi's Sarcoma Who Opt for Alternative Therapy," International AIDS Conference, Paris, France, 1986.

• In a further report on the men in the macrobiotic AIDS study, Dr. Levy reported in 1988: "The large majority of subjects reported a decrease in AIDS-related symptoms, particularly fatigue (23/29) and diarrhea (17/19). The lymphocyte number in the subgroup of nineteen subjects with Kaposi's sarcoma alone tended to increase with time after diagnosis. Only two of this group of nineteen lost more than 10 percent of their body weight during their participation in the study, which ranged from several months to more than three years. Nine of the nineteen with KS have died, seven are alive more than three years after diagnosis with KS." Source: Elinor M. Levy, Letter to the American Cancer Society, March 3, 1988.

• After initial observations, the macrobiotic AIDS test group was expanded to twenty men. "As a group, the men have had significant improvement in their total T-cell numbers, notably in T4 counts, although T4/T8 ratios have not changed significantly," Dr. Martha Cottrell reported. "Those with Kaposi's sarcoma have shown the best survival rates, three going five years or longer. The approach has demonstrated effective in managing their condition while minimizing opportunistic infections and use of toxic drugs. They are all working full time and enjoying a quality of life atypical of most AIDS patients. Most of all, they are relatively free of the sense of hopelessness, helplessness, and victimization which tends to take hold of other AIDS patients. Thus the physical benefits—prolonging life and improving the immunocompetence—seem complemented by a range of psychological benefits." Source: Martha Cottrell, M.D., Letter to the American Cancer Society, March 14, 1988. See also Tom Monte, *The Way of Hope* (New York: Warner Books, 1990).

• In Africa investigators have observed a significant correlation between AIDS and upper-class status. This strongly suggests a possible association with environmental factors. Urban centers throughout Africa have been increasingly influenced by Western technology, including the typical American diet of refined sugars and flours, meats, eggs, dairy products, food additives, and other foods. In the highly Westernized city of Kinshasa, capital of the Republic of the Congo, this dietary pattern is far more typical of urban people in the upper income bracket.

"It seems plausible that the rapid modernization of Africa's urban population, particularly of the upper class, may have set the stage for compromised immunity and thereby predisposed them to the pathogenic effects of the AIDS virus," concluded Martha Cottrell, M.D., who gave seminars on diet and AIDS in West Africa.

The typical upper-class diet, based on the haute cuisine of France and Belgium, includes imported red meats, eggs, white sugar, baked white-flour products, dairy foods, hydrogenated oils, and imported fruits and vegetables. "Heavy reliance on imported products has introduced high levels of artificial preservatives and agricultural chemicals to the urban elite's food supply. Clearly this is not the kind of diet one would expect to support resistance to infectious diseases."

By contrast, the native lower-class diet includes locally grown fruit, cassava meal (a starchy root vegetable), avocado, red onions, and small amounts of fish, game, and insects. "In sum, the typical diet of low-income Kinshasans is basically low in protein, low in fat, and high in complex carbohydrates and fiber. By nutritional standards, this type of dietary pattern would clearly favor strong immunity."

Source: Michio Kushi and Martha Cottrell, M.D., *AIDS, Macrobiotics, and Natural Immunity* (New York and Tokyo: Japan Publications, 1990), 216–17.

• When AIDS first appeared in 1981, macrobiotic educator Michio Kushi began recommending thorough chewing as a key dietary measure to help prevent the development of immune deficiency. He noted that the yang, contractive properties of saliva, which are promoted during chewing, could help neutralize the extreme yin, expansive quality of the AIDS virus. Now medical studies for this theory have emerged. Saliva contains substances that prevent the AIDS virus from infecting white blood cells. In a study, researchers tested saliva from three healthy men, thirty-five, forty, and forty-two years old. Tests indicated the men were not carriers of the AIDS virus and were not known to be at high risk for infection. In laboratory dishes, the men's saliva prevented the AIDS virus from infecting lymphocytes, a type of white blood cell that is among the immune system cells attacked by the AIDS virus in the body. The dental researchers said the finding might help explain why no cases have been documented in which the AIDS virus was transmitted from person to person through saliva, such as through kissing or sharing toothbrushes. The scientists concluded that saliva is well known to contain substances that kill bacteria and fungi and so might also be able to block the AIDS virus. Source: P. C. Fox et al., "Saliva Inhibits HIV-1 Infectivity," *Journal of the American Dental Association* (1988) 116:635–37.

• Retinoids (foods and substances high in vitamin A) and carotenoids (foods and substances high in beta-carotene, a precursor to vitamin A) can stimulate some human immune responses, including heightened antitumor cell activity, increased natural killer (NK) cell response, and activated lymphocytes. In 1990 researchers at the University of Arizona reported that retinoids and carotenoids appear to have different effects on the immune system. Retinoids act on the differentiation process of immune cells, increasing mitogenesis of lymphocytes and enhancing phagocytosis of monocytes and macrophages as well as acting as antioxidants reducing loss of immunological functions due to free radicals. Carotenoids increase T-helper cell numbers and natural killer cells. "Restoring the number of these cells may be useful in acquired immunodeficiency syndromes such as AIDS, where immune cells are in low numbers and defective in nature," the researchers noted. The scientists recommended that clinical trials begin to study the role of these dietary agents in AIDS patients. Foods naturally high in these nutrients include orange and yellow vegetables such as carrots, squash, parsnips, and rutabaga. Source: R. H. Prabhala et al., "Immunomodulation in Humans Caused by Beta-carotene and Vitamin A," *Nutritional Research* 10:1473–86.

• In 1989 researchers in Germany reported that vegetarians appeared to have stronger immune systems than people eating the modern high-fat, high-sugar diet. Epidemiologists at the German Cancer Research Center had previously found that vegetarians had a lower risk of developing cancer than people consuming a standard diet and theorized that his might partly be due to a more active immune system. In a study of twenty-two vegetarians and matched controls, they found that the activity of lymphocytes or NK cells in vegetarians was 100 percent higher than the activity of similar cells obtained from nonvegetarians: "The results of this study suggest that NK cell activity of a vegetarian is about twice as high as that of an omnivorous person. This is in line with the idea that the reduced cancer risk of vegetarians is possibly partially related to the better natural defense system which they seem to have." Source: Margarete Malter et al., "Natural Killer Cells, Vitamins, and Other Blood Components of Vegetarian and Omnivorous Men," *Nutrition and Cancer* 12:271–78.

• Kaposi's sarcoma has recently been observed in organ-transplant patients as well as in some cancer patients undergoing chemotherapy. "This implies that KS primarily affects those patients with [already] compromised immune systems," concluded Dr. Martha Cottrell. Source: Michio Kushi and Martha Cottrell, M.D., *AIDS, Macrobiotics, and Natural Immunity* (New York and Tokyo: Japan Publications, 1990), 125.

DIAGNOSIS

Modern society diagnoses AIDS by blood tests that show the presence of antibodies to the HIV in the body. However, since people may not symptomatize for years, millions of men and women are believed to be carrying the HIV virus without knowing it. When symptoms appear, it is often too late for them to begin to reverse it. From the modern medical view, AIDS is considered incurable and the most that can be done is to prolong life through drugs such as AZT and to minimize pain and suffering. From the macrobiotic view, AIDS or a tendency toward loss of natural immunity can be evaluated through traditional Oriental physiognomic methods.

While not everyone conforms to the same profile, people susceptible to AIDS often share the following characteristics: 1) general fatigue, physically and mentally, with a tendency to become inactive and seek more comfortable situations and surroundings; 2) development of frequent colds and infections accompanied by light fever; 3) skin rashes, similar to allergic reactions; 4) intestinal disorders, including gas, constipation, and frequent diarrhea; 5) feeling of nausea; 6) irregular appetite, fluctuating from insatiable to almost no appetite, and frequent cravings for sweets, fruit, pastries, and similar foods; 7) night perspiration; 8) chronic hypoglycemia, including a tendency to be more mentally depressed, irritable, and pessimistic, particularly in the late afternoon; feelings of exhaustion at night or while sleeping; peripheral parts of the body being colder than normal; and cravings for simple sugars; 9) liver infection; 10) swelling of lymph glands; 11) abnormal balance of blood components, with a dramatic decrease in white blood cells, especially lymphocytes, as shown by the ratio of T-4 to T-8 helper cells; 12) pneumoncystis carinii accompanied by a chronic low-temperature fever that may continue for several months, leading to a difficulty in breathing; and 13) the appearance of KS or cancerous lesions on the skin.

Visually, a person with AIDS or carrying the AIDS virus appears to have little vitality or energy, the face is red or purply (a color that may show an infectious condition), the movement or action is slow, the texture of the skin is milky, the skin easily ruptures, the intestines are loose, and diarrhea may arise frequently. About half of the AIDS cases I have seen had hepatitis or other liver disorders. In another 20 to 30 percent, the spleen or lymph nodes are swollen and expanded and lymphoma arises. Eighty percent or more have hypoglycemia, or chronically low blood sugar, from longtime consumption of dairy products, poultry, eggs, and other fatty foods that gather and harden the pancreas. Hormones can't release properly, and to relax they constantly crave sweets, fruits, and other strong yin products. Pre-AIDS conditions, in my experience, are mononucleosis, chronic fatigue syndrome, and Epstein-Barr virus.

DIETARY RECOMMENDATIONS

The primary cause of AIDS-related cancers and other immune-deficiency diseases is long-time consumption of excessive yin foods and beverages, along with other extreme yin influences including drugs and medication, exposure to artificial electromagnetic fields, and other factors that lower natural immunity to disease. All sugar, chocolate, honey, sweets, spices, herbs, soft drinks, wine, alcohol, fruit, juice, coffee, chemicalized tea, and other stimulants, foods of tropical origin, and oily, greasy foods of all kinds must be minimized. Because they are excessively mucous-producing, all flour products are to be avoided, except for occasional consumption of nonyeasted, unleavened whole wheat or rye bread if craved. Chemicalized and artificially produced and treated foods and beverages are to be completely eliminated. Even unsaturated vegetable oil is to be completely avoided or minimized in cooking for a one- or two-month period. All ice-cold foods and drinks should be avoided. While AIDS is caused by more yin conditions, it is important not to yangize too quickly. If you try to strengthen yourself by taking too much good-quality yang, such as whole grains, sea salt, sea vegetables, etc., the opposite problem may arise, including tightness and rigidity. The idea is to achieve balance, reducing yin, with a slight more emphasis on yang.

• **Whole Grains:** Fifty to sixty percent of daily consumption, by volume, should be whole-cereal grains. The first day prepare plain pressure-cooked short-grain brown rice. On following days, prepare brown rice pressure-cooked with 20 to 30 percent millet, then rice with 20 to 30 percent barley, then rice with 20 to 30 percent aduki beans or lentils, and then plain rice again. A delicious morning porridge can be made by taking leftover rice, adding a little more water to soften, and seasoning with a little miso at the end and simmering for two to three minutes more. Except for morning porridge, which may be soft, the grain should be cooked in a ratio of 2 parts grain to 1 part water. For seasoning, cook with a postage stamp–sized piece of kombu instead of salt, though in some cases sea salt may be used, depending on the person's condition. Other grains can be used occasionally, including whole wheat berries, rye, corn, and whole oats, though oats should be avoided for the first month. Buckwheat and seitan should be minimized. Good-quality sourdough bread may be enjoyed two to three times a week, and noodles, both udon and soba, may also be taken. Avoid all hard baked products until the condition improves, including cookies, cakes, pie, crackers, muffins, and the like.

• **Soup:** Five to 10 percent soup, consisting of one or two cups or bowls per day of soup cooked with wakame sea vegetable and various land vegetables such as onions and carrots and seasoned with miso or shoyu. Occasionally a small volume of shiitake mushroom may be added to the soup. The miso may be barley miso, brown rice miso, or soybean (hatcho) miso and should be naturally aged two to three years. To satisfy a desire for a sweet taste, millet soup with sweet vegetables such as squash, cabbage, onions, and carrots may be prepared often. Grain soups, bean soups, and other soups may be taken from time to time.

• **Vegetables:** Twenty to 30 percent vegetables, cooked in a variety of forms, with plenty of hard, green leafy vegetables, which are good for the liver and detoxification; round vegetables such as squash, cabbage, and onions, which are good for the spleen and immune system; and root vegetables such as daikon, carrot, and burdock, which are strengthening to the intestines and the blood and lymph as a whole. As a rule of thumb, the following dishes may be prepared, though the frequency may differ from person to person: nishime-style vegetables, three to four times a week; squash-aduki-kombu dish, three times a week; dried daikon, one cup, three times a week; carrots and carrot tops or daikon and daikon tops, three times a week; boiled salad, five to seven times a week; pressed salads, five to seven times a week; raw salad and salad dressing, avoid; steamed greens, five to seven times a week; sautéed vegetables, two times a week using water the first month instead of oil, then occasionally a small volume of sesame oil may be brushed on the skillet, *kinpira,* sautéed in water, two-thirds of a cup, two times a week, then oil may be used after three weeks; dried tofu, tofu, tempeh, or seitan with vegetables, two times a week.

• **Beans:** Five percent small beans, such as aduki beans, lentils, chickpeas, or black soybeans, may be used daily, cooked together with sea vegetables such as kombu or with onions and carrots. Other beans may be used altogether two to three times a month. For seasoning, a small volume of unrefined sea salt or shoyu or miso can be used. Bean products, such as tempeh, natto, and dried or cooked tofu, may be used occasionally, but in moderate volume. Avoid making the tofu too creamy and use firm, rather than soft, tofu.

• **Sea Vegetables:** Five percent or less sea vegetable dishes, including wakame and kombu, daily when cooking grain, in soup, etc. A sheet of toasted nori may also be taken daily. A small dish of hijiki or arame should be prepared two times a week. All other sea vegetables are optional.

• **Condiments:** Condiments to be available on the table are *gomashio* (sesame salt), on the average made with 1 part salt to 18 parts sesame seeds (reduced to 1:16 after two months); kombu, kelp, or wakame powder; umeboshi plum; and tekka, though all other regular macrobiotic condiments may be used if desired. These condiments may be used daily on grains and vegetables, but the volume should be moderate to suit individual appetite and taste. Umeboshi (one half to one plum a day) and tekka (one quarter to one third teaspoon a day) are good for restoring immune ability.

• **Pickles:** Pickles, made at home in a variety of ways, are to be eaten daily, one tablespoon in all, though salty pickles are to be minimized.

• **Animal Food:** Though animal food is to be avoided, a small volume of white-meat fish may be eaten once every week or two weeks. The fish should be prepared steamed, boiled, or poached and garnished with daikon or ginger. After two months, fish may be eaten once or twice a week and may be prepared with other cooking styles, such as broiling, grilling, and baking. Strictly avoid blue-meat and red-meat fish and all shellfish. For energy and vitality, koi koku may be taken if desired, one bowl for no more than three days in a row. For anemia, small dried fish may be taken, sautéed in a little water or oil with shoyu at the end, two small pieces a day. Make plenty and keep in a jar.

• **Fruit:** None the best, the less the better, including temperate-climate as well as tropical, until the condition improves. If cravings develop, a small volume of cooked fruit with a pinch of salt or dried fruit may be taken. Avoid all fruit juices and cider.

• **Sweets and Snacks:** Avoid all sweets and desserts, including good-quality macrobiotic desserts, until the condition improves. Just a little sugar, chocolate, carob, honey, maple syrup, or soy milk will bring out KS and other symptoms. To satisfy a sweet tooth, use sweet vegetables every day in cooking, drink sweet vegetable drink (see special drinks below), and use sweet vegetable jam. Mochi, rice balls, vegetable sushi, and other grain-based snacks may be eaten frequently. Limit rice cakes, popcorn, and other dry or baked snacks, as they may increase fat beneath the skin and prevent discharge. In the event of cravings, a small volume of grain-based sweeteners such as barley malt or rice syrup may be taken.

• **Nuts and Seeds:** Nuts and nut butters are to be avoided due to their high amount of fat and protein, except for chestnuts. Unsalted, roasted seeds such as squash seeds and pumpkin seeds may be consumed as a snack, up to one cup altogether per week. Sunflower seeds may be taken only in the summer.

• **Seasonings:** Seasonings, such as unrefined sea salt, shoyu, and miso, are to be used moderately in order to avoid unnecessary thirst. Avoid mirin and garlic. If you become particularly thirsty after a meal or between meals, you should cut back on these seasonings until the normal level of thirst returns.

• **Beverages:** Beverages and other dietary practices can follow the general recommendations in Part I, including bancha twig tea as the main beverage. Strictly avoid the beverages on the "infrequent" and "avoid" list, including all aromatic, stimulant beverages, and refrain from grain coffee for the first two to three months after starting this new way of eating.

The most important thing in connection with dietary practice is chewing very well, until all food becomes liquid in the mouth and well mixed with saliva. Chew very, very well, at least 50 times, preferably 100 times, per mouthful. It is also important to avoid overeating and eating within three hours of sleeping.

As noted in the introduction to Part II, persons who have received or who are currently undergoing medical treatment may need to make further dietary modifications.

SPECIAL DRINKS AND PREPARATIONS

I have devised several special condiments to strengthen the immune system. Along with sweet vegetable drink, these may need to be taken, depending on the individual case. Please see a qualified macrobiotic teacher for guidance. Amounts and frequencies given here are averages; this will differ from person to person.

• **Sweet Vegetable Drink:** Take one to two small cups every day for the first month, then every other day the second month, and then several times a week after that as desired

• **Lotus Root: Carrot-Kombu-Aduki Condiment:** Chop one half cup lotus root, add one third cup kombu, one third cup carrots, one third cup cooked aduki beans, and combine with five times as much water. Cook for thirty minutes and add a little salt at the end. Drink the liquid and eat the food substances (if soft) from this mixture every day, one to two cups, for twenty days.

• **Baked Kombu-Shiitake-Sesame Condiment:** Bake *kombu* in a dry skillet, crush into powder, and put aside. This will constitute 50 percent of the condiment. Bake dried shiitake mushroom, by volume about 25 percent of total mixture, and on a dry surface, chop and set aside. Roast black sesame seeds, about 25 percent by volume, and crush in a suribachi. Mix all the ingredients together and crush once more. Take one teaspoon every day for ten days. This condiment may be eaten as is, or sprinkled on grain or in tea. Then take every other day for ten days and then occasionally as desired every three or four days for one to one and one half months.

• **Umeboshi Plums:** Take often, every day or every other day for several weeks, and then gradually less often or as needed.

HOME CARES

• **Body Scrub:** Scrubbing the whole body, including the abdominal region and the spinal region, with a towel that has been immersed in hot water and squeezed out is very helpful for better circulation of blood, lymph, and other body fluids, as well as for activating physical and mental energies.

• **Compress Guidelines:** For a small number of AIDS cases, a compress may be needed to help gradually draw out excess mucus and fat. Please see a qualified macrobiotic teacher for guidance on the proper use and frequency of a compress or plaster. Several types are used depending on the person's condition. Precede the compress or plaster with application of a towel that has been soaked in hot water and squeezed out over the affected area for about three to five minutes to stimulate circulation.

• **Medical Attention:** In the event the lymph glands become swollen due to the cancer spreading through the lymph system, or other lack of improvement, medical attention may be necessary. Again, a qualified macrobiotic teacher, nutritionist, or medical associates or professionals should be consulted.

OTHER CONSIDERATIONS

• Be active, walk, exercise, but don't exhaust yourself. The purpose is to improve circulation and energy flow, not build yourself up like a wrestler.

• Swimming is good, especially in sea water.

• Wear a hat outside or stay in the shade to avoid the direct rays of the sun.

• A mountainous or forest region is better than the seashore for recovery.

• Take a walk every day and begin to reconnect with the natural environment.

• Avoid or limit watching television, using computers, or exposure to other artificial electromagnetic fields.

• Sing a happy song each day.

• From time to time meditate, contemplate, pray, or visualize, especially healthy, positive thoughts and images.

• Practice safe sex. During intercourse, mucus and other fluids and energies, including HIV virus, are discharged and exchanged. Natural infection easily arises as a result unless both partners are eating very well.

• Strictly avoid all drug use.

• Maintain a clean, orderly environment and observe sanitary conditions.

• If circumstances allow, temporarily move to or arrange to visit a more northern or cooler climate, where the incidence of AIDS is less and the spread less rapid. In such a climate, we naturally tend to eat in a slightly more yang way—more salt, more grain, more longtime cooking, etc.—which helps alkalinize the body and restore natural immunity. Similarly, AIDS flourishes in more humid conditions than dry ones and more in rainy seasons than in dry ones.

PERSONAL ACCOUNTS

AIDS and Kaposi's Sarcoma

Frank's ailments came to a head in early 1985. Doctors told him he had parasitic infections and AIDS-related complex, including KS. His T-cell count was consistently below normal, and he went on disability. His doctor told him it was time to make out his will but, interestingly, also suggested that he look into macrobiotics. The physician, Roger Enlow, used to be the director of Gay Lesbian Health concerns for the city of New York and had met my son, Larry Kushi, a medical researcher, at a scientific convention and learned about diet as a possible factor in AIDS and other conditions. The doctor told Frank he shouldn't be eating dairy products or red meat.

Frank began to look into macrobiotics, reading various books and attending meetings of HEAL, a macrobiotic-oriented support group. He also attended awareness workshops and worked on his emotions: "What I really liked about macrobiotics is the global sense of everything—the world perspective, the big picture on everything," he recalled. "And that really helped me get out of my little egocentric, dualistic world view."

Frank's condition began to improve with the new way of eating. His weight, which five years earlier had peaked at 230, dropped to 155, and he felt great. His skin became clearer, his eyes began to shine, and his energy level went up. All this happened within the first five months. The T-cell counts went back up to normal ranges. Still, some physicians he visited were skeptical. "I have had to exercise my patient rights with medical specialists who wanted to dominate my course of healing," Frank explained. "Once I literally got up and took off the examination gown. This guy was examining me and wanted to do a bone-marrow biopsy. So he walked in after knowing me ten minutes, with a huge needle, and was going to go in my back. . . . I said, 'Wait a minute. Hold on! I really don't think this is necessary.' And it turned out it wasn't necessary. There was a simple blood test that could have told them basically the same thing."

Frank found that he did not miss the foods he was used to, such as meat, ice cream, liquor, marijuana, and coffee. As a copywriter for a market research company, his work took him all around the country, and frequently he would eat out with businessmen. Some of these executives were stunned when he took out rice balls to eat instead of having steak and salad and martinis. Once at one of the poshest restaurants in Baltimore, Frank told the waiter he was on a special diet and the head chef, a Frenchman, came in and prepared him an incredible plate of brown rice, fish cooked with sesame oil, and a big plate of vegetables without butter. "The businessman almost died because I got royal treatment from this chef, who had a great deal of respect for people who ate natural food," Frank observed.

In 1986 Frank began to write up his experiences for the *New York Native*, a gay publication, which was considered a breakthrough in raising public awareness about diet and AIDS. "I'm not going to take any chances or be foolish in my way of living. The time to heal, the time to live, is now," Frank noted.

Source: Profile by Mark Mead in Michio Kushi and Martha Cottrell, M.D., *AIDS, Macrobiotics, and Natural Immunity* (New York and Tokyo: Japan Publications, 1990).

PART III

Practical Approaches

29

General Dietary Recommendations

The following dietary guidelines are a summary of material presented in Part I, Chapter 5. They are intended for use by reasonably healthy individuals or families. Modifications for persons with cancer are discussed in the individual chapters in Part II and summarized in the following chapter. Persons with sicknesses other than cancer may safely follow these standard guidelines for grains, soup, vegetables, beans, sea vegetables, and beverages. However, they should minimize or avoid animal food, fruit, salad, and sweets until they have consulted an experienced macrobiotic teacher or medical professional for evaluation of their health condition and dietary recommendations suited to their personal situation. Chapter 31, "Making a Smooth Transition," should also be read carefully to help implement these guidelines. In the lists of foods that follow, *regular* use means suitable for daily use or use five times a week; *occasional* means two or three times a week; *infrequent* means two or three times a month; and *avoid* means refrain completely or limit. The guidelines are for a four-season temperate climate, and the volumes are per day, not per meal. See Appendix II for tropical and polar guidelines. Foods in the principal categories (whole-cereal grains, beans, nuts and seeds, seasonings, oil) are listed in the order of general recommended intake, most to least; foods in the supplemental categories (vegetables, fruits, snacks, etc.) are alphabetized.

WHOLE-CEREAL GRAINS

The principal food of each meal is whole grain, comprising from 50 to 60 percent of the total volume of the meal. Cooked whole grains are preferred to flour products. Whole-cereal grain and grain products include:

Regular Use

Short-grain brown rice
Medium-grain brown rice
Long-grain brown rice (for hot climates)
Whole barley
Pearl barley (hato mugi)
Millet
Corn
Whole-wheat berries

Buckwheat
Whole oats
Rye

Occasional Use

Sweet brown rice
Wild rice
Mochi (pounded sweet rice)
Cracked wheat (bulgur)
Steel cut oats
Rolled oats
Corn grits
Rye flakes
Couscous
Quinoa
Amaranth
Teff
Basmati rice (infrequently)

Occasional Use: Flour Products

Whole wheat noodles and pasta
Udon noodles
Somen noodles
Soba noodles (buckwheat)
Unyeasted whole wheat bread
Unyeasted whole-rye bread
Fu (puffed wheat gluten)
Seitan (wheat gluten)

SOUPS

One or two cups or bowls of soup seasoned with miso, shoyu, or sea salt is recommended every day, making up about 5 percent of daily intake. Prepare soups with a variety of ingredients, including sea vegetables, seasonal vegetables, grains, and beans. Occasionally soups may include small pieces of white-meat fish or seafood.

VEGETABLES

About one-quarter (25 to 30) percent of daily food intake includes fresh vegetables prepared in a variety of ways, including steaming, boiling, or sautéing (with a small amount of unrefined sesame or corn oil). In general, up to one-third of vegetables may be eaten in the form of pickles or salad. The rest should be cooked. In selecting vegetables, observe these guidelines:

Regular Use: Green and Whit Leafy Vegetables

Bok choy

Carrot tops
Chinese cabbage
Chives
Collard greens
Dandelion leaves
Kale
Leeks
Mustard greens
Parsley
Scallions
Turnip greens
Watercress

Regular Use: Round Vegetables

Acorn squash
Broccoli
Brussels sprouts
Buttercup squash
Butternut squash
Cabbage
Cauliflower
Hokkaido pumpkin
Hubbard squash
Onion
Pumpkin
Red cabbage
Rutabaga
Turnip

Regular Use: Root Vegetables

Burdock
Carrots
Daikon
Jinenjo (mountain potato)
Lotus root
Parsnips
Radishes

Occasional Use

Beets
Celery
Coltsfoot
Cucumbers
Endive
Escarole
Garlic

Green beans
Green peas
Iceberg lettuce
Jerusalem artichoke
Kohlrabi
Lambs-quarters
Mushrooms
Patty pan squash
Romaine lettuce
Salsify
Shiitake mushroom
Snap beans
Snow peas
Sprouts
Summer squash
Wax beans
Winter melon
Zucchini

Vegetables to Avoid or Limit

Asparagus
Avocado
Curly dock
Eggplant
Fennel
Ferns
Green and red peppers
Plantain
Potatoes
Purslane
Shepherd's purse
Sorrel
Spinach
Sweet potatoes
Taro (albi potato)
Tomatoes
Yams

BEANS

A small portion (about 5 to 10 percent) of daily intake includes cooked beans or bean products. The most suitable include:

Regular Use

Aduki beans
Chickpeas (garbanzos)

Lentils (green or brown)
Black soybeans
Tofu (fresh soybean curd)
Dried tofu
Natto (fermented soybeans)
Okara (residue in making tofu)
Tempeh (fermented soybeans)

Occasional Use

Black-eyed peas
Black turtle beans
Great northern beans
Kidney beans
Lentils (red)
Lima beans
Mung beans
Navy beans
Pinto beans
Split peas and whole dried peas
Yellow soybeans

SEA VEGETABLES

These important foods are served in small quantities and are included in various cooked dishes, comprising about 5 percent of daily intake.

Regular Use

Toasted *nori* sheet
Kombu
Wakame

Occasional Use

Arame
Hijiki

Optional Use

Agar-agar
Dulse
Irish moss
Mekabu
Ocean ribbons
Sea palm

FISH AND SEAFOOD

For those in good health, once or twice a week a small amount of white-meat fish or seafood may be eaten.

Occasional Use

Carp
Cod
Chirimen iriko (tiny dried fish)
Clams
Eel
Flounder
Haddock
Halibut
Iriko (small dried fish)
Littlenecks
Oysters
Red snapper
Scallops
Smelt
Sole
Trout
Other white-meat fish

Avoid or Limit

Red-meat or blue-skinned fish such as salmon, swordfish, bluefish, tuna, etc., which are high in fat and oil. Seafood high in cholesterol such as lobster, crab, and shrimp should be limited.

FRUIT

Fruit is preferably eaten cooked, dried, or dried and cooked, though fresh fruit may be consumed several times a week, especially in warmer weather, by those in usual good health.

Occasional Use: Temperate-Climate Fruit

Apples
Apricots
Blackberries
Blueberries
Cantaloupe
Cherries
Cranberries
Currants
Grapefruit
Grapes
Honeydew melon
Oranges
Peaches
Pears
Plums

Prunes
Raspberries
Strawberries
Tangerines
Watermelon

Avoid: Tropical Fruits

Bananas
Coconut
Dates
Figs
Kiwis
Mangoes
Papayas

NUTS AND SEEDS

A small volume of roasted seeds or nuts (with or without sea salt or shoyu) may be enjoyed as snacks. It is preferable to minimize the use of nuts and nut butters, as they are difficult to digest and high in fats.

Occasional Use

Sesame seeds
Sunflower seeds
Pumpkin seeds
Chestnuts
Almonds
Filberts
Peanuts
Pecans
Spanish peanuts
Walnuts

Avoid: Tropical Nuts

Brazil nuts
Cashews
Hazelnuts
Pistachio

SNACKS AND DESSERTS

Delicious snacks and desserts using all natural ingredients may be prepared from time to time.

Occasional Use

Mochi

Noodles
Popcorn (homemade and unbuttered)
Puffed whole-cereal grains
Rice balls
Rice cakes
Seeds
Vegetable sushi (homemade)

Sweets for Regular Use

A sweet taste can be achieved with the following vegetables:
Cabbage
Carrots
Daikon
Onions
Parsnips
Squash
Sweet vegetable drink (see recipe chapter)
Sweet vegetable jam (see recipe chapter)

Other Sweets for Occasional Use

Amasake
Barley malt
Brown rice syrup
Chestnuts
Hot apple cider
Hot apple juice

Avoid: Refined Sweeteners

Sugar (white, raw, brown, turbinado)
Molasses
Corn syrup
Saccharine and other artificial sweeteners
Nutrasweet
Fructose
Chocolate
Carob
Honey
Maple syrup

BEVERAGES

Spring or well water may be used for teas and drinks.

Regular Use

Bancha twig tea (kukicha)

Bancha stem tea
Roasted barley tea
Roasted brown rice tea
Spring water
Well water

Occasional Use

Carrot juice
Celery juice
Dandelion tea
Grain coffee (100 percent grain)
Kombu tea
Mu tea
Sweet vegetable drink (see recipe chapter)
Umeboshi tea

Infrequent Use

Beer
Green tea
Sake
Soy milk (with kombu)
Sprouted barley powder tea
Temperate-climate fruit juice
Vegetable juice

Avoid

Aromatic beverages
Black tea
Coffee
Cold drinks (with ice cubes)
Decaffeinated coffee
Distilled water
Hard liquors
Herbal teas
Mineral water and all bubbling waters (carbonated)
Stimulant beverages
Sugared and soft drinks
Tap water
Wine

CONDIMENTS

Main Use

Green nori flakes
Gomashio (roasted sesame seeds and salt)

Seaweed powder with or without toasted sesame seeds
Shiso leaf powder
Tekka
Umeboshi plums

Other Condiments

Brown rice vinegar
Cooked miso with scallions
Nori condiment
Shio kombu
Shiso leaf powder with toasted sesame seeds
Umeboshi plum with scallions
Umeboshi vinegar

SEASONINGS

Naturally processed, unrefined sea salt is preferable to refined table salt or gray sea salt. Miso and shoyu may also be used as seasonings. Use only naturally processed, nonchemicalized varieties. In general, seasonings are used moderately and used in cooking, not added at the table.

Regular Use

Barley miso
Brown rice miso
Soybean miso (hatcho miso)
Shoyu (natural soy sauce)
Unrefined white sea salt

Occasional Use

Ginger
Horseradish
Mirin
Rice vinegar
Umeboshi paste
Umeboshi plum
Umeboshi vinegar
Garlic
Lemon

Avoid

All unnatural, artificial, or chemically processed seasonings
Ginseng
Herbs
Iodized salt
Mayonnaise

Soy mayonnaise
Spices (cayenne, cumin, etc.)
Wine, or apple-cider, or balsamic vinegar

COOKING OIL

For cooking oil, use only naturally processed, high-quality, cold-pressed un-refined vegetable oil. Oil should be used in moderation for fried rice, fried noodles, and sautéing vegetables. Generally, two to three times a week is reasonable. Occasionally, oil may be used in deep-frying grains, vegetables, fish, and seafood or in making tempura.

Regular Use

Sesame oil (dark or light)
Corn oil
Mustard seed oil

Occasional Use

Safflower oil
Sunflower oil
Soybean oil
Olive oil
Peanut oil
Canola oil
Other traditional oils

Avoid

Butter or margarine (including soy margarine)
Coconut oil
Lard, shortening, and all animal fats
Palm oil
Refined, chemically processed vegetable oils

PICKLES

To help digest grains and other food, a small volume of pickles, about one tablespoon, should be taken daily.

Regular Use (Types)

Bran
Brine
Miso
Miso Bran
Pressed
Sauerkraut

Takuan
Shoyu
Umeboshi

Avoid (Types)

Dill
Garlic
Herbs
Spices
Vinegar (apple-, wine-, etc.)

FOODS TO AVOID FOR BETTER HEALTH

In addition to some of the items noted above, the following foods should be reduced or avoided.

Animal Products

Red meat (beef, lamb, pork)	Poultry
Cured meat (ham, bacon, salami, etc.)	Sausage (hot dogs, etc.)
	Wild game
Eggs	

Dairy Products

Butter	Margarine
Cheese	Milk (whole, raw, skim, buttermilk, etc.)
Cream	
Ice cream	Sour cream
Kefir	Whipped cream
	Yogurt

Processed Foods

Polished (white) rice	Foods processed with
Refined (white) flour	Additives
Canned foods	Artificial coloring
Dyed foods	Artificial flavoring
Frozen foods	Chemicals
Genetically altered foods	Emulsifiers
Instant foods	Preservatives
Irradiated foods	Stabilizers
Sprayed foods	

Vitamins and Supplements

Vitamin pills (synthetic or natural)	Mineral supplements

B-complex
B_1
B_2
B_6
B_{12}
Biotin
C
Choline
E
Folic acid
Inositol
Niacin
Niacinamide
PABA
Pantothenic acid

Bone meal
Calcium
Dolomite
Iron
Selenium
Zinc
Lecithin capsules
Bee pollen
Bran tablets
Brewer's yeast
Desiccated liver
Diet pills
Ginseng tablets or pills
Herbal tablets
Papaya tablets
Other similar products

30

Guidelines for People with Cancer

When properly applied, the Cancer Prevention Diet can help to restore an excessively yin or yang condition to one of more natural balance. However, slight modifications are needed in every case. Below is a summary of the common types of cancer and the general dietary adjustments for the category in which they fall. Specific nutritional advice for each cancer is given in the individual chapters in Part II under the section "Dietary Recommendations." Cancer patients should consult an experienced macrobiotic counselor or medical associate to make sure the evaluation of their condition is accurate and to help formulate a diet suited to their unique case and personal needs.

Kind of Food	More Yin Cancer	Combination of Both	More Yang Cancer
	Brain (outer regions)	Bladder/Kidney	Bone
	Breast	Liver	Brain (inner regions)
	Esophagus	Lung	Colon
	Leukemia	Melanoma	Ovary
	Lymphoma and Hodgkin's disease	Spleen	Pancreas
	Mouth (except tongue)	Stomach (lower)	Prostate
	Skin	Tongue	Rectum
	Stomach (upper)	Uterus	
Grains		Minimize buckwheat	Minimize buckwheat
Soup	Slightly stronger flavor (more miso or shoyu)	Moderate flavor	Milder flavor (less miso or shoyu)

Kind of Food	More Yin Cancer	Combination of Both	More Yang Cancer
Vegetables	Slightly greater emphasis on root varieties (burdock, carrot, turnip, etc.)	Greater emphasis on ground varieties (cauliflower, acorn and butternut squash, pumpkin)	Greater emphasis on leafy green varieties (daikon, carrot, or turnip greens, kale, watercress, etc.)
Beans	A little more strongly seasoned, use less often	Moderately seasoned and moderate volume	More lightly seasoned, may use regularly
Sea Vegetables	Longer cooking, slightly thicker taste	Moderate cooking, medium taste	Quicker cooking, lighter taste
Pickles	More long-time pickles	More medium-time pickles	More short-time pickles
Condiments	Stronger use	Moderate use	Lighter use
Animal Food	Occasional small volume of white fish or dried fish, only if craved	Avoid completely or minimize	Avoid completely
Salad	Avoid raw salad, occasional boiled salad	Limit raw salad, frequent boiled or pressed salad	Occasional raw, frequent boiled or pressed salad
Fruit Dessert	Avoid completely	Small amount of dried or cooked fruit (locally grown and seasonally), if craved	Small amount of dried or cooked fruit (locally grown and seasonal), if craved, occasional fresh fruit in small volume
Seeds and Nuts	Occasional roasted seeds, avoid nuts	Occasional roasted seeds, limit nuts	Occasional roasted seeds, avoid nuts
Oil	Sesame only, as little as possible. Apply with brush to prevent burning. No raw oil.	Sesame or corn only, as little as possible. Apply with brush to prevent burning. No raw oil.	Sesame or corn for cooking, small amount occasionally for sautéing. No raw oil.
Beverage	Longer-cooked, thicker-tasting tea.	Medium-cooked, medium-tasting tea	Shorter-cooked, lighter-tasting tea

31

Making a Smooth Transition

The transition to a more natural diet and way of life should present no serious conflict. However, sometimes we approach the process too ambitiously and go to great lengths to avoid the foods to which we were previously accustomed. If we rush things and try to change overnight, we are bound to make mistakes and within a short period will revert to our former lifestyle or go on to sample something else. This desire for instant satisfaction is part of the modern consumer mentality, and we can make the mistake of approaching the Cancer Prevention Diet in this way as well as anything else.

In selecting natural foods, we begin to appreciate crops that have matured in the fields and weathered the elements in contrast to those that have been produced in a factory and artificially aged. Similarly, we must respect our own biological rhythms and personal rates of growth. In many cases, it has taken ten, twenty, or thirty years or more of poor eating for the cancerous condition to develop. Depending upon our own unique situation, it will take several months and, in some cases, a few years to recover our normal digestive, respiratory, circulatory, excretory, and nervous functions. The healing process should not be artificially hurried.

When starting the new way of eating, it is best to begin with just a few basic preparations, such as pressure-cooked brown rice, miso soup, a few vegetable dishes, one sea vegetable, and bancha tea. Then, day by day, week by week, we can gradually widen our selection of natural foods and introduce new cooking styles. In the meantime, we can still be eating some of the same types of foods we have been eating in the past, including salads and fruit, flour products, and seafood. Rather than eliminating certain categories of food from our diet, it is better initially to reduce their intake and then switch to a better quality of intermediary food until a taste and appreciation for the new foods are developed.

The important thing is to begin to change in the right direction. Ideally the rate of change should be more like walking long distances, where we gradually build up our endurance, rather than like sprinting or marathon running, where we get off to a fast start but inevitably get worn out. If we throw away all of our old food the first day and memorize the yin and yang tables like a catechism, we will soon either leave the diet as abruptly as we adopted it or become missionaries, preaching to the nutritionally unconverted. Such behavior is childish and violates the macrobiotic way of life, which respects all lifestyles and understands opposites as complementary aspects of the whole.

On the other hand, there is a danger of taxiing so slowly down the dietary runway that our plane never takes off. Sometimes we can remain in a holding pattern for years, never realizing that we are still on the ground. We are conscious of the importance of proper food and eat a little brown rice and a little miso soup, but we never really experience looking at things from a healthy perspective. If we adopt a middle way between proceeding too quickly and too slowly, we will soon find ourselves pleasantly aloft.

Of course, these reflections on making a smooth transition apply to people already in relatively healthy shape. Those with cancer or other serious conditions may need to adopt a strict form of the diet at once without the luxury of integrating it into their previous way of eating. However, in practice the reduction in pain and discomfort quickly convinces the person of the value of the new approach.

As far as obtaining natural foods, growing our own grains and vegetables, of course, is best if the situation allows. We should all try to cultivate a garden, even if it is a very small one in an urban environment. Next best is to obtain food at an organic farmers market or a natural foods co-op so that we can actually experience some of the living energy of the food before it reaches the market shelf or dinner table. In most North American and European cities, there are now natural foods and health food stores, which supply most of the staple items in the Cancer Prevention Diet as well as a regular supply of fresh, seasonal produce. It is important to shop around and learn what each store offers in terms of quality, availability, service, and price. Buying in bulk saves on packaging and is more ecological and less expensive. Ethnic markets, such as Oriental, Latin America, Afro-American, and Middle Eastern food shops, are also potential sources of basic items, such as grains and beans, and often have a wider selection of vegetables than elsewhere. Even the local supermarket often has a natural foods section and suitable locally grown produce. For those people who do not have access to any of these sources or who are confined, a list of whole foods distributors and mail order stores can be obtained from the Kushi Foundation.

As far as possible, we should try to make our own bread, tofu, pickles, and traditionally processed foods. Homemade dishes have a much fresher quality, are more delicious, and contribute to the peaceful energy of the home. Each week, each month, or each season of the year, we can try our new food preparation or style of cooking and slowly build up a reservoir of experience that can become translated into well-balanced recipes and menus.

During the transition period, there will be times when we crave the taste, texture, odor, and other characteristics of previous foods and drinks, especially those we had in childhood. Often, when eating such foods, we suffer from feelings of guilt. These feelings should be put aside and a more relaxed attitude developed. Instead of feeling as if we have committed a sin, we should reflect and try to understand why such cravings arose. Usually, during the first weeks or months of the new diet, these cravings reflect a natural discharge process. As our condition improves, the toxins and mucus that have accumulated in our bloodstream and internal organs are eliminated from the body through the bowels, urination, perspiration, and other excretory functions. As they leave the body, the discharged food particles often impress themselves in our consciousness and we experience them as cravings. At other times, after our condition has stabilized, these occasional cravings signify that our diet is imbalanced in the opposite yin or yang direction from the food to which we are attracted. Thus if we are attracted to fruit juice or ice cream, our diet is probably too salty, overcooked, and generally yang. If we are attracted to fish, eggs, or other animal products, we are consuming too many sweets, liquids, and other strong yin foods. These promptings are one of the body's way of alerting us to a disequilibrium in our way of eating.

Rather than suppress these natural urges, it is better to acknowledge them and take a tiny volume of the previous type of food from time to time until such cravings lessen and finally go away, as they ultimately will. During the transition period, the following table may serve as a guide in substituting better-quality foods for the previous items that we miss.

Cravings	Replacement	Goal
Meat	Fish, seafood	Grains, beans, seitan, tempeh, tofu
Sugar, molasses, chocolate, carob, and other highly refined sweeteners	Honey, maple syrup	Rice syrup, barley malt, and ultimately natural sweeteners from whole grains and vegetables
Dairy food, cheese, milk, cream, butter	Organic dairy food, in small volume; nuts and nut butters; soy milk	Traditional soy products such as miso and tofu; tahini and other seed butters
Tropical and semitropical fruits and juices such as orange, grapefruit, and pineapple; artificial juices and beverages	Organic fruits and fruit juices	Organic temperate-climate fruit (fresh, dried, and cooked) and juices in small volume and in season
Coffee, black tea, soft drinks, diet drinks	Herb teas, green tea, mineral water	Bancha twig tea, grain coffee, and other traditional nonaromatic teas

During the transition period, instead of coffee or decaffeinated coffee, use grain coffee. To keep awake, take bancha tea with a little barley malt. In the beginning, some people find it difficult to eat brown rice. In this case, take other whole grains and gradually introduce brown rice, or take white rice cooked together with barley or millet and barley and gradually over the next few weeks add a small volume of brown rice. During this time, as the body begins to rebalance, brown rice will become more appetizing and can be used regularly. Ordinarily, of course, we don't use white rice, but in this case it may temporarily be used until the intestines and other organs are able to digest whole grains.

In addition to cravings, the discharge process is often accompanied by some abnormal physical manifestations that may last from three to ten days and, in some cases, up to four months, until the quality of the blood fully changes. If our native constitution is strong and well structured, such reactions are usually negligible. However, if our embryonic and childhood development suffered from chaotic dietary habits, if we have ingested many chemicals, drugs, or medications, or if we have had surgery or an abortion, these discharge reactions will be more pronounced.

Whatever the case may be, we should not worry if these reactions occur. They are part of the natural healing process and signify that our systems are regenerating themselves, dislodging and throwing off the excess that has accumulated over many years. These reactions may be generally classified as follows.

General Fatigue

A feeling of general fatigue may arise among people who have been eating an excessive amount of animal protein and fat. The energetic activity that they have previously experienced was the result of the vigorous caloric discharge of these excessive foods rather than a more healthy, balanced, and peaceful way of activity. Often these people initially experience physical tiredness and slight mental depression until the new diet starts to serve as an energy supply for activity. Such a period of fatigue usually ends within a month.

Pains and Aches

Pains and aches may sometimes be experienced, especially by people who have been taking excessive liquid, sugar, fruits, or any other extremely yin quality food and beverages. These pains and aches—such as headaches and pains in the area of the intestines, kidneys, and chest—occur because of the gradual contraction of abnormally expanded tissues and nerve cells. These aches and pains disappear—either gradually or suddenly—as soon as these abnormally expanded areas return to a normal condition. This usually takes between three and fourteen days, depending upon the previous condition.

Fever, Chills, Coughing

As the new diet starts to form a more sound quality of blood, previous excessive substances—excessive volume of liquid, fat, and many other things—

begin to be discharged. If at this time the functions of the kidneys, urinary system, and respiratory system have not yet returned to normal, this discharge sometimes takes the form of fever, chills, or coughing. These are temporary and disappear in several days without any special treatment.

Abnormal Sweating and Frequent Urination

As in the symptoms described above, unusual sweating may be experienced by some people from time to time, for a period of several months, and other people may experience unusually frequent urination. In their previous diets, these people have been taking excessive liquid in the form of water, various beverages, alcohol, fruits, fruit juices, or milk or other dairy food. By reducing these excessive liquids and fats accumulated in the form of liquid, the body returns to a normal, balanced, healthy condition. When metabolic balance has been gradually restored, these discharges will cease.

Skin Discharge and Unusual Body Odors

Among the forms of elimination is the discharge of unusual odors from the entire body surface, through breathing, urination, or bowel movements and often, in the case of women, through vaginal discharges. This usually occurs among people who were previously taking excessive volumes of animal fat, dairy food, and sugar. In addition, some people experience—for only short periods—skin rashes, reddish swelling at the tips of the fingers and toes, and boils. These types of elimination arise especially among people who have taken animal fat, dairy food, sugar, spices, chemicals, and drugs and among those who have had chronic malfunctions of the intestines, kidneys, and liver. However, these eliminations naturally heal and usually disappear within a few months without any special attention.

Diarrhea or Constipation

People who had been chronically disturbed intestinal conditions, caused by previous improper dietary habits, may temporarily experience either diarrhea (usually for several days) or constipation (for a period lasting up to twenty days). In this case, diarrhea is a form of discharge of accumulated stagnated matter in the intestines, including unabsorbed food, fat, mucus, and liquid. Constipation is the result of a process of contraction of the intestinal tube, which was abnormally expanded due to the previous diet. As this contraction restores normal elasticity to the intestinal tube, the normal elimination of the bowels resumes.

Decrease of Sexual Desire and Vitality

There are some people who may feel a weakening of sexual vitality or appetite, not necessarily accompanied by a feeling of fatigue. The reason for such a decline is that the body functions are working to eliminate imbalanced factors from all parts of the body and excessive vitality is not available to be used for sexual activity. Also, in some cases, the sexual organs are being actively healed by the new quality of blood and are not yet prepared to resume normal activity. These conditions, however, last only for a short period, usually a few weeks and, at most, a few months. As soon as this recovery period is over, healthy vitality and desire for sexual activity return.

Temporary Cessation of Menstruation

In a few women, there may be a temporary cessation of menstruation. The reason for this cessation is that in the healing of the entire body, once again the vital organs need to receive energy first. Less vital functions, including reproductive activities, are healed later. The period of cessation of menstruation varies with the individual. However, when menstruation begins anew, it is healthy and natural, and begins to adjust to the normal twenty-eight-day lunar cycle and presents no discomfort, as was previously often the case. Mental clarity and emotional clarity are strengthened as well as physical flexibility.

Mental Irritability

Some people who have been taking stimulants, drugs, and medications for long periods experience emotional irritability after changing their dietary practices. This irritability reflects adjustments taking place in the blood and various body functions, following the change to the different quality of food, and generally passes within one week to several weeks, depending upon how deeply affected the body systems were by the previous habitual use of drugs and medications. The consumption of sugar, coffee, and alcohol for long periods, as well as long-time smoking, also produces temporary emotional irritability when the new diet is initially practiced.

Other Possible Transitory Experiences

In addition to the above conditions, some people may experience other manifestations of adjustment, such as bad dreams at night or a feeling of coldness. These too will pass.

In many instances, the discharge process is so gradual that none of these more visible temporary conditions arises. However, when they do appear, the symptoms vary from person to person, depending upon their inherited constitution and physical condition, and usually require no special treatment, naturally ceasing as the whole body readjusts to normal functioning. In the possible event that the symptoms are severe or uncomfortable, the discharge process can be slowed down by modifying the new diet to include continuous consumption of some previous food in small volume—about 10 to 30 percent of the meal—until balance is restored. The important thing is to understand that the discharge mechanism is part of the normal healing process and these symptoms are not to be suppressed by taking drugs or medications, resorting to vitamin or mineral supplements, or going off the diet altogether in the mistaken belief that it is deficient. If there is any uncertainty or question about proper practice that arises during this transition period, a qualified macrobiotic counselor or medical professional should be contacted.

As mentioned earlier, introductory macrobiotic cooking classes are essential for proper orientation to the new way of eating. In addition, it is important to have a community of support consisting of other individuals or families who are eating in this way or in the general direction of more natural foods. Dishes and recipes can then be exchanged and experiences shared in the spirit of adventure and discovery.

Variables in cooking such as salt, oil, pressure, time, and liquid are always changing with the seasons and our own development and take time to master. Another factor connected with unsatisfactory cooking is the use of electricity or microwave. Some families either have recently installed expensive ranges or ovens or live in an apartment where they come furnished with the kitchen. We have found that when people, especially cancer patients, switch to gas heat they invariably get improved results, and a peaceful energy replaces the chaotic vibration of the previously prepared food. Although it may appear uneconomical in the short run to invest in another stove, the change in food quality and improved health will be well worth it in the long run. Even a small portable camping stove with one or two propane burners can be set up conveniently in a corner of the kitchen for this purpose.

All of these factors will contribute to a smoother transition and more delicious and satisfying meals.

32

Recipes

This chapter includes many of the basic recipes for the dietary recommendations in this book. People with cancer should be careful to follow the guidelines in the individual chapters in Part II and may need to restrict their use of oil, animal food, fruit, salad, dessert, and other items. Those in good health may wish to consult a macrobiotic cookbook with a wider selection of recipes, such as *Aveline Kushi's Complete Guide to Macrobiotic Cooking* (New York: Warner Books, 1985), Alex and Gale Jack's *Amber Waves of Grain: American Macrobiotic Cooking* (New York and Tokyo: Japan Publications, 1992) or Edward and Wendy Esko's *Macrobiotic Cooking for Everyone* (New York and Tokyo: Japan Publications, 1980).

FOOD SELECTION

For variety, these aspects of day-to-day cooking can be changed:

1. The selection of foods within the following categories: grains, soups, vegetables, beans, sea vegetables, condiments, pickles, and beverages;
2. The methods of cooking: boiling, steaming, sautéing, frying, pressure cooking, etc.;
3. The ways of cutting vegetables;
4. The amount of water used;
5. The amount of seasoning and condiments used;
6. The kind of seasoning and condiments used;
7. The length of cooking time (do not overcook or pressure-cook vegetables);
8. The use of higher or lower flame in cooking foods;
9. The combination of foods and dishes;
10. The seasonal cooking adjustments.

PREPARATION

Macrobiotic cooking is unique. The ingredients are simple and cooking is the key to producing meals that are nutritious, tasty, and attractive. The cook has the ability to change the quality of the food. More cooking, the use of pressure, salt, heat, and time, makes the energy of food more concentrated, while quick cooking and little salt preserve the lighter quality of the food. A good cook controls the health of those for whom he or she cooks by varying the cooking styles.

Methods of Cooking and Food Preparation

Regular Use

Boiling
Oil-sautéing
Pickling
Pressing
Pressure cooking
Steaming
Soup
Waterless
Water-sautéing

Occasional Use

Baking
Broiling
Deep-frying
Raw
Stir-frying
Tempura

GRAINS

PRESSURE-COOKED BROWN RICE

1 cup organic brown rice
1¼ to 1½ cups spring water per cup
  of rice

pinch of sea salt per cup of
  rice

Gently wash and quickly place rice (short- or medium-grain) in a pressure cooker and smooth out surface of rice so it is level. Slowly add spring water down side of pressure cooker so surface of rice remains calm and even. Add sea salt. Place cover on pressure cooker and bring up to pressure slowly. When pressure is up, place a flame deflector underneath and turn flame to low. Cook for 50 minutes. When rice is done, remove pressure cooker from burner and allow to stand for about 5 minutes before reducing pressure and opening. With a bamboo rice paddle, lift rice from pot one spoonful at a time and smooth into wooden bowl. Distribute more cooked rice at bottom and less cooked rice at top evenly in bowl. The rice will have a delicious, nutty taste and impart a very peaceful feeling.

Note: Each cup of uncooked rice makes about 3 cups of cooked rice. Allow about 1 cup per person. In general, you will want to start with 3 or more cups of uncooked rice and store the remainder. Leftover rice will keep for several days. After rice cools off, place in a closed container in the refrigerator. Warm up by placing rice in a cheesecloth or piece of unbleached muslin, placing in a ceramic saucepan or on top of a steamer that fits into a pot or saucepan, add ¼ to ½ inch of water, and bringing to a boil. After rice has heated for a few minutes, remove from cloth and serve.

Variation: One-third of an *umeboshi* plum may be added instead of salt for each cup of uncooked rice. Long-grain rice may occasionally be used in summer.

BOILED RICE

1 cup brown rice　　　　　　　　　*pinch of sea salt*
2 cups spring water

Wash rice and place in heavy pot or saucepan. Add water and salt. Cover with a lid. Bring to a boil, lower flame, and simmer for about 1 hour or until all water has been absorbed. Remove and serve.

Note: It is highly recommended that cancer patients eat pressure-cooked brown rice. It is sweeter and more energizing than boiled rice. Healthy persons should also eat primarily pressure-cooked rice. However, they may have boiled rice occasionally, especially lightly roasted rice.

BROWN RICE WITH MILLET

2 cups brown rice　　　　　　　*2-inch piece of kombu or pinch of*
½ cup millet　　　　　　　　　　*sea salt*
4½ cups spring water

Wash the grains and place in pressure cooker with kombu, or place over fire and, when the water is warm, add a pinch of sea salt. Put on the cover and bring up to pressure. Cook for about 45 minutes. Let set for 5 minutes. Bring down the pressure and gently remove from the pot.

BROWN RICE WITH BARLEY

2 cups brown rice　　　　　　　*2-inch piece of kombu or pinch of*
½ cup barley　　　　　　　　　　*sea salt*
4 cups spring water

Wash the grains and place in pressure cooker with kombu, or place over fire, and when the water is warm, add a pinch of sea salt. Put on the cover and bring up to pressure. Cook for about 45 minutes. Let set for 5 minutes. Bring down the pressure and gently remove from the pot.

SOFT BROWN RICE (Rice Kayu)

1 cup brown rice
5 cups spring water

pinch of sea salt

Wash rice and pressure-cook or boil as in previous recipes. However, not all of the water will be absorbed. Rice should be creamy and some of the grains should be visible after cooking. In case water boils over while pressure cooking, turn off flame and allow to cool off. Then turn on flame again and continue to cook until done.

Note: Makes a nourishing and appetizing breakfast cereal. Especially recommended for cancer patients and others who have difficulty swallowing or holding food down.

Variation: Vegetables such as daikon or Chinese cabbage or an *umeboshi* plum may be added while cooking. Also, a one-inch square of dried *kombu* is highly recommended.

GENUINE BROWN RICE CREAM

1 cup brown rice
10 cups spring water

½ umeboshi plum or a pinch of sea
salt per cup of rice

Dry-roast rice in a cast-iron or stainless-steel skillet until golden brown. Place in pot, add water and plum or salt, and bring to a boil. Cover, lower heat, and place flame deflector beneath pot. Cook until water is one-half of original volume. Let the rice cool and place in cheesecloth or unbleached muslin, tie, and squeeze a creamy liquid out of the pulp through the cloth. Heat the cream again, then serve. Add salt if needed. The remaining pulp is also very good to eat and can be made into a small ball and steamed with grated lotus root or carrot.

Note: Makes a delicious breakfast cereal and is also good for those who have difficulty eating. The lives of many people who otherwise could not eat have been saved with rice cream. The love, care, and energy of the cook can be imparted to the food with his or her hands.

Variation: Garnish with scallions, chopped parsley, nori, gomashio, or roasted sunflower seeds.

FRIED RICE

4 cups cooked brown rice
1 tablespoon dark sesame oil
1 medium onion sliced diagonally or
  diced

1 to 2 tablespoons shoyu

Brush skillet with sesame oil. Let heat for a minute or less, but do not let oil start to smoke. Add onion; place rice on top. If rice is dry, moisten with a few drops of water. Cover skillet and cook on low flame for 10 to 15 minutes. Add shoyu and cook for another 5 minutes. There is no need to stir. Just mix before serving.

Note: Those in good health may have fried rice several times a week, though the amount of oil may need to be reduced depending on the individual's condition. Cancer patients may need to restrict their oil and may use 2 to 3 tablespoons of water to replace the oil. Check dietary recommendations carefully.

Variation: Use scallions, parsley, or a combination of vegetables such as carrots and onion, cabbage and mushroom, and daikon and daikon leaves.

RICE WITH BEANS

1 cup brown rice
¹/₁₀ to ⅛ cup of beans per cup of rice

1½ to 2 cups spring water
pinch of sea salt

Wash rice and beans. Cook beans ½ hour beforehand following basic recipes in bean section below. Allow beans to cool; add with cooking water and sea salt to rice. Bean water counts as part of the total water in the recipe. Pressure-cook for 45 to 50 minutes and serve as with plain rice.

Note: Cancer patients should generally use only aduki, chickpeas, or lentils. Those in good health may use a variety of other beans as well. Grains and beans cooked together make for a substantial meal and save the time and fuel needed for cooking each dish separately.

RICE AND VEGETABLES

1 cup brown rice
¼ cup dried daikon
½ cup carrots (*finely diced or small matchsticks*)
⅛ cup burdock (*finely diced or cut into small matchsticks*)

1½ to 2 cups spring water per cup of rice
pinch of sea salt per cup of rice

Place washed rice in pressure cooker and mix with vegetables. Add water and salt, cover, and cook as for plain rice.

Variation: A small amount of shoyu may be added with salt before cooking. Other vegetables that go well with rice are sweet rice, green beans, green peas and carrots, etc. Soft vegetables such as onion and green leafy vegetables tend to become mushy and should be avoided for this dish. Rice and vegetables may also be cooked with sesame seeds, with walnuts, or with lotus seeds, as well as with aduki beans or black soybeans.

RICE BALLS WITH NORI SEA VEGETABLE

1 sheet toasted nori
pinch of sea salt
dish of spring water

1 cup cooked brown rice
½ to 1 umeboshi plum

Roast a thin sheet of nori by holding the shiny side over a burner about 10 to 12 inches from the flame. Rotate for 3 to 5 seconds until color changes from black to green. Fold nori in half and tear into two pieces. Fold and tear again. You should now have four pieces that are about 3 inches to a side. Add pinch of salt to a dish of water and wet your hands. Form a handful of rice into a solid ball. Press a hole in the center with your thumb and place a small piece of umeboshi inside. Then close hole and compact ball again until solid. Cover rice ball with nori, one piece at a time, until it sticks. Wet hands occasionally to prevent rice and nori from sticking to them, but do not use too much water.

Note: Rice balls make a tasty, convenient lunch or snack because they can be eaten without utensils. They are great to take along when traveling and keep fresh for a few days. Use less or no umeboshi when making rice balls for children.

Variation: Rice can be made into triangles instead of balls by cupping your hands into a V-shape. Balls or triangles can be rolled in toasted sesame seeds and eaten with nori. Small pieces of salt or bran pickles, vegetables, pickled fish, or other condiments can be inserted inside instead of umeboshi. Instead of nori sheets, use roasted crushed sesame seeds, shiso leaves, pickled rice leaves, dried wakame sheets, or green leafy vegetable leaves.

WHOLE OATS

1 cup whole oats   pinch of sea salt per cup of oats
5 to 6 cups spring water

Wash oats and place in pot. Add water and salt. Cover and bring to a boil. Reduce flame and simmer on a low flame for several hours or overnight until water is absorbed. Use a flame deflector to prevent burning. Makes an excellent cereal.

Note: Whole oats are very strengthening for cancer patients and are to be preferred to steel cut oats or rolled oats.

Variation: Cooking time can be reduced by pressure-cooking following the basic brown rice recipe. For a very nourishing and peaceful dish, combine 1½ cups barley, 1 cup whole oats, and ½ cup partially cooked beans. Add 3 pinches of sea salt, about 4 cups of water, and pressure-cook as usual.

SWEET RICE

1 cup sweet rice   pinch of sea salt
1½ to 2 cups spring water

Wash rice, add water and salt, and cook in pressure cooker following basic rice recipe.

Note: Sweet rice is more glutinous than regular rice and should be used only occasionally. It may also be added in small volume to regular rice for a sweeter taste.

MOCHI

Mochi is sweet rice served in cakes or squares. They are made by pounding cooked sweet rice with a heavy wooden pestle in a wooden bowl. Pound until grains are crushed and become very sticky. Wet pestle occasionally to prevent rice from sticking to it. Form rice into small balls or cakes, or spread on a baking sheet that has been oiled and dusted with flour and allow to dry. Cut into pieces and roast in a dry skillet, bake, or deep-fry. For occasional use and special celebrations.

RYE

1 cup rye   *pinch of sea salt*
1¼ to 1½ cups spring water

Cook the same as basic pressure-cooked brown rice, or boil, in which case 2 cups of water are used.

Note: Since rye is hard and requires a lot of chewing, it is usually mixed with other grains or consumed in flour form as rye bread. For a delicious, chewy dish, add 1 part rye to 3 parts brown rice. Rye may be dry-roasted in a skillet for a few minutes prior to cooking to make it more digestible.

CORN

Prepare fresh corn on the cob by steaming or boiling in a saucepan for 10 minutes or until done. Instead of butter or margarine, season with a little bit of umeboshi plum.

WHEAT

1 cup wheat berries   *pinch of sea salt*
1¼ to 1½ cups spring water

Cook following basic pressure-cooked brown rice recipe or boiled-rice recipe. Boiled wheat will usually take longer to cook than rice.

Note: Wheat is difficult to digest in whole form and must be thoroughly chewed. It also requires longer cooking time. Soaking wheat berries 3 to 5 hours beforehand reduces cooking time and makes a softer, more digestible dish. For a tasty combination, combine 1 part wheat berries and 3 parts rice or other grain.

NOODLES AND BROTH

4 cups spring water
1 package soba or udon noodles
1 piece of kombu, 2 to 3 inches long

2 dried shiitake mushrooms
2 to 3 tablespoons shoyu

Boil water. Oriental noodles already contain salt, so no salt needs to be added to the water. Add noodles to water and boil. After about 10 minutes, check to see if they are done by breaking the end of one noodle. Buckwheat cooks faster than whole wheat, and thinner noodles cook faster than thicker ones. If the inside and outside are the same color, noodles are ready. Remove noodles from pot, strain, and rinse with cold water to stop them from cooking and prevent clumping. To make the broth, place kombu in pot, add the 4 cups of spring water and mushrooms that have been soaked, their stems cut off, and sliced. Bring to boil. Reduce flame and simmer for 3 to 5 minutes. Remove kombu and mushrooms. Add shoyu to taste for 3 to 5 minutes. Place cooked noodles into the broth to warm up. Do not boil. When hot, remove and serve immediately. Garnish with scallions, chives, or tasted nori.

Note: Soba buckwheat noodles are very strengthening. In summer they can be cooked and enjoyed cold. Udon wheat noodles are much lighter. Western-style whole-grain noodles and pasta may also be used regularly. These include whole wheat spaghetti, shells, spirals, elbows, flat noodles, lasagna, etc. Use pinch of salt in water when cooking.

FRIED NOODLES

1 package soba or udon noodles
1 tablespoon sesame oil

2 cups cabbage
1 to 2 tablespoons shoyu
½ cup sliced scallions

Cook noodles as in previous recipe, rinse under cold water, and drain. Oil skillet and put in cabbage. Place noodles on top of vegetables. Cover and cook on low flame for several minutes until noodles become warm. Add shoyu and mix noodles and vegetables well. At the very end of cooking, add scallions. Serve hot or cold.

Note: If you cannot take oil, use 2 tablespoons of water for sautéing.

Variation: Many combinations of vegetables may be used, including carrots and onions, scallions and mushrooms, and cabbage and tofu.

WHOLE WHEAT BREAD

8 cups whole wheat flour
¼ to ½ teaspoon sea salt
spring water

2 tablespoons sesame oil (optional)

Mix flour and salt, add oil, and sift thoroughly together by hand. Form a ball of dough by adding just enough water and knead 300 to 350 times. Oil two bread pans with sesame oil and place dough in pans. Place damp cloth over pans and let sit for 8 to 12 hours in a warm place. After dough has risen, bake at 300°F for 15 minutes and then 1¼ hours longer at 350°F.

Note: Flour products, including bread, are not recommended for regular use by cancer patients.

Variation: A delicious sourdough starter for bread can be made by combining 1 cup of flour and enough water to make a thick batter. Cover with damp cloth and allow to ferment for 3 to 4 days in a warm place. After starter has soured, add 1 to 1½ cups of starter to bread dough, knead, and proceed as above. For rye bread, use 3 cups rye flour to 5 cups whole-wheat flour.

RICE KAYU BREAD

2 cups brown rice   *8 cups spring water*

Pressure-cook rice in water for 1 hour or more. Take out rice and allow to cool in large bowl. While still slightly warm, add to rice:

2 teaspoons sesame oil (optional)   *enough whole-wheat flour to form*
½ teaspoon sea salt   *into a ball of dough*

Add oil and salt to rice and mix well. Add enough flour to make soft ball of dough. Knead 300 to 350 times, adding flour to ball from time to time to keep from getting too sticky. Place dough in two oiled bread pans, shape into loaves, cover with damp cloth, set in warm place, and let rise 8 to 12 hours. Bake at 300°F for 30 minutes and 350°F for another hour, or until golden brown.

Note: This bread is better for cancer patients than whole-wheat bread but should still be used sparingly.

SOUPS

BASIC VEGETABLE MISO SOUP

3-inch piece of dry wakame sea   *1 quart spring water*
*   vegetable*   *1¼ teaspoons miso*
1 cup thinly sliced onions   *scallions, parsley, ginger, or water-*
                                       *   cress*

Rinse wakame quickly in cold water and soak for 3 to 5 minutes and slice into ½-inch pieces. Place wakame and onions in pot and add water. Bring to a boil, cover flame, and simmer for 10 to 20 minutes or until tender. Reduce flame to very low, but not boiling or bubbling. Place miso in a bowl or *suribachi*. Add ¼ cup of broth and puree until miso is completely dissolved in liquid. Add puréed miso to soup. Simmer for 3 to 5 minutes and serve. Garnish with scallions, parsley, ginger, or watercress.

Note: Be careful to reduce the flame while the miso is cooking in order to preserve the beneficial enzymes in miso. As a general rule, use about ½ teaspoon of miso for each cup of water in the broth. Soup shouldn't taste too salty or too bland.

Variation: Barley or brown rice miso is highly recommended. Hatcho (100 percent soybean) miso is strong, but not salty, and also may be used to help restore health. Other misos may be used occasionally. In terms of aging, select miso that has fermented 2 years or more. All types of miso may be eaten year-round and slightly modified in proportion according to the season or condition of health. Vegetables may be varied often. Other basic combinations include wakame, onions, tofu; onions and squash; cabbage and carrots; and daikon and daikon greens. If your health allows for oil, you may brush 1 teaspoon or less of unrefined vegetable oil, especially dark sesame oil, sauté the vegetables first, and then add to the wakame in the pot.

MISO SOUP WITH DAIKON AND WAKAME

1½ cups daikon	*3 teaspoons miso*
1 quart spring water	*chopped scallion*
3-inch piece of wakame	

Wash and slice daikon into ½-inch slices and add to water. Cook for 5 minutes. Meanwhile, soak wakame for 3 to 5 minutes and chop into small pieces. Add wakame to pot and cook over low flame until vegetables are soft. Dilute and add miso to stock. Simmer for 3 minutes. Garnish with chopped scallion.

Note: Daikon is particularly helpful to eliminate excess mucus, fat, protein, and water from the body. Cooking time of *wakame* depends on how soft or hard it is.

MILLET AND SWEET VEGETABLE SOUP

1 cup millet	*1-inch piece of wakame*
½ cup butternut or buttercup squash, chopped finely	*small piece of shiitake mushroom*
½ cup carrots, chopped finely	*miso (½ teaspoon per person) or shoyu (several drops)*
½ cup cabbage, chopped finely	
½ onion, chopped finely	

Combine ingredients except miso or shoyu with 3 times as much water, bring to a boil, reduce heat, and let simmer for about 30 minutes or until done. Toward the end of cooking, season lightly with miso or shoyu and simmer for another 3 to 4 minutes.

SHOYU BROTH

2 shiitake mushrooms
3-inch piece of kombu sea
  vegetable
4 cups spring water

2 cakes of tofu, cubed
2 to 3 tablespoons shoyu
1/4 cup sliced scallions
nori

Soak shiitake 10 to 20 minutes. Place kombu and shiitake in water (including soaking water) and boil for 3 to 4 minutes. Take kombu and shiitake out and save for another recipe. Add tofu and boil until tofu comes to the surface. Do not boil tofu too long or it will become too hard. Tofu in soup is best enjoyed soft. Add shoyu and simmer for 2 to 3 minutes. Garnish with scallions and nori.

Variation: This clear broth soup can be made with chopped watercress and other vegetables instead of tofu. The shiitake, too, is optional, but very good for cancer patients.

LENTIL SOUP

1 cup lentils
2 onions, diced
1 carrot, diced
1 small burdock root, diced

1 quart spring water
1/4 to 1/2 teaspoon sea salt
1 tablespoon chopped parsley

Wash lentils. Layer vegetables starting with onions, then carrot, burdock, and lentils on top. Add water and pinch of salt. Bring to a boil. Reduce flame to low, cover, and simmer for 45 minutes. Add chopped parsley and remaining salt. Simmer 20 more minutes and serve. Shoyu may be added for flavor.

Variation: For those who can use oil, vegetables may first be sautéed and then cooked with lentils as above.

ADUKI BEAN SOUP

1-inch square of dried kombu
1 cup aduki beans
1 quart spring water
1 medium onion, sliced
1/2 cup sliced carrots

1/4 to 1/2 teaspoon sea salt
shoyu to taste (optional)
scallions or parsley

Soak kombu 5 minutes and slice. Wash beans, place in pot, and add water. Bring to a boil. Reduce flame and simmer for 1¼ hours or until beans are 80 percent done. Take out cooked beans or use other pot. Put onion on bottom, then carrots, then aduki beans and kombu on top. Add salt. Cook for 20 to 25 minutes more until vegetables are soft. At very end, add shoyu to taste. Garnish with scallions or parsley and serve.

Variation: Instead of carrots and onion, winter squash may be used. This is particularly recommended for kidney, spleen, pancreas, and liver troubles.

CHICKPEA SOUP

3-inch piece of kombu
1 cup chickpeas soaked overnight
4 to 5 cups spring water
1 onion, diced
1 carrot, diced
1 burdock stalk, quartered

¼ to ½ teaspoon sea salt
scallions, parsley, or bread crumbs

Place kombu, chickpeas, and water in pressure cooker and cook for 1 to 1½ hours. Bring pressure down. Place beans in another pot. Add vegetables and salt. Cook for 20 to 25 minutes on medium-low flame. Garnish with scallions, parsley, or bread crumbs.

BARLEY SOUP

½ cup barley
¼ cup lentils
1 celery stalk
3 onions, diced

1 carrot
5 to 6 cups spring water
¼ to ½ teaspoon sea salt

Wash barley and lentils. Layer vegetables in pot starting with celery on bottom, then onions, carrot, lentils, and barley on top. Add water just enough to cover and bring to a boil. Add sea salt just before boiling. Lower flame and simmer until barley becomes soft and milky. Check taste. You may add a drop of shoyu for flavor and garnish with nori or parsley.

Note: Barley broth is very nourishing for cancer patients. The amount of barley may be increased and other variations of vegetables may be used.

Variation: You may cook barley before using for soup, adding ½ cup barley to 1½ cups water. Cook 20 to 30 minutes, then follow recipe.

BROWN RICE SOUP

3 shiitake mushrooms
3-inch piece kombu
1 quart spring water
2 cups cooked brown rice
¼ cup diced celery

1 to 2 tablespoons shoyu
scallion

Boil mushrooms and kombu in water for 2 to 3 minutes. Remove and slice into thin strips or pieces. Place them back in water, add rice, and bring to a boil. Lower flame and cook for 30 to 40 minutes. Add celery and simmer for 5 minutes. Add shoyu to taste and simmer for final 5 minutes, garnish with scallion, and serve.

Variation: You may also add miso for a wonderful, warming soup.

CORN SOUP

4 ears fresh corn
1 celery stalk, diced
2 onions, diced

5 to 6 cups spring water or
kombu stock
¼ teaspoon sea salt
shoyu to taste
chopped, parsley, watercress or
scallions and nori

Strip kernels from corn with knife. Place celery, onions, and corn in pot. Add water and pinch of salt. Bring to a boil, lower flame, cover, and simmer until celery and corn are soft. Add rest of salt and shoyu to taste if desired. Serve with chopped parsley, watercress, or scallions and nori.

KOMBU SEA VEGETABLE STOCK

Wipe kombu with a dried brush quickly to remove dust. Minerals are lost by wiping, so, if not dusty, place immediately in pot containing cold spring water. Boil 3 to 5 minutes. Remove kombu and use in other dishes or dry out and use as a condiment or side dish. Use stock for miso, grain, bean, or vegetable soups.

SHIITAKE MUSHROOM STOCK

Soak 5 to 6 shiitakes in water for 30 minutes. Add shiitake and its soaking water to 1 to 2 quarts of spring water and bring to a boil. Boil 5 to 10 minutes. Remove shiitake and save for the soup (in which case be sure to remove stems) or use in another recipe. Kombu may also be combined with shiitake to make a stock.

FRESH VEGETABLE STOCK

Save vegetable roots, stems, tops, and leaves for a nutritious soup stock. Boil in 1 to 2 quarts spring water for 5 to 10 minutes. Remove vegetable pieces and compost or discard.

VEGETABLES

Nishime Dish (Waterless Cooking)

Use a heavy pot with a heavy lid or cookware specifically designed for waterless cooking. Soak a 3-inch piece of kombu until soft and cut into 1-inch-square pieces. Place kombu in the bottom of the pot and cover with water (about 1 to 2 inches). Add sliced vegetables. For nishime preparations, vegetables are cut in large size. It is usually a combination of two or three such as carrot/burdock/kombu or burdock/lotus root/kombu. Onions, hard winter squash, or cabbage may also be used. The vegetables are layered in the pot after cutting, on top of the kombu, or placed in sections around the pot. Sprinkle a few pinches of sea salt or shoyu over the vegetables. Cover and set flame on high until a lot of steam is generated. Lower the flame and cook peacefully for 15 to 20 minutes. If the water should evaporate too quickly during cooking, add more water to the bottom of the pot. When each vegetable has become soft and edible, add a few drops of shoyu and gently shake the pot (rather than stirring). Remove cover, turn off flame, and let the vegetables sit for about 2 minutes. You may serve the vegetable juice along with the dish, as it is very delicious.

Nishime combination suggestions:

1. Carrot, burdock, and kombu
2. Burdock, lotus root, and kombu
3. Daikon, lotus root, and kombu
4. Carrot, parsnip, and kombu
5. Turnip, shiitake mushroom, and kombu
6. Squash, onion, and kombu

Sautéing

There are two basic ways of sautéing; with oil and with water. In the first, cut the vegetables into small pieces such as matchsticks, thin slices, or shaved slices. Lightly brush skillet with dark or light sesame oil. Heat oil, but before oil begins to smoke add vegetables and a pinch of sea salt to bring out their natural sweetness. Occasionally turn over or move vegetables with chopsticks or wooden spoon to ensure even cooking. However, do not stir. Sauté for 5 minutes on medium flame, followed by 10 minutes on low flame. Gently mix from time to time to avoid burning. Season to taste with sea salt or shoyu and cook 2 to 3 minutes longer.

The second method combines water and oil. Vegetables may be prepared either in small pieces or in large, thick pieces. Sauté as above in lightly oiled skillet for about 5 minutes. Then add enough cold water to cover the vegetables halfway or just enough to cover the surface of the skillet. Add a pinch of sea salt, cover, and cook until almost tender. When 80 percent done, season with sea salt or shoyu and cook 3 to 4 minutes more. Remove cover and simmer until water evaporates.

Note: Sautéing with oil is not recommended for many cancer patients or others who need to avoid or reduce oil. However, for those in good health, sautéed vegetables may be prepared daily. For those who cannot use oil, use 1 to 2 tablespoons of water instead. Leftover bean juice—the liquid remaining after cooking beans—may also be used to sauté in from time to time and is very delicious.

Variation: Delicious combinations include burdock and carrots; onion and carrots; cabbage, onion, and carrots; parsnips and onions; mushrooms and celery; broccoli and cauliflower; Chinese cabbage, mushrooms and tofu; and kale and seitan. Soft vegetables take only 1 to 2 minutes to sauté, while cooking time for root vegetables will be longer. Other unrefined vegetable oils may be used in this way. However, only sesame and corn oil are recommended for regular use.

Boiling

Place about ½ to 1 inch of cold spring water in pot; add a pinch of sea salt. Bring to a boil and add vegetables. Vegetables should be tender but crisp.

Note: In order to keep a green color, cook watercress, parsley, scallions, and other green leafy vegetables at a high flame for only 1 to 2 minutes. In order to preserve the taste, it is also better not to add salt after boiling. Shoyu may be added at end of cooking for flavor.

Variation: For an especially sweet taste, place a 3-inch piece of kombu on bottom of pot when cooking round vegetables such as carrots or daikon. Vegetables may be seasoned with shoyu or miso instead of salt. Tasty combinations of boiled vegetables include broccoli and cauliflower; cabbage, corn, and tofu; and carrots, onions, and green peas.

Steaming

Place ½ inch of spring water in pot. Insert a vegetable steamer inside pot or a wooden Japanese steamer on top of pot. Place sliced vegetables in steamer and sprinkle with a pinch of sea salt. Cover and bring water to boil. Steam until tender but slightly crisp. Greens will take only 1 to 2 minutes, other vegetables 5 to 7 minutes depending on type, size, and thickness.

Note: Lightly steamed greens can be eaten every day. These include leafy tops of turnip, daikon, and carrot; watercress; kale; mustard greens; Chinese cabbage; and parsley.

Variation: If you don't have a steamer, place ½ inch of water in bottom of pot. Add vegetables and pinch of sea salt. Bring to a boil, lower flame to medium, and steam until tender. Save vegetable water for soup stock or sauces.

Other Cooking Styles

Vegetables may be prepared in a variety of other styles, including baking, broiling, and tempuraing (deep-frying). However, these are not generally recommended for cancer patients.

ADUKI, KOMBU, AND SQUASH

1 cup aduki beans
2 3-inch strips of kombu

1 hard winter squash
spring water
sea salt

Wash and soak aduki beans with kombu. Remove kombu after soaking and chop into 1-inch-square pieces. Place kombu at bottom of pot and add chopped hard winter squash such as acorn, butternut, or hokaido. Add adukis on top of squash. Cover with water and cook over a low flame until beans and squash are soft. Sprinkle lightly with sea salt. Cover and let cook for 10 to 15 minutes. Turn off flame and let sit for several minutes before serving.

Note: This dish is helpful in regulating blood sugar levels, especially in those who are hypoglycemic or diabetic or have pancreatic or liver disorders. It is naturally sweet and delicious and will reduce the craving for sweets. May be prepared 1 to 2 times per week.

Variation: You may cook aduki beans 50 to 70 percent, then add on top of squash, and proceed as above.

DRIED DAIKON WITH KOMBU AND SHOYU

2 6-inch strips of kombu
½ cup dried daikon (long white radish)

shoyu to taste

Soak kombu and slice lengthwise into ¼-inch strips and place in bottom of heavy pot with a heavy lid. Soak daikon until soft. If daikon is very dark in color wash first. Place daikon on top of kombu in pot. Add enough kombu and daikon soaking water and spring water if needed to just cover top of daikon. Cover pot, bring to boil, lower flame, add shoyu, and simmer 30 to 40 minutes until kombu is tender. Cook away excess liquid.

Note: This dish helps to dissolve fat deposits throughout the body.

Variation: Fresh daikon has more power than dried. Slice fresh daikon and cook as above until very tender. If daikon is unavailable, red radish may be used, though the effect is not so strong.

DAIKON AND DAIKON LEAVES

Finely chop 1 daikon radish and the daikon leaves. Place in a pot with a small volume of spring water. Cover and cook with a high steam for about 10 minutes. Toward the end of cooking, add a small pinch of sea salt or few drops of shoyu and simmer for 2 to 4 minutes.

Note: You may lightly cook the root part first and the leafy part later on.

Variation: Carrots and carrot tops, turnips and turnip greens, or dandelion roots and dandelion leaves may be cooked in the same way.

STEAMED GREENS DISH

Wash and slice any of the following vegetables: turnip greens, daikon greens, carrot tops, kale, mustard greens, watercress, collard greens, Chinese cabbage, bok choy. Place the vegetables in a small amount of water, about ½ inch, or in a stainless steel steamer over 1 inch of boiling water. Cover and steam for 2 to 3 minutes, depending on the texture of the vegetables. At the end of cooking, lightly sprinkle shoyu over the vegetables. Transfer quickly into a serving dish. When served, the greens should still be fresh and bright.

SAUTÉED VEGETABLES

Cut carrots, onions, cabbage (finely cut), or other vegetables, including leafy green vegetables. Brush the bottom of the pan with dark sesame oil or use just a small amount of water. When oil or water is hot, sauté the vegetables quickly for a few minutes. Sprinkle with a pinch of sea salt or shoyu and add a little water if necessary. Simmer for a few more minutes. The vegetables should be crispy and colorful but cooked. Stirring is not necessary; just gently move from time to time with cooking chopsticks or a wooden paddle.

KINPIRA

Lightly brush sesame oil in a skillet and heat up. Place equal amounts of burdock and carrots (cut into matchsticks or shaves) into a skillet and add a pinch of sea salt. Sauté for 2 to 3 minutes. Add spring water to lightly cover the bottom of the skillet. Cover and cook until the vegetables are 80 percent done; it should take about 30 minutes or more. Add several drops of shoyu, cover, and cook for several minutes until all remaining water has cooked down. At the very end of cooking, add a few drops of ginger juice (squeezed from grated ginger).

Note: Onions, turnips, or lotus root can be substituted or used together with carrots and burdock.

DRIED TOFU, TOFU, OR TEMPEH WITH VEGETABLES (Stew)

Soak a 4-inch piece of kombu in 3 cups of water. Bring to a boil and cook for 3 to 5 minutes. Add either one of the following: soaked and sliced dried tofu or tempeh cubes along with sliced daikon, burdock, carrots, or lotus root, to the boiling water and cook for about 15 minutes. Add a pinch of sea salt or a dash of shoyu. Add a combination (2 or 3) of the following vegetables: onions, cabbage, Chinese cabbage, squash, Brussels sprouts, and cook for 3 to 5 minutes. If you use fresh tofu, add it with the lighter green vegetables toward the end of cooking. Chop finely 2 or 3 scallions and cook in for 1 minute and serve.

Note: All vegetables should be boiled and cooked until soft, but the leafy greens should still be fresh. A small amount of ginger may be added at the very end of cooking. A mild seasoning of miso may be added at the end of cooking instead of shoyu.

Variation: Cooked seitan may be used instead of tofu or tempeh. If so, you may not need to add any additional salt or shoyu, as seitan is usually salty.

BOILED SALAD

spring water

sea salt

1 cup sliced Chinese cabbage

½ cup sliced onion

½ cup thinly sliced carrots

½ cup sliced celery

1 bunch watercress

When making a boiled salad, boil each vegetable separately. All vegetables, however, may be boiled in the same water. Cook the mildest-tasting vegetables first, so that each will retain its distinctive flavor. Place 1 inch of water and a pinch of sea salt in a pot and bring to a boil. Drop Chinese cabbage slices into water and boil 1 to 2 minutes. All vegetables should be slightly crisp, but not raw. To remove vegetables from water, pour into a strainer that has been placed inside a bowl so as to retain the cooking water. Put the drained-off water back into the pot and reboil. Next boil the sliced onion. Drain as above, retaining water and returning to boil. Next boil sliced carrots followed by sliced celery. Last, drop watercress into boiling water for just a few seconds. In order for vegetables to keep their bright color, each vegetable should be allowed to cool off. Sometimes you can run under cold water while in the strainer, but it is not ideal. Mix vegetables together after boiling. A dressing of 1 umeboshi plum or 1 teaspoon of umeboshi paste may be added to ½ cup of water (vegetable stock from boiling may be used) and puréed in a bowl or *suribachi* for seasoning.

Note: A refreshing way to prepare vegetables in place of raw salad. Especially recommended for cancer patients who cannot have uncooked foods. This method just takes out the raw taste and preserves the crispy freshness.

PRESSED SALAD

Wash and slice desired vegetables into very thin pieces, such as ½ cabbage (may be shredded), 1 cucumber, 1 stalk celery, 2 red radishes, 1 onion. Place vegetables in a pickle press or large bowl and sprinkle with ½ teaspoon sea salt and mix. Apply pressure to the press. If you use a bowl in place of the press, place a small plate on top of the vegetables and place a stone or weight on top of the plate. Leave it for at least 30 to 45 minutes. You may leave it up to 3 to 4 days, but the longer you press the vegetables the more they resemble light pickles.

Note: This is a method to remove excess liquid from raw vegetables. For cancer patients, a boiled salad is preferable.

Variation: A press is not necessary when using soft vegetables. Just mix with salt and serve after 30 minutes.

RAW SALAD

A variety of vegetables may be used in this preparation rather than just lettuce. These include cabbage, grated carrots, radishes, cucumbers, celery, and watercress.

SALAD DRESSING SUGGESTIONS

Use homemade rather than store-bought dressings, which are usually high in oil, as well as herbs and spices.

1. 1 umeboshi plum or 1 teaspoon of umeboshi paste may be added to ½ cup spring water and puréed in a suribachi.

2. Dilute a few teaspoons of miso in warm water and heat up for several minutes. Add a few drops of rice vinegar.

3. Use condiments such as gomashio or shiso leaf powder.

4. Sprinkle on a few drops of umeboshi vinegar.

5. Add a few drops of shoyu and lemon juice.

PRESSED SALT PICKLES

2 large daikon and their leaves
¼ to ½ cup sea salt

Wash daikon and their leaves with enough cold water 2 to 3 times, making sure all dirt is removed, especially from the leaves. Set aside and let dry for about 24 hours. Slice the daikon into small rounds. Sprinkle sea salt on the bottom of heavy ceramic or wooden crock or keg. Next layer some of the daikon leaves, followed by a layer of daikon rounds. Then sprinkle with sea salt again. Repeat this until the daikon is used or the crock is filled. Place a lid or plate that will fit inside the crock on top of the daikon, daikon leaves, and salt. Place a heavy rock or brick on top of the lid or plate. Cover with a thin layer of cheesecloth to keep out dust. Soon water will begin to be squeezed out and rise to the surface of the plate. When this happens, replace heavy weight with a lighter one. Store in a dark, cool place for 1 to 2 weeks or longer. If water is not entirely squeezed out, add more salt. And make sure water is always covered or it will spoil. When ready, remove a portion, wash under cold water, slice, and serve.

Note: Pickles are a naturally fermented food and aid in digestion. A small volume may be eaten daily. However, commercial pickles such as dill pickles that have been made with vinegar and spices should be strictly avoided.

Variation: Pickles may also be made from Chinese cabbage, carrots, cauliflower, and other vegetables in this manner.

SHOYU PICKLES

Mix equal parts spring water and shoyu in a bowl or glass jar. Slice vegetables such as turnips or rutabaga and place in this liquid. Soak for 4 hours to 2 weeks, depending on the strength desired.

RICE BRAN PICKLES (NUKA)

Long Time (Ready in 3 to 5 Months)	Short Time (Ready in 1 to 2 Weeks)
10 to 12 cups nuka (rice bran) or wheat bran	10 to 12 cups nuka
1½ to 2 cups sea salt	⅛ to ¼ cup sea salt
3 to 5 cups spring water	3 to 5 cups spring water

Roast nuka or wheat bran in a dry skillet until it gives off a nutty aroma. Allow to cool. Combine roasted nuka or wheat bran with salt and mix well. Place a layer of bran mixture on the bottom of a wooden keg or ceramic crock. A single vegetable such as daikon, turnips, rutabaga, onion, or Chinese cabbage may be used. Slice vegetables into 2- to 3-inch pieces and layer on top of the nuka. If more than one type of vegetable is used, layer one on top of another. Then sprinkle a layer of nuka on top of the vegetables. Repeat this layering until the nuka mixture is used up or the crock is filled. Always make sure that the nuka mixture is the top layer. Place a wooden disk or plate to fit inside the crock, on top of the vegetables and nuka. Place a heavy weight, such as a rock or brick, on top of the plate. Soon water will begin to be squeezed out and rise to the surface of the plate. When this happens, replace heavy weight with a lighter one. Cover with a thin layer of cheesecloth and store in a cool room. To serve, take out pickled vegetables as needed and rinse under cold water to remove excess bran and salt. The same nuka paste may be used for several years. Just keep adding vegetables and a little more bran and salt.

BEANS AND BEAN PRODUCTS

ADUKI BEANS

1 cup aduki beans
2½ cups spring water per cup of beans

¼ teaspoon sea salt per cup of beans

Wash beans and place in pressure cooker. Add water, cover, and bring to pressure. Reduce flame to medium-low and cook 45 minutes. Remove pressure cooker from burner and rinse cold water over it to bring pressure down quickly. Open; add salt; cook uncovered until liquid evaporates.

Note: Most other types of beans can be pressure-cooked in this way. Chickpeas and yellow soybeans should first be soaked. Black soybeans should not be pressure-cooked because they clog up the gauge.

Variation: Beans may also be boiled by putting in a pot, adding 3½ to 4 cups of water per cup of beans, and cooking for about 1 hour and 45 minutes. When 80 percent cooked, add salt and cook for another 15 to 20 minutes until liquid is evaporated. To reduce cooking time, add flavor, and make beans more digestible, lay a 3-inch piece of kombu under beans at the beginning. A small volume of vegetables may also be cooked along with beans, such as chopped squash, onions, or carrots.

LENTILS

1 cup lentils
2½ cups spring water

¼ teaspoon sea salt

Wash lentils and place in pot. Add water, cover, and bring to a boil. Reduce flame to medium-low. After 30 minutes, add salt and cook another 15 to 20 minutes. Remove cover and allow liquid to cook off.

Variation: Chopped onions and celery go well with lentils and may be cooked together.

CHICKPEAS

1 cup chickpeas
3 cups spring water

½ teaspoon sea salt

Wash beans and soak overnight. Place beans and soaking water in pressure cooker. Add more water if necessary. Bring to pressure, turn down flame to medium-low, and cook 1 to 1½ hours. Take off burner and allow pressure to come down. Remove lid, add salt, and return to burner. Cook uncovered for another 45 to 60 minutes.

Variation: Diced onion and carrots may be added to beans during last hour of cooking.

COLORFUL SOYBEAN CASSEROLE

2 cups yellow soybeans
2 3-inch pieces kombu
1 shiitake mushroom
5 large pieces dried lotus root
6 dried tofu

1 carrot, sliced
1 burdock, sliced
1 stalk of celery, sliced
1 dried daikon, shredded
soaking water
1½ tablespoons shoyu
1 teaspoon kuzu

Soak soybeans overnight in 2½ cups of cold water per cup of soybeans. Next day, place beans and soaking water in pressure cooker and bring to pressure. Soak kombu, shiitake, lotus root, and dried tofu for 10 minutes. After beans have cooked 70 to 80 percent (approximately 15 minutes) reduce pressure, open, and layer kombu, shiitake, lotus root, and dried tofu on top. Bring back to pressure and cook 10 more minutes. Reduce pressure, open, skim off hulls from beans, and take out vegetables and put on separate plates. Meanwhile, cut up carrot, burdock, celery, and dried daikon. Slice up cooked kombu and put in bottom of a large saucepan in a little water. On top of kombu add soft vegetables such as celery, shiitake, daikon, and tofu; then root vegetables including carrots, burdock, and lotus root; and finally soybeans and any original water remaining in pressure cooker. Add 1½ tablespoons shoyu; cover; cook 30 minutes. Add 1 teaspoon of kuzu to make creamy and a little grated ginger for flavoring. Soybeans should be very tender and sweet.

Note: This dish is extremely nourishing and highly recommended for cancer patients. However, those with yin cancer should be careful not to use more than one shiitake mushroom. Those with a yang cancer or healthy persons may use 5 to 6 shiitakes.

Variation: Depending on availability, some vegetables may be omitted or added. Also, seitan makes this dish especially delicious.

BLACK SOYBEANS

2 cups black soybeans
1 teaspoon sea salt

spring water
shoyu

Wash beans quickly and soak overnight in cold water, adding ¼ to ½ teaspoon sea salt per cup of beans. The salt will prevent the skins from peeling. In the morning, place beans and soaking water in pot. If necessary, add additional water to cover surface of beans. Bring to a boil, reduce heat, and simmer uncovered. When a dark foam rises to the surface, skim and discard. Continue in this way until no more foam rises. Cover beans and cook for 2½ to 3 hours.

Add water to cover surface of beans if necessary. Toward end of cooking, uncover and add a little shoyu to give the skins a shiny, black color. Cook away excess liquid. Shake pot up and down to coat beans with remaining juice, and serve.

Note: This dish is particularly beneficial for the sexual organs and to relieve an overly yang condition caused by excess meat or fish. Avoid pressure-cooking black beans, since they may clog the valve.

MISO

Miso (fermented soybean paste) is highly recommended for daily use. There are now many types of miso available. For daily miso soup, we recommend using traditionally made organic or natural miso that has fermented 2 to 3 years. Barley miso, brown rice miso, or hatcho miso (all soybean) may be used. Short-time misos, including red miso and white and yellow misos, may be used occasionally for sauces, dressings, and special dishes. Instant miso is suitable for traveling, but not for daily home use. As a rule of thumb, about ¼ to ½ teaspoon of miso is used per cup of soup. Also, because miso contains beneficial enzymes that can be destroyed by too high a heat, it is usually recommended not to boil the soup but, after adding the miso, to let it simmer for 3 to 4 minutes over a low flame.

TOFU

Tofu is soybean curd made from cooked soybeans and nigari (crystallized salt). It is high in protein and is used in soups, vegetable dishes, dressings, and other dishes. It can be made at home (see *Aveline Kushi's Complete Guide to Macrobiotic Cooking* for recipe) or purchased inexpensively at the natural foods store. Obtain an organic-quality tofu if available. Firm usually holds up better than silken in most dishes.

TEMPEH

Tempeh is a traditional fermented soyfood originating in Indonesia. In the last decade it has become increasingly popular in the Far East and West and is now available in many natural foods stores. Tempeh is crisp, delicious, and nourishing and may be steamed, boiled, baked, or sautéed. It is enjoyed with a wide variety of grains, vegetables, and noodles and may be used in soups, salads, or sandwiches. Tempeh should always be cooked before eating. Tempeh may also be made at home. A special culture is available in many natural foods stores or may be obtained through mail order.

CABBAGE-ROLL TEMPEH

2 strips kombu
several outer layers of cabbage

8 ounces tempeh
2 onions

Soak kombu one hour or more. Steam cabbage until soft. Cut the tempeh into 2-inch rectangles and steam or boil. Place on cabbage leaves and roll up. Slice soaked kombu and onions thinly. Layer kombu and onions on bottom of pot. Add water and cabbage rolls. Add sea salt to taste if desired. Cook until very soft.

Note: Avoid cooking with salt or shoyu when serving tempeh to children. Tempeh is very energizing and salt could make them overactive.

NATTO

Natto is a fermented soy product that aids digestion and strengthens the intestines. It looks like baked beans connected by long slippery strands and has a unique odor. Natto is available in macrobiotic specialty stores or can be made at home. Natto is usually eaten with a little shoyu, mixed with rice, or served on top of buckwheat noodles.

SEA VEGETABLES

WAKAME

2 cups soaked wakame
1 medium onion, sliced

soaking water
2 teaspoons shoyu

Rinse wakame quickly under cold water and soak 3 to 5 minutes. Slice into 1-inch pieces. Put onion in pot and wakame on top. Add soaking water to cover vegetables. Bring to boil, lower flame, and simmer for 30 minutes or until wakame is soft. Add shoyu to taste and simmer 10 to 15 more minutes.

Note: Wakame is the chief vegetable added to miso soup. It also makes a tasty side dish or can be used as an alternative in most recipes calling for kombu.

KOMBU

1 12-inch strip kombu
1 onion, halved, then quartered
1 carrot, cut in triangular pieces

spring water
1 tablespoon shoyu

Soak kombu 3 to 5 minutes, slice in half, and then slice diagonally into 1-inch pieces. Place in pot and add vegetables and enough soaking water to cover vegetables halfway. Add one tablespoon shoyu. Bring to a boil. Reduce the flame to low and simmer for 30 minutes. Add additional shoyu to taste if desired, and cook for 5 to 10 more minutes.

Note: Kombu is delicious as a side dish or can be used as a stock for soups.

Adding a 3-inch piece of kombu beneath beans will speed up cooking, add flavor, and make beans more digestible. When cooking with kombu, oil is usually not used.

HIJIKI AND ARAME

2 cups soaked hijiki or arame
spring water
1 medium onion, sliced

1 carrot, sliced in matchsticks
3 to 4 tablespoons shoyu

Wash hijiki quickly under cold water. Place in bowl, cover with water, and soak 5 to 10 minutes. Drain water and save. Slice hijiki in 1- to 2-inch pieces. Place hijiki on top of other vegetables in pot. Add enough soaking water to cover top of hijiki. Bring to a boil; cover; reduce flame to low. Add one tablespoon shoyu. Cook on low flame for 45 to 60 minutes. Season with additional shoyu to taste and simmer for 20 more minutes until liquid evaporates. Mix vegetables only at end and serve.

Note: Hijiki is thicker and coarser in texture than arame. Arame is milder, softer, has less of a briny taste, takes less time to cook, and is usually the sea vegetable preferred by those new to macrobiotic cooking.

Variation: Both hijiki and arame can be cooked with lotus root, daikon, and other vegetables; combined with grains or tofu; added to a salad; or put into a pie crust and baked as a roll. For those who can use oil, a strong, rich dish can be created by adding a little oil at the beginning of cooking.

NORI

Nori comes in thin sheets and can be used for wrapping rice balls (see recipe in grain section). It is also used to make vegetable sushi and makes an attractive garnish for soups, noodles, and salads. Toast lightly by holding nori, shiny side up, 10 to 12 inches from flame and rotating about 3 to 5 seconds until the nori changes from black to green.

DULSE

Dulse may be eaten dry as a snack or dry-roasted and ground into a powder in a *suribachi* to make a condiment. Dulse can also be used to season soups at the very end of cooking, salad, and main dishes.

AGAR-AGAR

This whitish sea vegetable forms into a gelatin when cooked and is used to make vegetable aspics and delicious fruit desserts. See recipe for kanten in dessert section.

SAUCES, DRESSINGS, AND SPREADS

KUZU SAUCE

1 tablespoon kuzu   *1½ cups vegetable stock or water*

Dilute kuzu (a white starch) in small volume of cold water and add to pot containing stock or water. Bring to a boil, lower flame, and simmer 10 to 15 minutes. Stir constantly. Add shoyu to taste. Serve over vegetables, tofu, noodles, grains, or beans.

Variation: Arrowroot powder may be used instead of kuzu. Avoid thickeners such as corn starch.

BECHAMEL SAUCE

1 medium onion, diced   *3 cups spring water or kombu stock*
1 teaspoon sesame oil   *or vegetable soup stock*
½ cup whole-wheat pastry flour or   *1 tablespoon shoyu*
brown rich flour

Sauté onion in lightly oiled skillet until transparent. Stir in flour and sauté 2 to 3 minutes until each piece of onion is coated. Gradually add water or stock and stir continually to prevent lumping. Bring to a boil, lower flame, and simmer 2 to 3 minutes. Add shoyu to taste and cook 10 to 12 minutes more until thick and brown. Serve over millet, buckwheat, or seitan.

Note: This savory sauce can be mucous-producing and should only be used occasionally by those in good health. Cancer patients should avoid it altogether.

UMEBOSHI DRESSING

2 umeboshi plums   *½ teaspoon sesame oil*
¼ to ½ teaspoon grated onion   *½ cup spring water*

Purée umeboshi and onion in *suribachi*. Add slightly heated oil and mix. Add water and mix to smooth consistency. Serve on salad.

Note: Cancer patients can make this dressing without oil by adding a little bit more water.

Variation: Umeboshi paste may be used instead of plums. Use 1 teaspoon of paste per plum. Also, chives and scallions may be substituted for onions and the mixture used as a dip for crackers or chips.

TOFU DRESSING

½ teaspoon puréed umeboshi plum   *8 ounces tofu*
¼ onion, grated or diced   *chopped scallions or parsley*
2 teaspoons spring water

Purée *umeboshi*, onion, and water in *suribachi*. Add tofu and purée until creamy. Add water to increase creaminess if desired. Garnish with scallions or parsley. Serve with salad.

TAHINI DRESSING

2 umeboshi plums   *2 tablespoons tahini*
½ small onion grated or diced   *½ to ¾ cup spring water*

Purée umeboshi, onion, and tahini in *suribachi*. Add water and purée until creamy. Serve with salad.
   Note: Tahini is high in oil and generally not recommended for cancer patients.

MISO-TAHINI SPREAD

6 tablespoons tahini   *1 tablespoon barley or rice miso*

Dry-roast tahini in a skillet over medium-low flame until golden brown. Stir constantly to prevent burning. In *suribachi* stir tahini with miso. Delicious with bread or crackers.
   Variation: Add chopped scallions.
   Note: This spread is high in oil and should be avoided by most cancer patients.

CONDIMENTS

SHOYU

   Shoyu refers to traditional, naturally made soy sauce as distinguished from the commercial, chemically processed soy sauce found in many Oriental restaurants and supermarkets. In natural foods stores there is now also available a wheatless soy sauce, known as genuine or real tamari. It is stronger in flavor. Shoyu, however, is recommended for regular use and should be used primarily in cooking and not added to rice or vegetables at the table.

GOMASHIO (Sesame Salt)

Dry-roast 1 part sea salt. Wash and dry-roast 16 to 18 parts sesame seeds. Add seeds to sea salt and grind in a *suribachi* until about two-thirds of the seeds are crushed. Used to season grains, noodles, vegetables, salad, or soup at the table. Use about 1 teaspoon per day.

ROASTED SEA VEGETABLE POWDER

Use either wakame, kombu, dulse, or kelp. Roast sea vegetable in oven until nearly charred (approximately 10 to 15 minutes at 350°F) and crush in a *suribachi*.

Note: For more yin cancer, this powder can be used more frequently in larger amounts (up to 1 teaspoon per day). For more yang cancer, slightly less volume is advisable (about ½ teaspoon per day). For cancers caused by a combination of both, an in-between volume is recommended.

UMEBOSHI PLUMS

Umeboshi are special plums (imported from Japan and now also grown in the United States) that have been dried and pickled with sea salt and aged from one to three years. They usually come with shiso (beefsteak) leaves, which contribute to their distinctive red color. Umeboshi may be eaten by themselves or used to enhance grains and vegetables. They may also be pureed for making a tart and tangy dressing, sauce, or tea. The umeboshi contains a harmonious balance of more yin factors, such as the natural sourness of the plum, and more yang factors created by the salt, pressure, and aging used in their preparation. Umeboshi are excellent for strengthening the intestines and may be used regularly by persons with all types of cancer. Some natural foods stores also sell umeboshi paste without the pits. The paste is not as strong or balanced, and cancer patients are advised to use the whole plums.

TEKKA (Root Vegetable Condiment)

⅓ cup finely minced burdock	½ teaspoon grated ginger
⅓ cup finely minced carrot	¼ cup sesame oil
⅓ cup finely minced lotus root	⅔ cup hatcho miso

Prepare vegetables, mincing as finely as possible. Heat oil in a skillet and sauté vegetables. Add miso. Reduce flame to low and cook 3 to 4 hours. Stir frequently until liquid evaporates and a dry, black mixture is left.

Note: Tekka is very strengthening for the blood but should be used sparingly because of its strong contractive nature. For many yin cancers, it can be used daily (about ½ teaspoon). For more yang cancer or cancer caused by a combination of yin and yang, use small volume only on occasion.

SHOYU-NORI CONDIMENT

Place dried nori or several sheets of fresh nori in ½ to 1 cup of spring water and simmer until most of the water cooks down to a thick paste. Add shoyu several minutes before end of cooking for a light to moderate taste.

Note: This special condiment helps the body recover its ability to discharge toxins. It may be eaten by persons with all types of cancer. For more yang cancer, use a slightly smaller volume (approximately ½ teaspoon per day). For more yin cancer, use up to 1 teaspoon daily. Those with cancers caused by a combination of both may eat an in-between volume.

SHIO-KOMBU CONDIMENT

1 cup sliced kombu   *½ cup shoyu*
½ cup spring water

Soak kombu until soft and chop into 1-inch-square pieces. Add sliced kombu to water and shoyu. Bring to a boil and simmer until the liquid evaporates. Cool off and place in a covered jar to keep for several days.

Note: This condiment is very high in minerals and aids in the discharge of toxins. Cancer patients may eat several pieces daily. If it is too salty, reduce the amount of shoyu.

SAUERKRAUT

A small amount of sauerkraut made from organic cabbage and sea salt may be used as a condiment occasionally.

VINEGAR

Brown rice vinegar, sweet brown rice vinegar, and umeboshi vinegar may be used moderately. Avoid red-wine or apple-cider vinegars.

GINGER

Fresh grated gingerroot may be used occasionally in a small volume as a garnish or flavoring in vegetable dishes, soups, pickled vegetables, and especially with fish or seafoods.

HORSERADISH

May be used occasionally by those in good health to aid digestion, especially for fish and seafood.

CARP AND BURDOCK SOUP (Koi Koku)

1 fresh carp
burdock in weight at least equal to
*   that of fish*
½ to 1 cup used bancha tea leaves and
*   twigs wrapped in cheesecloth sack*

miso to taste
1 tablespoon grated ginger
spring water and bancha (kukicha)
*   tea*
chopped scallions

Select a live carp and express your gratitude for taking its life. Ask fishseller to carefully remove gallbladder and yellow bitter bone (thyroid) and leave the rest of the fish intact. This includes all scales, bones, head, and fins. At home, chop entire fish into 1- to 2-inch slices. Remove eyes if you wish. Meanwhile, chop at least an equal amount of burdock (ideally 2 to 3 times the weight of fish) into thinly shaved slices or matchsticks. This quantity of burdock may take a while to prepare. When everything is chopped up, place burdock and fish in pressure cooker. Tie old bancha (kukicha) twig leaves and stems from your teapot in cheesecloth. It should be the size of a small ball. Place this ball in pressure-cooker on top or nestled inside fish. The tea twigs will help soften the bones while cooking. Add enough liquid to cover fish and burdock, approximately ⅓ bancha tea and ⅔ spring water. Pressure-cook 1 hour. Bring down pressure; take off lid; add miso to taste (½ to 1 teaspoon per cup of soup) and grated ginger. Simmer for 5 minutes. Garnish with chopped scallions and serve hot.

Note: This delicious, invigorating soup is excellent for restoring strength and vitality and opening the electromagnetic channel of energy in the body. It may be eaten occasionally by all cancer patients, even those who otherwise shouldn't eat animal products. It is also good for mothers who have just given birth or who are breast-feeding. In cold weather it is particularly warming. Be careful, however, to eat only a small volume (1 cup or less) at a time. Otherwise you will become too yang and be attracted to liquids, fruits, sweets, and other strong yin. Soup will keep for a week in the refrigerator or several months in the freezer where it can be taken out from time to time as needed.

Variation: For those whose oil isn't restricted, the burdock may be sautéed for a few minutes in sesame oil at the start, prior to cooking with the fish. Soup may also be made by boiling in lidded pot for 4 to 6 hours or until all bones are soft and dissolved. As liquid evaporates, more water or bancha tea should be added. If carp is unavailable, substitute another more yin fish such as perch, red snapper, or trout. If burdock is scarce, use carrots instead, or use half burdock and half carrots.

DESSERTS AND SNACKS

COOKED APPLES

Wash apples and peel, unless organically grown, in which case skins may be eaten. Slice and place in a pot with a small amount of water to keep from burning (about ¼ to ½ cup). Add pinch of sea salt and simmer for 10 minutes, or until soft.

Note: Those with yin cancer should avoid desserts completely. Those with yang cancer may have a small volume of cooked fruit on occasion if craved.

Variation: Purée in a Foley food mill to make applesauce. Other fruits may be cooked in this way.

ROASTED SEEDS

Dry-roast sesame, sunflower, pumpkin, or squash seeds by placing several cups of seeds in a skillet. Turn on flame to medium-low and gently stir with wooden roasting paddle or spoon for 10 to 15 minutes. When done, seeds should be darker in color, crisp, and give off a fragrant aroma. Seeds may be lightly seasoned with shoyu while roasting.

Note: Cancer patients may occasionally have roasted seeds in small volume.

KANTEN (Gelatin)

3 apples, sliced	*pinch of sea salt*
2 cups spring water	*agar-agar flakes*
2 cups apple juice	

Wash and slice fruit and place in pot with liquid and salt. Add agar-agar flakes in amount according to directions on package (varies from several teaspoons to several tablespoons). Stir well and bring to boil. Reduce flame to low and simmer 2 to 3 minutes. Place in shallow dish or mold and put in refrigerator to harden.

Note: This delicious natural gelatin is not recommended for some cancer patients because of the high fruit and fruit juice content.

Variation: Kanten may also be made with other temperate-climate fruits, including strawberries, blueberries, peaches, or melon. Nuts and raisins may be added to the fruit. Vegetable aspics may be made in this same way with vegetable soup stock instead of fruit juice and vegetable pieces instead of fruit. Aduki beans and raisins are a delicious combination.

AMASAKE (Sweet Rice Beverage)

4 cups sweet brown rice

8 cups spring water
½ cup koji

Wash rice, drain, and soak in 8 cups of water overnight. Place rice in pressure cooker and bring to pressure. Reduce flame and cook for 45 minutes. Turn off heat and allow to sit in pressure cooker for 45 minutes. When cool enough, mix koji into rice by hand and allow to ferment 4 to 8 hours. During fermentation, place mixture in a glass bowl, cover with wet cloth or towel, and place near oven, radiator, or other warm place. During fermentation period, stir the mixture occasionally to melt the koji. After fermenting, place ingredients in a pot and bring to boil. When bubbles appear, turn off flame. Allow to cool. Refrigerate in a glass bowl or jar.

Note: Amasake may be served hot or cold as a nourishing beverage or used as a natural sweetener for making cookies, cakes, pies, or other desserts. As a beverage, first blend the amasake and place in a saucepan with a pinch of sea salt and spring water in volume to desired consistency. Bring to a boil and serve hot or allow to cool off.

Note: Cancer patients may have amasake occasionally as a beverage, especially to satisfy craving for a sweet taste.

RICE PUDDING

½ cup almonds
3 to 4 tablespoons tahini
¾ cup spring water
3½ cups cooked brown rice

1½ cups apple juice
¼ teaspoon sea salt
⅓ to ½ cup spring water

Boil almonds and tahini in ¾ cup water and purée in a blender. Place mixture and other ingredients in pressure cooker and cook for 45 minutes. After pressure has come down, take out and place mixture in a baking dish or covered casserole, and bake at 350°F for 45 to 60 minutes.

Note: A tasty dessert for those in good health but best avoided by cancer patients.

SWEET VEGETABLE JAM

Cut finely a large equal volume of onions, cabbage, carrots, and hard winter squash such as butternut or buttercup. Place the cut vegetables into a large pot and add 1½ times water. Bring to a boil, then reduce the flame to low, and cook for 4 to 5 hours or until the vegetables cook down into a jam. Add a pinch of sea salt and cook another 20 minutes. Remove sweet vegetable jam and put into a jar. For storage, this jar may be refrigerated for about a week. Sweet vegetable jam can be used as a spread to satisfy sweet cravings. It may be used, for example, on rice cakes or on steamed sourdough bread.

HOMEMADE TAHINI

Roast black sesame seeds in a dry skillet. In a *suribachi* grind them with a little salt until about half-crushed. Use as a spread on rice cakes or steamed sourdough bread.

WAKAME SNACK

Take a small piece (2 to 3 inches) of wakame and chew it raw. It is a little salty, so don't use every day, but occasionally or for several days in a row.

KUZU WITH BARLEY MALT

For a sweet taste, mix a teaspoon of kuzu in cold water, heat in a pan with 1 cup spring water, stir until dissolved, about 5 minutes, and then add a few drops of barley malt and simmer for another minute.

BEVERAGES

BANCHA TWIG TEA (Kukicha)

Bancha twig tea is the usual daily beverage in most macrobiotic households. The organic or natural quality bancha twig tea in the natural foods store has usually been dry-roasted. To make tea, add 2 tablespoons of roasted twigs to 1½ quarts of spring water and bring to a boil. Lower flame and simmer for several minutes. Place tea strainer in cup and pour out tea. Twigs in strainer may be returned to teapot and used several times, adding a few fresh twigs each time.

BROWN RICE TEA

Dry-roast uncooked brown rice over medium flame for 10 minutes or until a fragrant aroma develops. Stir and shake pan occasionally to prevent burning. Add 2 to 3 tablespoons of roasted rice to 1½ quarts of spring water. Bring to a boil, reduce flame, and simmer 10 to 15 minutes.

Variation: Teas may be made from other whole grains in this way.

ROASTED BARLEY TEA

Prepare same way as roasted brown rice tea above. This tea is especially good for melting animal fat from the body. Roasted barley tea also makes a very nice summer drink and may also aid in the reduction of fever.

MU TEA

Mu tea is a medicinal tea made with a variety of herbs, including ginseng. Mu #9 is excellent for strengthening the female sex organs and for stomach troubles and may also be used therapeutically by men. *Mu* tea is sold prepackaged in most natural foods stores. Stir package in 1 quart of water and simmer for 10 minutes. Except for medicinal purposes, macrobiotic cooking does not recommend ginseng, which is extremely yang, and fragrant and aromatic herbs, which are too yin, for ordinary daily consumption.

SWEET VEGETABLE DRINK

Chop finely: ¼ cup onions, ¼ cup carrots, ⅓ cup cabbage, and ¼ cup sweet winter squash such as butternut or buttercup. Add to 4 cups boiling water and allow to boil for 2 to 3 minutes. Reduce flame to low, cover, and let simmer for 20 minutes. Strain out vegetables and drink the broth hot, warm, or at room temperature. (The vegetables may be saved and used in soups and stews.)

Note: No seasoning is used in this recipe. Sweet vegetable broth may be kept in the refrigerator, but warm it up again before drinking or let it come back to room temperature.

33

Menus

The following weekly menu is a sample of the kinds of meals that might be prepared by an individual or family in relatively good health. It is set for the end of the summer and early autumn, so seasonal adjustments would be recommended for other times of the year.

Breakfast	Lunch	Dinner
	SUNDAY	
Miso Soup	Udon and Broth	Pressure-cooked Brown
Soft Brown Rice with	Steamed Brussels	Rice
Kombu and Shiitake	Sprouts	Colorful Soybean
Mushroom	Garden Salad	Casserole
Bancha Tea	Bancha Tea	Steamed Mustard
		Greens
		Hijiki with Onion
		Cooked Peaches
		Bancha Tea
	MONDAY	
Miso Soup	Seitan Stew	Pressure-cooked Brown
Soft Barley with	Boiled Peas and	Rice with Millet
Shiitake	Mushrooms	Aduki Beans with
Mushroom	Grain Coffee	Kombu and Winter
Bancha Tea		Squash
		Corn Soup
		Arame with Carrots,
		Burdock, and Onions
		Bancha Tea

TUESDAY

Miso Soup with Millet
Whole Oatmeal
Bancha Tea

Corn on the Cob with
   Umeboshi Paste
Pressed Salad
Arame
Bancha Tea

Pressure-cooked Brown
   Rice with Barley
Lentil Soup
Boiled Kale, Broccoli
   and Carrots
Watermelon
Bancha Tea

WEDNESDAY

Soft Brown Rice with
   Winter Squash
Rice Kayu Bread
Bancha Tea

Fried Rice with Scal-
   lions and Chinese
   Cabbage
Navy Beans with
   Kombu
Bancha Tea

Pressure-cooked Brown
   Rice
Whole Wheat Lasagna
   with Tofu Filling
Boiled String Beans
   and Onions
Steamed Watercress
Bancha Tea

THURSDAY

Miso with Daikon and
   Wakame
Soft Millet
Bancha Tea

Whole Oats with Bar-
   ley and Chickpeas
Steamed Kale
Fresh Cantaloupe
Grain Coffee

Pressure-cooked Brown
   Rice with Aduki
   Beans
Squash Soup
Boiled Mustard Greens
Cabbage Roll Tempeh
Arame with Dried
   Daikon
Bancha Tea

FRIDAY

Barley Miso Soup
Steamed Rye Bread
Bancha Tea

Fried Soba
Boiled Celery
Natto
Bancha Tea

Steamed Scrod with
   Ginger Sauce
Pressure-cooked Brown
   Rice
Boiled Carrots and
   Onions
Steamed Parsley
Blueberry Pie
Roasted Barley Tea

SATURDAY

Shoyu Broth
Whole Oatmeal
Bancha Tea

Rice Ball with Nori
Boiled Salad
Bancha Tea

Pressure-cooked Brown
   Rice with Rye
Millet Soup with Sweet
   Vegetables
Kidney Beans with
   Kombu
Steamed Cabbage
Bancha Tea

MENU FOR CANCER PATIENTS

The following is an example of a weekly meal plan for someone with cancer. It does not include pickles, condiments, and special drinks and side dishes, which should also be prepared. It does not include oil, which may be used in some cases or which may be used after the first month in others. Also the use of whole oats, seitan, soba, fruit, and desserts may be limited in some cases. These foods are indicated with an asterisk (*). Please check the dietary recommendations for each particular illness and make adjustments before implementing this general meal plan.

Breakfast	*Lunch*	*Dinner*
	SUNDAY	
Miso Soup	Udon Noodles	Pressure-cooked Brown
Mochi	Millet Soup with Sweet	Rice
Steamed Kale	Vegetables	Aduki-Squash-Kombu
Bancha Tea	Boiled Salad	Carrots and Carrot
	Brown Rice Tea	Tops
		Kinpira
		Pressed Salad
		Bancha Tea
	MONDAY	
Miso Soup	Corn on the Cob	Pressure-cooked Brown
Soft Rice	*Seitan Stew	Rice with Millet
Dried Daikon with	Arame	Lentil Soup
Kombu	Boiled Salad	Nishime-Style Vegeta-
Bancha Tea	Bancha Tea	bles with Tempeh
		Steamed Watercress
		*Amasake Pudding
		Bancha Tea
	TUESDAY	
Miso Soup	Rice Balls with Nori	Pressure-cooked Brown
Soft Rice with Millet	Tofu with Water-	Rice with Barley
*Steamed Rice	sautéed Vegetables	Shoyu Broth
Kayu Bread	Daikon and Daikon	Aduki-Squash-Kombu
Bancha Tea	Tops	Steamed Collard
	Barley Tea	Greens
		Pressed Salad
		Bancha Tea
	WEDNESDAY	
Miso Soup	*Soba Noodles	Pressure-cooked Brown
Soft Rice with Barley	Millet Soup with Sweet	Rice with Chickpeas
Dried Daikon with	Vegetables	Nishime-Style
Kombu	Kinpira	Vegetables
Bancha Tea	Bancha Tea	Steamed Bok Choy
		Pressed Salad
		* Apple Kanten
		Bancha Tea

THURSDAY

Miso Soup
Soft Rice with
  Chickpeas
Bancha Tea

Corn on the Cob
Leftover Rice
Hijiki
Steamed Broccoli and
  Cauliflower
Bancha Tea

Pressure-cooked Brown
  Rice
Shoyu Broth
Aduki-Squash-Kombu
Boiled Salad
Bancha Tea

FRIDAY

Miso Soup
Soft Rice
Steamed Chinese
  Cabbage
Hato Mugi (Pearl Bar-
  ley) Tea

Rice Ball with Nori
Corn Chowder
Nishime-Style
  Vegetables
Bancha Tea

Pressure-cooked Brown
  Rice with Millet
Colorful Soybean
  Casserole
Carrots and Carrot
  Tops
Pressed Salad
Bancha Tea

SATURDAY

Miso Soup
*Whole Oatmeal
*Steamed Sourdough
  Bread
Steamed Kale
Bancha Tea

Whole Rye
Dried Tofu with
  Vegetables
Pressed Salad
Bancha Tea

Pressure-cooked Brown
  Rice with Barley
Aduki Bean Soup
Water-sautéed
  Vegetables
Boiled Salad
Bancha Tea

34

Kitchen Utensils

Pressure Cooker

A pressure cooker is an essential item in preparing the Cancer Prevention Diet, especially in preparing brown rice and other whole grains. Stainless steel is recommended.

Cooking Pots

Stainless steel and cast iron are recommended, although Pyrex, stoneware, or unchipped enamelware may also be used. Avoid aluminum or Teflon-coated pans.

Metal Flame Deflectors

These are especially helpful when cooking rice and other grains as they help distribute heat more evenly and prevent burning. Avoid asbestos pads.

Suribachi (Grinding Bowl)

A *suribachi* is a ceramic bowl with grooves set into its surface. It is used with a wooden pestle and is needed in preparing condiments, puréed foods, salad dressings, and other items. A six-inch size is generally fine for regular use.

Flat Grater

A small enamel or steel hand-style grater that will grate finely is recommended.

Pickle Press

Several pickle presses or heavy crocks with a plate and weight should be available for regular use in the preparation of pickles and pressed salads.

Steamer Basket

The small stainless steel steamers are suitable. Bamboo steamers are also fine for regular use.

Wire Mesh Strainer

A large strainer is useful for washing grains, beans, sea vegetables, and some other vegetables and draining noodles. A small, fine mesh strainer is good for washing smaller items such as millet or sesame seeds.

Vegetable Knife

A sharp, high-quality Oriental knife with a wide rectangular blade allows for the more even, attractive, and quick cutting of vegetables. Stainless steel and carbon steel varieties are recommended.

Cutting Board

It is important to cut vegetables on a clean, flat surface. Wooden cutting boards are ideal for this purpose. They should be wiped clean after each use. A separate board should be used for the preparation of dishes containing animal foods.

Foley Hand Food Mill

This utensil is useful for puréeing, especially when preparing baby foods or dishes requiring a creamy texture.

Glass Jars

Large glass jars are useful for storing grains, seeds, nuts, beans, or dried foods. Wood or ceramic containers, which allow air to circulate, are better but may be difficult to locate.

Shoyu Dispenser

This small glass bottle with a spout is very helpful in controlling the quantity of shoyu used in cooking.

Tea Strainer

Small, inexpensive bamboo strainers are ideal, but small mesh strainers may also be used.

Vegetable Brush

A natural-bristle vegetable brush is recommended for cleaning vegetables.

Utensils

Wooden utensils such as spoons, rice paddles, and cooking chopsticks are recommended since they will not scratch pots and pans or leave a metallic taste in your foods.

Bamboo Mats

Small bamboo mats may be used in covering food. They are designed to allow heat to escape and air to enter so that food does not spoil quickly if unrefrigerated.

Electrical Appliances

Avoid all electrical appliances as far as possible when preparing foods or cooking. Electricity produces a chaotic vibration that is transmitted to the energy of the food. Instead of toasting bread, steam or bake it. Instead of using an electric blender, use a *suribachi* to purée sauces and dressings. Occasionally, however, an automatic blender may be used to grind the soybeans for making tofu or when cooking for a party or large numbers of people. Use common sense.

35

Home Remedies and Cares

The following home remedies are based on traditional macrobiotic Oriental medicine and folk medicine, modified and adjusted for more practical use in modern society. Similar remedies have been used for thousands of years to help alleviate various imbalances caused by faulty diet or unhealthy lifestyle activities. They should be followed only after complete understanding of their uses. If there is any doubt as to whether these remedies should be used, please seek out of an experienced macrobiotic counselor or medical professional for proper guidance.

Bancha Stem Tea

Used for strengthening the metabolism in all sicknesses. Use one tablespoon of tea to one quart of water, bring to a boil, reduce flame, and simmer four to five minutes.

Body Scrub

Body scrubbing can be done before or after a bath or shower or anytime. All you need is a sink with hot water and a medium-sized cotton bath towel. Turn on the hot water. Hold the towel at either end and place the center of the towel under the stream of hot water. Wring out the towel, and while it is still hot and steamy begin to scrub with it. Do one section of the body at a time. For example, begin with the hands and fingers and work your way up the arms to the shoulders, neck, and face, then down to the chest, upper back, abdomen, lower back, buttocks, legs, feet, and toes. Scrub until the skin becomes slightly red or until each part becomes warm. Reheat the towel by running it under hot water after scrubbing each section or as soon as the towel starts to cool.

Brown Rice Cream

Used in cases when a person in a weakened condition needs to be nourished and energized or when the digestive system is impaired. Dry-roast brown rice evenly until all the grains turn a yellowish color. To 1 part rice, add a tiny amount of sea salt and 3 to 6 parts water, and pressure-cook for at least two hours. Squeeze out the creamy part of the cooked rice gruel through a cheese-cloth sanitized in boiling water. Eat with a small volume of condiment such as umeboshi plum, gomashio, tekka, kelp, or other sea vegetable powder.

Brown Rice Plaster

When the swelling of a boil or infection is not opened by the taro plaster, the rice plaster can be used to help reduce the fever around the infected area. Hand-grind 70 percent cooked brown rice, 30 percent raw leafy vegetables, and a few crushed sheets of raw nori in a *suribachi*—the more grinding the better. (If the mixture is very sticky, add water.) Apply the paste to the affected area. If the plaster begins to burn, remove it, since it is no longer effective. To remove, rinse with warm water to remove direct paste.

Buckwheat Plaster

Purpose: Draws retained water and excess fluid from swollen areas of the body.

Preparation: Mix buckwheat flour with enough hot water to form a hard, stiff dough, and then combine thoroughly with 5 to 10 percent fresh grated ginger. Apply in a half-inch layer to the affected area; tie in place with a bandage or piece of cotton linen.

Special Consideration for Cancer Cases: A buckwheat plaster should be applied in cases where a patient develops a swollen abdomen due to retention of fluid. If this fluid is surgically removed, the patient may temporarily feel better but on some occasions may suddenly become much worse after several days, so it is better to avoid such a drastic procedure.

This plaster can be applied anywhere on the body. In cases where a breast has been removed, for example, the surrounding lymph nodes, the neck, and in some cases, the arm often become swollen after several months. To relieve this condition, apply ginger compresses to the swollen area for about five minutes, then apply a buckwheat plaster, and place a salt pack (see instructions below) on top of the plaster to maintain a warm temperature. Replace the buckwheat plaster every four hours. After removing the plaster, you may notice that fluid is coming out through the skin or that the swelling is starting to go down. A buckwheat plaster will usually eliminate the swelling after only several applications or at most after two or three days.

Burdock Tea

Used for strengthening vitality. To 1 portion of fresh burdock shavings, add 10 times the amount of water. Bring to a boil, reduce flame, and simmer for ten minutes.

Carrot-Daikon Drink

To help eliminate excessive fats and dissolve hardening accumulation in the intestines. Grate one tablespoon each of raw daikon and carrot. Cook in two cups of spring water for five to eight minutes with a pinch of sea salt or seven to ten drops of shoyu.

Chlorophyll Plaster

This plaster will help take out fevers and relieve burns. Chop several green leafy vegetable leaves such as collards or kale very finely. Place in a *suribachi* and grind. Ten to 20 percent white flour may be added to the green paste to give it bulk. Spread the paste on a towel, about one-half-inch thick, and apply to the affected area. Leave it on for two to three hours.

Daikon-Radish Drink

Drink No. 1: Serves to reduce a fever by inducing sweating. Mix half a cup of grated, fresh daikon with one tablespoon of shoyu and one quarter teaspoon of grated ginger. Pour hot bancha tea or hot water over this mixture, stir, and drink while hot.

Drink No. 2: Induces urination. Use a piece of cheesecloth to squeeze the juice from the grated daikon. Mix two tablespoons of this juice with six table-spoons of hot water to which a pinch of sea salt or one teaspoon of shoyu has been added. Boil this mixture and drink only once a day. Do not use this preparation more than three consecutive days without proper supervision and never use it without first boiling.

Drink No. 3: Helps dissolve fat and mucus. In a teacup place one tablespoon of fresh grated daikon and one teaspoon shoyu. Pour hot bancha tea over mixture and drink. It is most effective when taken just before sleeping. Do not use this drink longer than five days unless otherwise advised by an experienced macrobiotic counselor.

Dandelion Root Tea

Used to strengthen the heart and small intestine function and increase vitality. One teaspoon of root to one cup of water. Bring to a boil, reduce flame, and simmer ten minutes.

Dentie

Helps to prevent tooth problems, promotes a healthy condition in the mouth, and stops bleeding anywhere in the body by contracting expanded blood capillaries. Bake an eggplant, particularly the calix or cap, until black. Crush into a powder and mix with 30 to 50 percent roasted sea salt. Use daily as a tooth powder or apply to any bleeding area—even inside the nostrils in case of nosebleed—by inserting squeezed, wet tissue dipped in dentie into the nostril.

Dried Daikon Leaves

Used to warm the body and to treat various disorders of the skin and female sex organs. Also helpful in drawing odors and excessive oils from the body. Dry fresh daikon leaves in the shade, away from direct sunlight, until they turn brown and brittle. (If daikon leaves are unavailable, turnip greens may be substituted.) Boil four to five bunches of leaves in four to five quarts of water until the water turns brown. Stir in a handful of sea salt and use in one of the following ways: 1) Dip cotton linen into the hot liquid and wring lightly. Apply to the affected area repeatedly, until the skin becomes completely red. 2) Women experiencing problems in their sexual organs should sit in a hot bath to which the daikon-leaves liquid described above has been added along with one handful of sea salt. The water should come to waist level, with the upper portion of the body covered with a towel. Remain in the water until the whole body becomes warm and sweating begins. This generally takes about ten minutes. Repeat as needed, up to ten days. Following this bath, douche with warm *bancha* tea, ½ teaspoon of sea salt, and juice of half a lemon or similar volume of brown rice vinegar.

Ginger Compress

Purpose: Stimulates blood and body fluid circulation, helps loosen and dissolve stagnated toxic matter, cysts, tumors, etc.

Preparation: Place a handful of grated ginger in a cheesecloth and squeeze out the ginger juice into a pot containing one gallon of very hot water. Do not boil the water or you will lose the power of the ginger. Dip a cotton hand towel into the ginger water, wring it out tightly, and apply, very hot but not uncomfortably hot, to the area of the body to be treated. A second, dry towel can be placed on top to reduce heat loss. Apply a fresh hot towel every two to three minutes until the skin becomes red.

Special Considerations for Cancer Cases: The ginger compress should be prepared in the usual manner. However, it should be applied for only a short time (about five minutes maximum) to activate circulation in the affected area and should be immediately followed by a taro potato or potato plaster. If a ginger compress is applied repeatedly over an extended time, it may accelerate the growth of the cancer, particularly if it is a more yin variety. The ginger compress should be considered only as a preparation for the taro plaster (see instructions below) in cancer cases, not as an independent treatment, and applied for several minutes only. Please seek more specific recommendations from a qualified macrobiotic adviser.

Ginger Sesame Oil

Activates the function of the blood capillaries, circulation, and nerve reactions. Also relieves aches and pains. Mix the juice of grated, fresh ginger with an equal amount of sesame oil. Dip cotton linen into this mixture and rub briskly into the skin of the affected area. This is also helpful for headache, dandruff, and hair growth.

Grated Daikon

A digestive aid, especially for fatty, oily, heavy foods and for animal food. Grate fresh daikon (red radish or turnip may be used if daikon is not available).

Sprinkle with shoyu and eat about one tablespoon. You may also add a pinch of grated ginger.

Green Magma Tea

Young barley grass powder available in many natural foods stores. Good for reducing and melting fats, cysts, and tumors arising from animal foods. Take one to two teaspoons and pour hot water over and drink. Consult an experienced macrobiotic counselor for length of time to use.

Kombu Tea

Good for strengthening the blood. Use one three-inch strip of *kombu* to 1 quart of water. Bring to a boil, reduce flame, and simmer for ten minutes. Another method is to dry kombu in a 350° F oven for ten to fifteen minutes, or until crisp. Grate one-half to one teaspoon of kombu into a cup and add hot water.

Kuzu Drink

Strengthens digestion, increases vitality, and relieves general fatigue. Dissolve a heaping teaspoon of kuzu powder in two teaspoons of water, then add to one cup of cold water. Bring the mixture to a boil, reduce the heat to the simmering point, and stir constantly until the liquid becomes a transparent gelatin. Stir in one teaspoon of shoyu and drink while hot.

Lotus-Root Plaster

Draws stagnant mucus from the sinuses, nose, throat, and bronchi. Mix grated, fresh lotus root with 10 to 15 percent pastry flour and 5 to 10 percent grated, fresh ginger. Spread a half-inch layer onto cotton linen and apply the lotus root directly to the skin. Keep on for several hours or overnight and repeat daily for several days. A ginger compress can be applied before this application to stimulate circulation and to loosen mucus in the area being treated.

Lotus-Root Tea

Helps relieve coughing and dissolves excess mucus in the body. Grate one-half cup of fresh lotus root, squeeze the juice into a pot, and add a small amount of water. Cook for five to eight minutes, add a pinch of sea salt or shoyu, and drink hot.

Mustard Plaster

Stimulates blood and body fluid circulation and loosens stagnation. Add hot water to dry mustard powder and stir well. Spread this mixture onto a paper towel and sandwich it between two thick cotton towels. Apply this "sandwich" to the skin area and leave on until the skin becomes red and hot and then remove. After removing, wipe off remaining mustard plaster from the skin with towels.

Nachi Green Tea

Helps dissolve and discharge animal fats and reduce high cholesterol levels. Place one half teaspoon of tea into the serving kettle. Pour one cup of hot water over the tea and steep for three to five minutes. Strain and drink one cup per day.

Salt Bancha Tea

Used to loosen stagnation in the nasal cavity or to cleanse the vaginal region. Add enough salt to warm bancha tea (about body temperature) to make it just a little less salty than sea water. Use the liquid to wash deep inside the nasal cavity through the nostrils or as a douche. Salt bancha tea can also be used as a wash for problems with the eyes, sore throat, and fatigue.

Salt Pack

Used to warm any part of the body. For the relief of diarrhea, for example, apply the pack to the abdominal region. Roast salt in a dry pan until hot and then wrap in thick cotton linen pillowcase or towel and tie with string or cord like a package. Apply to the troubled area and change when the pack begins to cool.

Salt Water

Cold salt water will contract the skin in the case of burns while warm salt water can be used to clean the rectum, colon, and vagina. When the skin is damaged by fire, immediately soak the burned area in cold salt water until the irritation disappears. Then apply vegetable oil to seal the wound from the air. For constipation or mucus or fat accumulation in the rectum, colon, and vaginal regions, use warm water (body temperature) as an enema or douche.

Sesame Oil

Used to relieve stagnated bowels or to eliminate retained water. Take one to two tablespoons of raw sesame oil with one-quarter teaspoon of ginger and shoyu on an empty stomach to induce the discharge of stagnated bowels. To eliminate water retention in the eyes, put a drop or two of pure sesame oil (preferably dark sesame oil) in the eyes with an eyedropper, ideally before sleeping. Continue up to a week, until the eyes improve. Before using the sesame oil for this purpose, it is important to boil and then strain it through a sanitized cheesecloth to remove impurities, and let cool.

Shiitake Mushroom Tea

Used to relax an overly tense, stressful condition and helps to dissolve excessive animal fats. Soak a dried black shiitake mushroom, then cut in quarters. Cook in two cups of water for twenty minutes with a pinch of sea salt or one teaspoon of shoyu. Drink only one-half cup at a time.

Shoyu Bancha Tea

Neutralizes an acidic blood condition, promotes blood circulation, and relieves fatigue. Pour one cup of hot bancha twig tea over one to two teaspoons of shoyu. Stir and drink hot.

Taro Potato (Albi) Plaster

Purpose: Often used after a ginger compress to collect stagnated toxic matter and draw it out of the body.

Preparation: Peel off taro potato skin and grate the white interior. Mix with 5 to 10 percent grated fresh ginger. Spread this mixture in a two-thirds to one-inch-thick layer onto a fresh cotton linen and apply the taro side directly to the skin. Change every four hours.

Taro potato can usually be obtained in most major cities in the United States and Canada from Chinese, Armenian, or Puerto Rican grocery stores or natural foods stores. The skin of this vegetable is brown and covered with "hair." The taro potato is grown in Hawaii as well as in the Orient. Smaller taro potatoes are the most effective for use in this plaster. If taro is not available, a preparation using regular white potato can be substituted. While not as effective as taro, it will still produce a beneficial result. Mix 50 to 60 percent grated white potato with 40 to 50 percent grated or mashed green leafy vegetables, mixing them together in a *suribachi*. Add enough wheat flour to make a paste and add 5 to 10 percent grated ginger. Apply as above.

Special Considerations for Cancer Patients: The taro plaster has the effect of drawing cancerous toxins out of the body and is particularly effective in removing carbon and other minerals often contained in tumors. If, when the plaster is removed, the light-colored mixture has become dark or brown, or if the skin where the plaster was applied also takes on a dark color, this change indicates that excessive carbon and other elements are being discharged through the skin. This treatment will gradually reduce the size of the tumor if applied repeatedly once or twice daily.

If the patient feels chilly from the coolness of the plaster, a hot ginger compress applied for five minutes while changing plasters will help relieve this. If chill persists, roast sea salt in a skillet, wrap it in a towel, and place it on top of the plaster. Be careful not to let the patient become too hot from this salt application.

Tofu Plaster

This treatment is more effective than an ice pack to draw out a fever. Squeeze the water from the tofu, mash it, and then add 10 to 20 percent pastry flour and 5 to 10 percent grated ginger. Mix the ingredients and apply directly to the skin. Change every two to three hours or sooner if plaster becomes hot.

Ume Extract

A concentrated form of umeboshi plums, available in some natural foods stores. Good for neutralizing an acid or nauseous condition and diarrhea in the stomach. Pour hot water or bancha tea over one quarter to one third teaspoon of ume extract.

Umeboshi Plum

Baked umeboshi plum or powdered backed whole umeboshi plum neutralizes an acidic condition and relieves intestinal problems, including those caused by microorganisms. Take one half to one umeboshi plum (baked is stronger than unbaked) with one cup bancha tea. If you bake and crush into a powder, add a teaspoon to one cup of hot water.

Ume-Sho-Bancha

Strengthens the blood and the circulation through the regulation of digestion. Pour one cup of bancha tea over the meat of one half to one umeboshi plum and one teaspoon shoyu. Stir and drink hot. Also helps relieve headaches in the front part of the head.

Ume-Sho-Bancha with Ginger

Helps to increase blood circulation. Same as above, but add one quarter teaspoon of grated ginger juice and pour one cup of hot bancha tea over. Stir and drink.

Ume-Sho-Kuzu Drink

Strengthens digestion, revitalizes energy, and regulates the intestinal condition. Prepare the kuzu drink according to the instructions for kuzu drink and add the meat of one half to one umeboshi plum. One-eighth teaspoon of fresh grated ginger may also be added.

White Potato Plaster

If taro potatoes are not available, this recipe may be used in place of a taro plaster. Grate a potato (green potatoes are the best). Mix 45 percent potato, 45 percent finely chopped greens (which have been mashed in a *suribachi*), and about 10 percent grated ginger. Mix well. If the potato is very watery, place it in a cheesecloth sack and squeeze out the excess water before combining it with the other ingredients. It may also be necessary to add white flour to the mixture. Use the same way as the taro plaster.

36

Prayers, Meditations, and Visualizations

PRAYERS

Daily Dedication for One Peaceful World

When we eat, let us reflect that we have come from food, which has come from nature by the order of the infinite universe, and let us be grateful for all that we have been given.

When we meet people, let us see them as brothers and sisters and remember that we have all come from the infinite universe through our parents and ancestors, and let us pray as One with all of humanity for universal love and peace on earth.

When we see the sun and moon, the sky and stars, mountains and rivers, seas and forests, fields and valleys, birds and animals, and all the wonders of nature, let us remember that we have come with them all from the infinite universe. Let us be thankful for our environment on earth, and live in harmony with all that surrounds us.

When we see farms and villages, towns and cities, arts and cultures, societies and civilizations, and all the works of humanity, let us recall that our creativity has come from the infinite universe, and has passed from generation to generation and spread over the entire earth. Let us be grateful for our birth on this planet with intelligence and wisdom, and let us vow with all to realize endlessly our eternal dream of One Peaceful World through health, freedom, love, and justice.

One Peaceful World Prayer

Having come from, being within, and going toward infinity,
May our endless dream be eternally realized upon this earth,
May our unconditional dedication perpetually serve for the creation of love and
    peace,
May our heartfelt thankfulness be devoted universally upon everyone, every-
    thing, and every being.

Prayer at Meal

From this infinite, this food has come to us,
By this food, we realize ourselves on this planet,
To this food we are grateful,
For nature and people who have brought this food, we are thankful,
This food becomes us.
By eating together we become one family on this planet,
Through this food, we all are one.
Let us love each other in this life,
Let us realize our endless dream.

Meditation and Prayer at the Meal

I am grateful to the meal now being offered to me.
I am grateful to people, nature, and the universe for having made this meal available to me.
I now reflect whether I truly deserve to have this meal.
I now pray that, through this meal, I may achieve a healthy body and peaceful mind.
I now resolve that, through this meal, I will continue to realize my dream of love and peace in our eternal journey of endless life.

MEDITATION

1. Find a quiet place and sit in a relaxed and comfortable position.

2. Raise your arms upward toward the ceiling and hold them there for several moments. Then tilt your head back so that you are looking up. Keep your head in this position for several seconds, and then lower your arms to their normal position. Return your head to its normal position a moment later. This simple stretching exercise helps straighten your spine and allows energy from the environment to flow more smoothly through your body. Do each step in a continuous sequence and repeat the entire procedure several times.

3. With your spine straight and your shoulders and elbows relaxed, let your hands rest comfortably in your lap with the palms facing up. Place your left hand, which corresponds to heaven (yang energy), on top of your right, which corresponds to the earth (yin energy). Lift your thumbs upward and touch the tips of both thumbs together, forming an arc or bridge. Your thumbs and index fingers should generally form a circle. This position creates unity and harmony between the left and right sides of the body and between the flow of heaven and earth's forces.

4. Close your eyes and begin to breathe naturally and quietly. Breathe in a normal, relaxed fashion. After making your breathing calm and quiet, begin to breathe more deeply, centering your breath in the lower abdomen. As you breathe in, let your abdomen expand, and as your breathe out, let it contract.

5. While you are breathing in this manner, let your mind become quiet,

relaxed, and free of distracting thoughts or images. Do not try to force distracting thoughts to go away, but simply let them dissolve. It may help to concentrate on your breathing. Sit this way for several minutes, breathing naturally and keeping your mind still and quiet.

6. To complete your meditation, slowly open your eyes and let your consciousness return to a normal waking state.

VISUALIZATION

To practice visualization, begin to meditate as in the exercise above. When you have reached step four, form an image of yourself as a healthy and happy person. Don't dwell on your illness; see yourself as you would like to be. Concentrate on this image for several minutes and then let your mind return to a peaceful, quiet state. Then complete your meditation as above.

Positive visualization reduces stress and inspires hope for the future. Your daily life can then become the process through which you actualize this positive, healthy image of yourself. Here are several other simple visualization exercises.

Visualization to Change Sickness to Health

Relax, close your eyes, and stabilize your breathing as in the above exercises.

In your mind, create an image of the infinite universe. See the heavens filled with billions and billions of galaxies and stars, solar systems and planets, cycling in perfect harmony.

Imagine the Earth bathed in the gentle, peaceful energy from all these celestial bodies.

Imagine this energy coming down and in to our planet in centripetal spiral waves and making it spin on its axis, coming up again from the center of the Earth in centrifugal waves that spiral in a complementary, outward, upward direction.

Imagine this energy of heaven and earth making the plants and animals grow, the grains blowing gently in the wind, the vegetables, beans, and other seeds pushing up from below ground, the seaweed swaying peacefully in the oceans, the salt and other minerals collecting in the sea, absorbing and gathering this vital energy.

Imagine eating a delicious, balanced meal made from these foods and that strong nourishing energy flowing through your body, from the digestive system, to the circulatory system, to the nervous system, to all organs, functions, tissues, and cells.

Imagine this energy creating fresh, new blood and lymph and gently melting away hardness, stagnation, and blockages that may have developed in the past.

Imagine your tumor or growth gradually shrinking and dissolving as this peaceful, harmonious energy is received.

Imagine yourself restored to health, surrounded by the love of family and friends.

Imagine yourself now completely well, guiding and helping other people with serious illness rediscover the laws of nature and the healing power of their own minds and bodies.

Imagine yourself five, ten, fifteen, twenty years, or more from now, experiencing ever greater realms of self-realization. Hold this image for a few minutes, let it subside naturally, and resume normal consciousness.

Visualization of Gratefulness

Reflect on your past way of life and eating, including all of the extreme foods you ate in the past. Be grateful for everything that has come before, good and bad.

Reflect on the wisdom of the body and how, despite your ignorance and foolishness, it constantly tried to warn you of imbalance through various symptoms and warnings, but how you failed to take notice. Be grateful for your wonderful body.

Reflect on how your body finally localized all of this incoming excess and stored it in one area as a tumor in order to let you continue to function relatively normally and live one, two, three, five years, or more. Be grateful for your sickness.

Reflect on who or what inspired you to change your way of life and way of eating, inspiring you to lead a more natural way of life. Be grateful for the ability to change.

Reflect that your tumor is no longer needed because now you have changed and are taking conscious responsibility for your health and sickness. Be grateful for your wonderful mind and spirit.

Reflect on the foods and drinks, and in some cases special home cares, that you will take to help dissolve your tumor or blockage and return to harmony with nature. Be grateful for the foods you receive each day.

Reflect on your bloodstream and lymph system, kidneys and bladder, lungs and large intestine, heart and small intestine, liver and gallbladder, stomach and spleen/pancreas, skin, and other organs and functions that will naturally help to eliminate accumulated excess from your body. Be grateful for your natural healing ability.

Reflect on how life will be six months, nine months, one year, two years, three years, five years from now when you are completely healthy and whole and see yourself getting stronger and healthier, cleaner and more peaceful during this time. Be grateful for this opportunity to change.

Reflect on hamburgers, soft drinks, ice cream cones, and all the other foods and experiences that hammered you and tested and raised your judgment. Be grateful to these because they are your teachers of life.

Reflect on cancer as one of the best things that ever happened to you, teaching you to take responsibility for your life and destiny and awakening you to the laws of the infinite universe. Be grateful to life as a whole and marvel at being alive on this beautiful planet. Hold this image for a few minutes, let it naturally subside, and return to normal awareness.

Visualization to Counterbalance Artificial Electromagnetic Energy

Sit quietly in any comfortable position, hold your hands on your lap or in the prayer position with palms touching, and stabilize your breathing.

Visualize a field of natural electromagnetic energy emanating from the chakras, or energy centers, in your body—extending from the spiral on the top of your head to the forehead, the throat, the heart, the solar plexus, the intestinal center, and the reproductive region.

Visualize energy in the form of shining white light, radiating from the chakras, extending eighteen to twenty-four inches in all directions, surrounding and protecting you from harmful (i.e., extreme yin or yang) influences.

Visualize each chakra as a miniature sun radiating light, and your entire body as an interconnected web of light and energy. Allow energy to circulate freely from the central energy channel to the periphery of the body, so that each organ, function, and cell is bathed in and illuminated by light. Then return from the periphery of the body back to the central energy channel. You should be completely relaxed, yet fully charged with energy.

Visualize artificial radiation from power lines, television, computers, and other sources harmlessly dissolving when it comes into contact with your energized aura and field.

Hold that image for several minutes, then let it naturally subside, and relax.

Visualization for Healing Planet Earth

Sit quietly in any comfortable position and hold your hands on your lap or in the prayer position with palms touching.

Stabilize your breathing.

Visualize the Earth as a bright tiny ball in the vastness of space.

Visualize that blue-green ball temporarily covered with a heavy, dark aura.

Visualize the way of life and health spreading from kitchen to kitchen, home to home, family to family, beginning with you.

Visualize people gradually recovering their health as they eat and live in a more natural direction.

Visualize more and more of the land devoted to growing grains and vegetables and less and less to raising cattle and other livestock.

Visualize the rivers and streams becoming cleaner and cleaner as natural farming and organic gardening spread.

Visualize the air becoming purer and purer as less industrial pollutants are released into the atmosphere.

Visualize the plants and animals thriving and returning to forests and woodlands, oceans and lakes.

Visualize human beings living peacefully on the planet, with no more war, crime, or violence; no more cancer, heart disease, or major sickness; no more poverty and injustice.

Visualize people of all colors, sexes, ages, and backgrounds living harmoniously in One Peaceful World, playing from morning till night, traveling freely, and respecting each other's customs, traditions, and ways of life.

Visualize the stagnated energy of the Earth from sickness, social disorder, and pollution of the environment melting into the general circulation of the energy as a whole. Visualize the Earth becoming lighter and more energized.

Visualize the dark aura around the Earth gradually dissolving and the Earth's aura—the ozone layer, Van Allen belt, aurora borealis—becoming brighter and brighter, lighter and lighter.

Visualize the Earth as a tiny ball in outer space surrounded by a radiant halo of energy spiraling through the Milky Way.

Visualize yourself as being at one with the Earth and all of life. Hold this image for a few minutes, let it subside naturally, and allow your consciousness to return to normal.

PALM HEALING

Palm healing is one of the most basic and simple healing techniques for anyone who wants better health the natural way. The art of sending energy—heaven and earth's force, yang and yin—through the hands has been used for centuries around the world. Here are several simple exercises that can help improve our health and well-being on a daily basis. For further information, including comprehensive care of different systems of the body and the immune function, see my book *Macrobiotic Palm Healing: Energy at Your Finger-tips* (with Olivia Oredson) (New York and Tokyo: Japan Publications, 1988).

Care for One Organ

In this exercise, we aim to improve the quality and quantity of energy flowing through an organ. For example, someone who has a blockage or tumor is the receiver, while a family member or friend is the giver.

1. The receiver may sit comfortably or lie down, eyes closed or partly open, breathing naturally. The giver sits at the side, with natural breathing, and begins with the hands in the prayer position (with palms touching).

2. Selecting one organ, the giver extends one palm, keeping the other hand in the lap, and briefly checks the energy of the organ, pausing about one-half to one inch above the surface of the body. Move the hand gently and slowly side to side over the organ, noticing any sensations such as magnetic density, electricity, warmth, and so on.

3. Now raise the palm six to ten inches above the organ and slowly approach again to about one-half to one inch. Gently bounce the hand in this way several times, noticing the energy as the hand gets closer.

4. Next, the giver gently rests the palm over the organ (or may hold the palm one-half to one inch above if desired). The other hand may be in the lap or held up to draw in heaven's force (yang energy) from above or held down to draw up earth's force (yin energy) from below. (Generally, in the case of cancer, draw in heaven's force to activate and supply energy or for tumors on the surface or front of the brain, mouth, esophagus, and upper digestive system, skin, leukemia, lymphoma, and cancers related to children, radiation, and AIDS. Draw in earth's force to disperse or reduce energy or for tumors of the lungs, liver, kidney, pancreas, colon, rectum, reproductive region, melanoma, bone, and inner or back regions of the brain.)

5. The giver follows the breathing of the receiver and the two breathe together in a natural, peaceful fashion. Chanting may be added, such as Su, the sound of peace and harmony, if desired. Mental imagery may be used also, visualizing a flow of healing energy through the organ. Continue two to five minutes and notice any perceptions experienced by the giver and the receiver.

6. Recheck the energy of the organ as in steps two and three. Is it the same as before, or has it changed?

7. Try other organs in the same way if desired. Take one to two minutes for each.

8. When finished, smooth down the whole body's energy with several long, smooth, head-to-toe movements of the palms about one-half to one inch over the person's body.

9. Remove the hands and relax. Giver and receiver may discuss their experiences.

SOUNDS FOR SPECIFIC ORGANS OF THE BODY

Since each organ has a different proportion of yin and yang, earth and heaven's energy flow, certain sounds benefit certain organs more than others, depending on their yin or yang qualities. Through many generations of experience, practitioners of traditional Far Eastern medicine arrived at the following understanding of specific sounds to benefic each organ.

Organ	Nourishing Sound
Lungs	Ha
Large intestine	Ah or ho
Heart	Shi ("sheee")
Small intestine	Toh or so
Spleen/pancreas	Hi ("heee")
Stomach	Iii ("eee")
Kidneys	Ji ("geee")
Bladder	Bo or bu
Liver	Ka or kan
Gallbladder	Da

We can strengthen specific organs through using their corresponding sounds in a number of ways:

1. While meditating or practicing palm healing or self-massage, chant the sound for the organ you wish to benefit. Chant ten to fifteen times, and place your palm on the corresponding organ if desired.

2. While giving palm healing to another person, chant the appropriate sound while you place your hand on a certain organ.

SONGS

Singing is beneficial to the lungs, circulatory system, immune function, and other organs and systems of the body. Any traditional songs will do, especially ones that are bright and happy. Here are several songs that are popular in macrobiotic homes around the world.

"One Peaceful World"
(Words and music by Edward Esko)

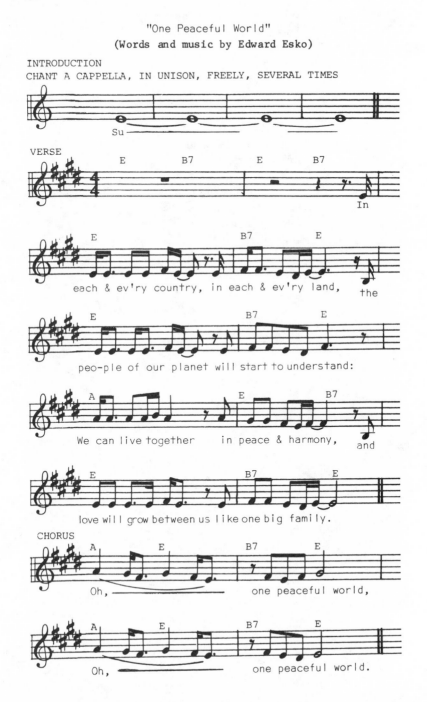

To the sun that shines above us,
To the earth that lies below,
To the universal spirit,
Our thankfulness shall go.
And the light will shine upon us,
Every single day.
When dreaming of tomorrow,
This is what we say.

Oh-Oh one peaceful world
Oh-Oh one peaceful world.
(Chorus)

In the east the sun is rising,
In the west it's going down.
And the two will join together,
In the new world comin' round.
Where unity will guide us,
In everything we do,
And dawn will soon be breakin'
On a world that's fresh and new.
(Chorus)

"Planetary Family"
(Words and music by Edward Esko and John Ineson)

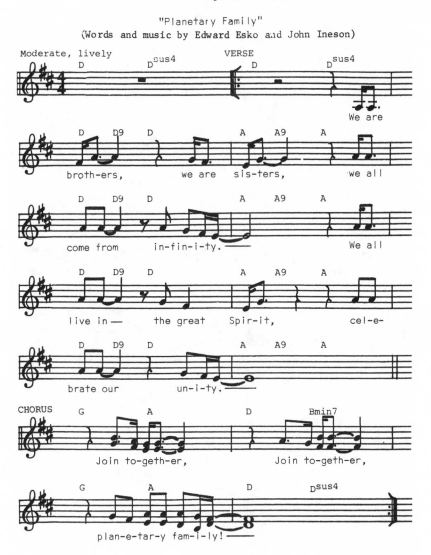

Some are white and some are yellow,
Skins of black and skins of brown
When we listen to our hearts beat,
They all make the same pure sound.

(Chorus)

All the boundaries of the nations
Can't be seen from outer space.
It is all just land and ocean,
A beautiful home for the human race.

(Chorus)

From Atlantic to Pacific,
From Suez to the North Sea,
From Tierra del Fuego,
To wherever you may be.

(Chorus)

From Jesus to Zoroaster,
From Moses to Mahavir,
From Buddha to Muhammad,
There is truth for us to hear.

(Chorus)

From Boston to Buenos Aires,
From Moscow to Tokyo,
The same sun shines upon us,
And around it we all go.

(Chorus)

From Sudan to Australia,
From Cape Can'veral to the Great Wall,
From Stonehenge to Mt. Fuji,
From the Rockies to the Taj Mahal.

(Chorus)

Glossary

Acid phosphatase test   Lab test measuring the amount of an enzyme produced in the prostate and released into the blood. High levels indicate possible multiple myeloma or metastatic prostate cancer.

Acupressure   Shiatsu massage, a healing art based on stimulating the flow of energy through the meridians of the body.

Acupuncture   Far Eastern medical art based on inserting needles in various parts of the body to relieve pain and release blocked energy.

Aduki bean   A small, dark red bean originally from Japan but also now grown in the United States.

Alkaline phosphatase test   Lab test measuring an enzyme in the blood and bone. High levels signify possible liver and pancreatic cancer or other serious condition.

Amasake   A sweetener or refreshing drink made from sweet brown rice and koji starter that is allowed to ferment into a thick liquid.

Angiogram   A medical procedure in which a radiosensitive dye or other material is injected into the arteries to diagnose cancer or other serious conditions in the inner organs, brain, heart, or limbs.

Arame   A thin, wiry black sea vegetable similar to hijiki.

Arrowroot   A starch flour processed from the root of an American plant. It is used as a thickening agent for making sauces, stews, gravies, or desserts.

Bancha tea   The stems and leaves from mature Japanese tea bushes, also known as kukicha. Bancha aids in digestion and is high in calcium. It contains no chemical dyes.

Benign tumor   A tumor that does not spread to other regions but remains confined to its original location.

Bioassay   A medical test in which living organisms are used, such as a carcinogenesis test.

Biopsy   Extraction of a sample of living tissue or fluid for microscopic examination and diagnosis.

Bok choy   A leafy green vegetable.

Bone scan   Medical procedure in which radiosotopes are introduced into the bone marrow for detection of bone cancer or metastasis.

Brown rice   Whole, unpolished rice. Comes in three main varieties: short-, medium-, and long-grain. Brown rice contains an ideal balance of minerals, protein, and carbohydrates.

Buckwheat A staple food in Russia and many European countries. This cereal food is eaten widely in the form of kasha, whole groats, and soba noodles.

Burdock A wild, hardy plant that grows throughout the United States. The long, dark root is valued in cooking for its strengthening qualities.

Cancer A disease of the whole body in which mucus and toxins accumulated over years of imbalanced eating are localized as tumors or a degenerating blood or lymph condition.

Carcinogen Any substance that augments cancer in humans or animals.

Carcinoma Cancer in an epithelial tissue, further differentiated into types such as squamous-cell, basal-cell, or adenocarcinoma.

Case-control study A medical study in which exposure data (such as food intake) are collected for individuals (cases) with a specific type of cancer and compared with similar data for a suitable noncancer group (controls).

CAT scan Computer-Assisted Transaxial device that takes cross-sectional X rays of the brain and torso.

Catheter A hollow tube for discharging fluids from a body cavity.

CBC Complete Blood Count, a computerized lab test that anlalyzes the constituents of the blood. The normal range for erythroctes (red blood cells) is 4.5 to 5 million per cubic millimeter; WBC (White Blood Count), 5,000 to 10,000; granulocytes, 2,000 to 4,000; differential count (ratio of mature to immature cells), 100; blasts (abnormal cells in marrow), less than 5 percent; hematocrit (percentage of red blood cells), 42 to 46 percent in men and 38 to 42 percent in women; hemoglobin, 13 to 16 grams per 100 milliliters; reticulocytes (young red blood cells), 0.5 to 1.5 percent of red blood cells.

CEA assay Lab test measuring the presence of Carcinoembryonic antigen in the blood. High levels indicate possible cancer in the digestive system, lung cancer, and other diseases.

Chemotherapy Treatment of cancer with chemicals or drugs.

Cholesterol A constituent of all animal fats and oils, which in excess can give rise to heart disease, cancer, and other illnesses.

Condition An individual's day-to-day or year-to-year state of health in contrast to constitution or characteristics acquired at birth.

Constitution An individual's characteristics determined before birth by the health and vitality of the parents, grandparents, and ancestors, especially by the food eaten by the mother during pregnancy.

Couscous Partially refined cracked wheat.

Cyst A sac containing fluid, mucous, or other material; a possible precancerous sign.

Daikon A long, white radish. Besides making a delicious side dish, daikon is a specific aid in dissolving fat and mucus deposits that have accumulated as a result of past animal food intake. Grated daikon aids in the digestion of oily foods. If unavailable, red radish may be substituted.

Dentie A black tooth powder made from sea salt and charred eggplant.

Disaccharide Double sugar such as sucrose (cane sugar) and lactose (milk sugar), which enters the bloodstream rapidly and can lead to imbalance.

Discharge The body's elimination of mucus, toxins, and other accumulations through normal or abnormal mechanisms ranging from urination and bowel movement to coughing and sneezing to cysts and tumors.

Do-in A form of Oriental self-massage based on harmonizing the energy flowing through the meridians.

Dulse A reddish-purple sea vegetable. Used in soups, salads, and vegetable dishes. Very high in iron.

Electromagnetic energy Natural energy from the environment that flows through all things. Includes atmospheric and celestial forces and the energy generated by the Earth's rotation and orbit.

Endoscope An instrument for viewing the interior of a body cavity.

Epidemiology The study of the occurrence and distribution of disease among human populations.

Estrogen A female hormone that regulates ovarian activity and that may be taken synthetically to control the birth cycle, menopause, or the development of breast, prostate, or other sex-related cancers.

Fiber The part of vegetable foods that is not broken down in the digestive process and facilitates the elimination of wastes through the intestine. Especially found in whole grains and legumes and to a lesser extent in vegetables and fruits.

Foley food mill A special steel food mill operated by a hand crank to make purées, sauces, dips, etc.

Gallium scan A total body scan in which radioactive gallium 67 is introduced into the veins. Used particularly to detect the spread of cancer to the lymph nodes.

Genmai miso Miso made from fermented brown rice, soybeans, and sea salt. Also referred to as brown rice miso.

GI series A diagnostic study of the gastrointestinal tract. Usually divided into upper and lower series. The upper observes abnormalities in the esophagus, stomach, and small intestine. The lower (also known as a barium enema) focuses on the large intestine.

Ginger A spicy, pungent, golden-colored root used in cooking and for medicinal purposes.

Ginger compress A compress made from grated gingerroot and water. Applied hot to an affected area of the body, it serves to stimulate circulation and dissolve stagnation.

Gluten The sticky substance that remains after the bran has been kneaded and rinsed from whole wheat flour. Used to make seitan.

Gomashio Sesame salt. A condiment made from roasted, ground sesame seeds and sea salt.

Hatcho miso A fermented soybean paste made from soybeans and sea salt and aged for two years. Used in making condiments, soup stocks, and seasoning for vegetable dishes.

Hijiki A dark brown sea vegetable, which, when dried, turns black. It has a wiry consistency and may be strong-tasting. Hijiki is imported from Japan but also grows off the coast of Maine.

Hokkaido pumpkin A round dark green or orange squash that is very sweet and harvested in the fall. Originally from New England, it was introduced to Japan and named after the island of Hokkaido.

Hysterectomy Total or partial surgical removal of the uterus.

Intravenous pylegram (IVP) A fluoroscopic X ray exam of the urinary system.

Iriko Small dried fish.

Jinenjo A light brown Japanese mountain potato that grows to be several feet long and two to three inches wide.

Kanten A jelled dessert made from agar-agar.

Kasha Buckwheat groats.

Kayu Cereal grain porridge that has been cooked with approximately five to ten times as much water as grain for a long period of time until it is soft and creamy.

Kelp A large family of sea vegetables that grow mainly in northern latitudes. Available packaged whole, granulated, or powdered.

Kinpira A sautéed burdock or burdock and carrot dish that is seasoned with shoyu.

Koji A grain inoculated with bacteria and used in making fermented foods such as miso, shoyu, amasake, natto, and sake.

Kokkoh Baby food porridge made from brown rice, sweet rice, barley, and kombu.

Kombu A wide, thick, dark green sea vegetable that grows in deep ocean water. Used in making soup stocks, condiments, and candy, and cooked with vegetables and beans.

Kukicha *Bancha* tea. Older stems and leaves of a tea bush grown in Japan.

Kuzu A white starch made from the root of a wild plant. Used in making soups, gravies, desserts, and for medicinal purposes. Also known as kudzu. If unavailable, arrowroot may be substituted.

Laboratory studies Medical tests in which food constituents or chemicals are analyzed for molecular structure, short-term effects on bacteria, yeast, or other biological systems, or long-term effects on animals.

Laparotomy Major abdominal surgery in which a biopsy may be taken of the inner organs.

Lotus root The root of water lily, which is brown-skinned with a hollow, chambered, off-white inside. Especially good for respiratory organs.

Malignant tumor A tumor with the ability to invade adjacent tissue or spread to distant body sites; life-threatening.

Mammogram X ray of the breast.

Mastectomy Surgical removal of the breast.

Meridian Channel or pathway of electromagnetic energy in the body. Oriental medicine, massage, and the martial arts are based on understanding the flow of energy through the meridians.

Metastasis The spread of cancer from a primary to a secondary site through the blood or lymph systems.

Millet A small yellow grain, originally native to China, other parts of Asia, and Africa. It can be used regularly in soups, vegetable dishes, and cereal form.

Miso Fermented soybean paste, used in soups, spreads, and for seasonings.

Mochi A rice cake or dumpling made from cooked, pounded sweet rice.

Monosaccharide Simple sugar such as glucose, fructose, and galactose. Both mono- and disaccharides enter the bloodstream quickly and can elevate blood sugar levels and cause hypoglycemic reactions.

Moxibustion Oriental medical technique of burning mugwort or other herb on the skin to release blocked energy and promote circulation.

Mucus Viscid liquid secreted by mucous glands and produced from eating foods high in fat and sugar, as well as flour products.

Mugi miso Soybean paste made from fermented barley, soybeans, sea salt, and water.

Mu tea A tea made from a variety of herbs that have the medicinal properties of warming the body and strengthening the female organs.

Natto   Soybeans that have been cooked and mixed with beneficial enzymes and allowed to ferment twenty-four hours.

Natural foods   Whole foods that are unprocessed and untreated with artificial additives or preservatives.

Nigari   Hard crystallized salt made from liquid droppings of dampened sea salt. Used in making tofu.

Nori   Thin sheets of dried sea vegetable. Black or dark purple when dried, they turn green when roasted over a flame. Used as a garnish, wrapped around rice balls, in making vegetable sushi, or cooked with shoyu and used as a condiment.

Okara   Coarse soybean pulp left over when making tofu. Can be put into soups.

Organic foods   Foods grown without the use of artificial chemical fertilizers, herbicides, and pesticides.

Palm healing   Healing method utilizing the palms of the hands to focus electromagnetic energy on various parts of the body.

Pap test   Medical test in which cell samples are taken from the cervix to detect possible cancer.

Physiognomy   The art of judging a person's health from the features of the face or the form of the body.

Polysaccharides   Complex sugars that gradually become absorbed during the digestive process. They include starch and cellulose found in large quantities in whole grains and vegetables.

Polyunsaturated fats   Essential fatty acids found in high concentration in grains, beans, and seeds and in smaller quantities in animal foods, especially fish.

Refined oil   Cooking oil that has been chemically processed to alter or remove color, taste, and odor.

Sarcoma   Cancer of bone, muscle, or connective tissue. Differentiated by site such as osteosarcoma, fibrosarcoma, etc.

Saturated fat   Animal fat primarily, which contributes to the formation of cholesterol and hardening of the arteries.

Sea salt   Salt obtained from the ocean and either sun-baked or kiln-baked. Unlike refined table salt, it is high in trace minerals and contains no chemicals, sugar, or iodine.

Seitan   Wheat gluten cooked in shoyu, kombu, and water.

Shiatsu   Traditional Oriental massage based on harmonizing the electromagnetic energy in the body and releasing blockages along the meridians.

Shiitake   A medicinal dried mushroom imported from Japan and now also grown in the United States. Scientific name is *Lentinus edodes*.

Shio kombu   Salty kombu. Pieces of kombu cooked for a long time in shoyu and used in small amounts as a condiment.

Shio nori   Pieces of nori cooked for a long time in shoyu and water and used as a condiment.

Shiso   Pickled beefsteak plant leaves.

Shoyu   Traditional, naturally made soy sauce as distinguished from refined, chemically processed soy sauce.

Soba   Noodles made from buckwheat flour or in combination with whole wheat flour.

Somen   Very thin, white, or whole wheat Japanese noodles.

Suribachi   A serrated, glazed clay bowl. Used with a pestle, called a *surikogi*, for grinding and puréeing foods.

Sushi   Rice rolled with vegetables, fish, or pickles wrapped in nori and sliced in rounds.

T'ai chi   A martial art developed in China based on fluid circular movements.

Taro   A potato that has a thick, hairy skin. Used in making taro potato plaster to draw toxins from the body. Also called albi.

Tekka   Condiment made from hatcho miso, sesame oil, burdock, lotus root, carrot, and gingerroot.

Tempeh   A traditional Indonesian soyfood made from split soybeans, water, and a special bacteria, which is allowed to ferment for almost a day. Available pre-packaged in some natural foods stores or can be made at home.

Tofu   Soybean curd made from soybeans and nigari. High in protein, used in soups, vegetable dishes, dressings, etc.

Tomogram   A cross-sectional view of an organ obtained by taking two X rays in a single plane.

Toxin   A poisonous product of animal or vegetable origin, which produces formation of antibodies.

Tumor   A swelling or growth of abnormal cells or tissues. May be benign or malignant.

Udon   Japanese noodles made from wheat, whole wheat, or whole wheat and un-bleached white flour.

Ultrasound   Diagnostic procedure using high-frequency sound echoes to produce an image of the body tissue.

Umeboshi   A salty pickled plum originally from Japan but now also made in the United States.

Unrefined oil   Vegetable oil that has been prepressed and/or solvent-extracted to retain the color, aroma, flavor, and nutrients of the natural substance.

Wakame   A long, thin green sea vegetable used in making soups, salads, and vegetable dishes.

Whole foods   Foods in their entire natural form that have not been refined or pro-cessed, such as brown rice, whole wheat berries, etc.

Yang   One of the two complementary and antagonistic forces that combine to produce all phenomena. Yang refers to the relative tendency of contraction, centripe-tality, fusion, heat, light, density, etc.

Yin   The antagonistic, complementary force to yang. Yin is the relative tendency of expansion, growth, centrifugality, diffusion, cold, darkness, etc.

Appendix I
Dietary Guidelines of
Major Scientific and
Medical Associations

U.S. SENATE SELECT COMMITTEE'S REPORT
DIETARY GOALS

In 1977, the U.S. Senate Select Committee on Nutrition and Human Needs issued *Dietary Goals for the United States*, a landmark report associating the modern diet with six of the leading causes of death, including heart disease and cancer. Summarizing its conclusions on the nation's way of eating, health, and future direction, the report stated:

> During this century, the composition of the average diet in the United States has changed radically. Complex carbohydrates—fruit, vegetables, and grain products—which were the mainstay of the diet, now play a minority role. At the same time, fat and sugar consumption have risen to the point where these two dietary elements alone now comprise at least 60 percent of total calorie intake, up from 50 percent in the early 1900s. In the view of doctors and nutritionists consulted by the Select Committee, these and other changes in the diet amount to a wave of malnutrition—of both over- and under-consumption—that may be as profoundly damaging to the Nation's health as the widespread contagious diseases of the early part of this century. The over-consumption of fat, generally, and saturated fat in particular, as well as cholesterol, sugar, salt, and alcohol, have been related to six of the leading causes of death: heart disease, cancer, cerebrovascular diseases, diabetes, arteriosclerosis, and cirrhosis of the liver.

The report listed six dietary goals:

1. Increase carbohydrate consumption to account for 55 to 60 percent of the energy (caloric) intake.

2. Reduce overall fat consumption from approximately 40 to 30 percent of energy intake.

3. Reduce saturated fat consumption to account for about 10 percent of total energy intake, and balance with polyunsaturated and monounsaturated fats, which should account for about 10 percent of energy intake each.

4. Reduce cholesterol consumption to about 300 milligrams a day.

5. Reduce sugar consumption by almost 40 percent to account for about 15 percent of total energy intake.

6. Reduce salt consumption by about 50 to 85 percent to approximately 3 grams a day.

The goals suggest the following changes in food selection and preparation:

1. Increase consumption of fruits and vegetables and whole grains.
2. Decrease consumption of meat and increase consumption of poultry and fish.
3. Decrease consumption of foods high in fat and partially substitute polyunsaturated fat for saturated fat.
4. Substitute nonfat milk for whole milk.
5. Decrease consumption of butterfat, eggs, and other high cholesterol sources.
6. Decrease consumption of sugar and foods that are high in sugar content.
7. Decrease consumption of salt and foods high in salt content.

Source: Select Committee on Nutrition and Human Needs, U.S. Senate, *Dietary Goals for the United States* (Washington, DC: U.S. Government Printing Office, 1977).

U.S. SURGEON-GENERAL'S REPORT *Healthy People*

In 1979 the U.S. Surgeon-General issued a report, *Healthy People*, that suggested degenerative disease could be relieved as well as prevented by dietary means and called for substantial increases in the consumption of whole grains, vegetables, and fresh fruit and reductions in meat, eggs, dairy food, sugar, and other processed foods. Citing medical studies on macrobiotic people in Boston, the report stated: " . . . Americans who habitually eat less fat-rich diets (vegetarians [macrobiotics] and Seventh-Day Adventists, for example) have less heart disease than other Americans; and that atherosclerotic plaques in certain arteries may be reversed by cholesterol-lowering diets."

The report concluded that while individual nutritional standards would be hard to establish because of varying conditions and personal needs, Americans would proably be healthier, as a whole, if they consumed:

• Only sufficient calories to meet body needs and maintain desirable weight (fewer calories if overweight).
• Less salt.
• Less sugar.
• Relatively more complex carbohydrates such as whole grains, cereals, fruits and vegetables.
• Relatively more fish, poultry, legumes (e.g., beans, peas, peanuts) and less red meat.

The Surgeon-General further warned against the processing of modern foods. "The American food supply has changed so that more than half of our diet now consists of processed foods rather than fresh agricultural produce. . . . Increased attention therefore also needs to be paid to the nutritional qualities of processed food."

Source: *Healthy People: The Surgeon General's Report on Health Promotion and Disease Prevention* (Washington, DC: Government Printing Office, 1979).

NATIONAL ACADEMY OF SCIENCES' REPORT
Diet, Nutrition, and Cancer

In 1982 the National Academy of Sciences issued *Diet, Nutrition, and Cancer*, a 472-page report in which the modern diet high in saturated fat, animal protein, sugar, and chemical additives was associated with a majority of cancers, including malignancies of the breast, colon, prostate, uterus, stomach, lung, and esophagus. The panel reviewed hundreds of current medical studies associating long-term eating patterns with the development of 30 to 40 percent of cancers in men and 60 percent in women. "Just as it was once difficult for investigators to recognize that a symptom complex could be caused by the lack of a nutrient," the panel noted, "so until recently has it been difficult for scientists to recognize that certain pathological conditions might result from an abundant and apparently normal diet." The report issued interim dietary guidelines calling for substantial decreases in meat, poultry, egg, dairy, and refined carbohydrate consumption and increased consumption of whole-cereal grains, vegetables, and fruits:

1. There is sufficient evidence that high fat consumption is linked to increased incidence of certain cancers (notably breast and colon cancer) and that low fat intake is associated with a lower incidence of these cancers. The committee recommends that the consumption of both saturated and unsaturated fats be reduced in the average U.S. diet. An appropriate and practical target is to reduce the intake of fat from its present level (approximately 40 percent) to 30 percent of total calories in the diet. The scientific data do not provide a strong basis for establishing fat intake at precisely 30 percent of total calories. Indeed, the data could be used to justify an even greater reduction. However, in the judgment of the committee, the suggested reduction (i.e., one-quarter of the fat intake) is a moderate and practical target, and is likely to be beneficial.

2. The committee emphasizes the importance of including fruits, vegetables, and whole-grain cereal products in the daily diet. In epidemiological studies, frequent consumption of these foods has been inversely correlated with the incidence of various cancers. Results of laboratory experiments have supported these findings in tests of individual nutritive and nonnutritive constituents of fruits (especially citrus fruits) and vegetables (especially carotene-rich and cruciferous vegetables).

These recommendations apply only to foods as sources of nutrients—not to dietary supplements of individual nutrients. The vast literature examined in this report focuses on the relationship between the consumption of foods and the incidence of cancer in human populations. In contrast, there is very little information on the effects of various levels of individual nutrients on the risk of cancer in humans. Therefore, the committee is unable to predict the health effects of high and potentially toxic doses of isolated nutrients consumed in the form of supplements.

3. In some parts of the world, especially China, Japan, and Iceland, populations that frequently consumed salt-cured (including salt-pickled) or smoked foods have a greater incidence of cancers at some sites, especially the esophagus and the stomach. In addition, some methods of smoking and pickling foods seem to produce higher levels of polycyclic aromatic hydrocarbons and N-nitroso compounds. These compounds cause mutations in bacteria and cancer in animals and are suspected of being carcinogenic in humans. Therefore, the committee recommends that the consumption of food preserved by salt-curing (including salt-pickling) or smoking be minimized.

4. Certain nonnutritive constituents of foods, whether naturally occurring or introduced inadvertently (as contaminants) during production, processing, and storage, pose a potential risk of cancer to humans. The committee recommends that efforts continued to be made to minimize contamination of foods with carcinogens from any source. Where such contaminants are unavoidable, permissible levels should continue to be established and the food supply monitored to assure that such levels are not exceeded. Furthermore, intentional additives (direct and indirect) should continue to be evaluated for carcinogenic activity before they are approved for use in the food supply.

5. The committee suggests that further efforts be made to identify mutagens in food and to expedite testing for their carcinogenicity. Where feasible and prudent, mutagens should be removed or their concentration minimized, when this can be accomplished

without jeopardizing the nutritive value of foods or introducing other potentially hazardous substances into the diet.

6. Excessive consumption of alcoholic beverages, particularly combined with cigarette smoking, has been associated with an increased risk of cancer of the upper gastrointestinal and respiratory tracts. Consumption of alcohol is also associated with other adverse health effects. Thus the committee recommends that if alcoholic beverages are consumed, it be done in moderation.

The report noted in conclusion: "The dietary changes now underway appear to be reducing our dependence on foods from animal sources. It is likely that there will be continued reduction in fats from animal sources and an increasing dependence on vegetable and other plant products for protein supplies. Hence, diets may contain increasing amounts of vegetable products, some of which may be protective against cancer."

Source: National Academy of Sciences, *Diet, Nutrition, and Cancer* (Washington, DC: National Academy Press, 1982).

AMERICAN CANCER SOCIETY GUIDELINES

In 1984 the American Cancer Society issued guidelines for the first time on diet and cancer, calling for increased consumption of high-fiber foods such as whole grains and fresh vegetables and fruit. In 1991 the society updated its recommendations, noting:

Evidence from numerous experimental and human population studies conducted during past years suggests that a large proportion of human cancers may be associated with what we eat and drink and certain other lifestyle factors. It is estimated that about one-third of the annual 500,000 deaths from cancer in the United States, including the most common sites such as breast, colon, and prostate, may be attributed to undesirable dietary practice. . . .

Recommendations:

1. Maintain a desirable body weight.
2. Eat a varied diet.
3. Include a variety of both vegetables and fruits in the daily diet.
4. Eat more high-fiber foods, such as whole-grain cereals, legumes, vegetables, and fruits.
5. Cut down on total fat intake
6. Limit consumption of alcoholic beverages, if you drink at all.
7. Limit consumption of salt-cured, smoked, and nitrite-preserved foods.

The guidelines noted:

• The consumption of vegetables and fruits is associated with a decreased risk of lung, prostate, bladder, esophagus, and stomach cancers.
• High fiber-containing vegetables, fruits, and cereals can be recommended as wholesome low-calorie substitutes for high-calorie fatty foods.
• For most healthy adults, a decrease in fat calories to 25 to 30 percent or less of total calorie intake can be achieved by changes in eating habits to reduce the consumption of fats, oils, and foods rich in fats, such as fatty meats, whole-fat dairy products, gravies, sauces, salad dressings, and high-fat desserts.

Source: *Nutrition and Cancer: Cause and Prevention* (New York: American Cancer Society, 1984) and *American Cancer Society Guidelines on Diet, Nutrition, and Cancer*, (1991).

AMERICAN MEDICAL ASSOCIATION GUIDELINES

Though not directed specifically at cancer, the American Medical Association issued dietary guidelines to reduce the overall risk of degenerative disease:

1. Eat meat no more than once a day and choose fish or poultry over red meat.
2. Bake or broil food rather than frying it and use polyunsaturated oils rather than butter, lard, or margarine.
3. Cut down on salt, MSG, and other flavorings high in sodium.
4. Eat more fiber, including whole-grain cereals, leafy green vegetables, and fruit.
5. Eat no more than four eggs a week.
6. For dessert or a snack, eat fruit rather than baked goods.

In a review of special diets, the nation's major medical association advised:

In the macrobiotic diet foods fall into two main groups, known as yin and yang (based on an Eastern principle of opposites), depending on where they have been grown, their texture, color, and composition. The general principle behind this diet is that foods biologically furthest away from us are better for us. Cereals, therefore, form the basis of the diet and fish is preferred to meat. Although fresh foods free of additives are preferred, no food is actually prohibited, in the belief that a craving for any food may reflect a genuine bodily need. In general, the macrobiotic diet is a healthful way of eating. However, extreme adherents of macrobiotics restrict fluid intake, and this could be harmful to health.

Source: *The American Medical Association Family Medical Guide* (New York: Random House, 1987).

NATIONAL RESEARCH COUNCIL'S REPORT
Diet and Health

In 1989 the NRC issued a 749-page report, *Diet and Health: The Implications for Reducing Chronic Disease,* calling for the nation to substantially reduce animal food consumption and increase intake of whole-cereal grains, fresh vegetables, and fruits.

After a comprehensive review of the epidemiologic, clinical, and laboratory evidence, the panel's nineteen experts concluded that the modern diet influences the risk of several major chronic diseases including atherosclerotic cardiovascular diseases, hypertension, cancers of the esophagus, stomach, large bowel, breast, lung, and prostate, dental caries, chronic liver disease, obesity, and noninsulin-dependent diabetes mellitus.

Conversely, the researchers found that a diet characterized by plant foods is associated with a lower risk of coronary heart disease, cancers of the lung, colon, esophagus, and stomach, diabetes mellitus, diverticulosis, hypertension, and gallstone formation. The committee recommended that the intake of carbohydrates be increased to more than 55 percent of total calories, especially complex carbohydrates as found in whole-cereal grains, legumes, breads, vegetables, and certain fruits. Regular consumption of green and yellow vegetables was also encouraged: "The committee notes that several countries with dietary patterns similar to those recommended in this report have about half the U.S. rates for diet-associated cancers. This suggests that the committee's dietary recommendations could have a substantial impact on reducing the risk of cancer in the United States."

In a review of alternative diets, the report noted:

[T]he U.S. population consumes relatively large amounts of meat and sugar, more refined than whole-grain products, and larger amounts of commercially processed than fresh foods. In contrast, most of the world's population today subsists on vegetarian or near-vegetarian diets for reasons that are economic, philosophical, religious, cultural, or ecological. Indeed, humans appear to have subsisted for most of their history on near-vegetarian diets.

Reviewing current studies of vegetarians, the panel found that they "had lower intakes of protein, preformed niacin, and vitamin B_{12} than nonvegetarians, but that their average intakes of all three nutrients were above the RDAs. All other nutrients were, on average, at the same level or higher in vegetarian than in nonvegetarian diets." These included calcium, vitamin A, vitamin C, and magnesium. The committee also found that vegetarian females of reproductive age (nineteen to thirty-four) had iron intake comparable to that of nonvegetarians and higher intakes of calcium, magnesium, phosphorus, vitamin A, riboflavin, vitamin B_{12}, vitamin C, vitamin B_6, and thiamine.

Recommendations:

• Reduce total fat intake to 30 percent or less of calories. Reduce saturated fatty acid intake to less than 10 percent of calories and the intake of cholesterol to less than 300 miligrams daily. The intake of fat and cholesterol can be reduced by substituting fish, poultry without skin, lean meats, and low- or nonfat dairy products for fatty meats and whole-milk dairy products; by choosing more vegetables, fruits, cereals, and legumes; and by limiting oils, fats, egg yolks, and fried and other fatty foods.

• Every day eat five or more servings of a combination of vegetables and fruits, especially green and yellow vegetables and citrus fruits. Also, increase intake of starches and other complex carbohydrates by eating six or more daily servings of a combination of breads, cereals, and legumes.

• Maintain protein intake at moderate levels.

• Balance food intake and physical activity to maintain appropriate body weight.

• The committee does not recommend alcohol consumption. For those who drink alcoholic beverages, the committee recommends limiting consumption to the equivalent of less than one ounce of pure alcohol in a single day. This is the equivalent of two cans of beer, two small glasses of wine, or two average cocktails. Pregnant women should avoid alcoholic beverages.

• Limit total daily intake of salt (sodium choloride) to six grams or less. Limit the use of salt in cooking and avoid adding it to food at the table. Salty, highly processed salty, salt-preserved, and salt-pickled foods should be consumed sparingly.

• Maintain adequate calcium intake.

• Avoid taking dietary supplements in excess of the RDA in any one day.

• Maintain an optimal intake of fluoride, particularly during the years of primary and secondary tooth formation and growth.

Source: National Research Council, *Diet and Health: Implications for Reducing Chronic Disease Risk* (Washington, DC: National Academy Press, 1989).

U.S. GOVERNMENT'S GUIDELINES

In newly revised *Dietary Guidelines for Americans*, the U.S. Department of Agriculture and Department of Health and Human Services called in 1990 for everyone to consume six to eleven servings of grains or grain products every day, including whole-grain breads, cereals, pasta, and rice. (This constitutes about 40 percent of the daily diet.) Vegetables constituted the second biggest category of foods, with three to five servings, including dark green leafy and deep yellow vegetables, dry beans and peas, and starchy vegetables such as potatoes and corn.

The guidelines also called for substantial reductions in fat, saturated fat, and cholesterol. In addition to calling for less animal food consumption (two to three servings a day), the report recommended that people "have cooked dry beans and peas instead of meat occasionally." Small amounts of dairy food (two to three servings a day) were allowed, especially low-fat yogurt and skim milk. The report called for people to use sugars only in moderation.

Source: U.S. Department of Agriculture and U.S. Department of Health and Human Services, *Dietary Guidelines for Americans* (Washington, DC: U.S. Government Printing Office, 1990).

THE NATIONAL CANCER INSTITUTE'S *China Health Study*

An international research project, touted as "the grand prix of epidemiology studies," challenged modern dietary assumptions in the early 1990s. Sponsored by the U.S. NCI and the Chinese Institute of Nutrition and Food Hygiene, the study correlated average food and nutrient intakes with disease mortality rates in sixty-five rural Chinese counties. The typical Chinese diet included a high proportion of cereals and vegetables and a low content of meat, poultry, eggs, and milk. Less than 1 percent of deaths were caused by coronary heart disease, and breast cancer, colon cancer, lung cancer, and other malignancies common in the West were comparatively rare. Among the researchers' chief findings:

• Fat consumption should ideally be reduced to 10 to 15 percent of calories to prevent degenerative disease, not 30 percent as usually recommended.

• The lowest risk for cancer is generated by the consumption of a variety of fresh plant products.

• Eating animal protein is linked with chronic disease. Compared to the Chinese, who derive 11 percent of their protein from animal sources, Americans obtain 70 percent from animal food.

• A rich diet that promotes early menstruation may increase a woman's risk of cancer of the breast and reproductive organs.

• Dairy food is not needed to prevent osteoporosis, the degenerative thinning of the bones that is common among older women.

• Meat consumption is not needed to prevent iron-deficiency anemia. The average Chinese consumes twice the iron Americans do, primarily from plant sources, and shows no signs of anemia.

Dr. T. Colin Campbell, a Cornell biochemist and principal American director of the project, noted: "Usually, the first thing a country does in the course of economic development is to introduce a lot of livestock. Our data are showing that this is not a very smart move, and the Chinese are listening. They're realizing that animal-based agriculture is not the way to go."

Source: Chen Junshi, T. Colin Campbell, Li Junyao, and Richard Peto, *Diet, Lifestyle, and Mortality in China* (Ithaca, NY: Cornell University Press, 1990), and Jane Brody, "Huge Study of Diet Indicts Fat and Meat," *New York Times*, May 8, 1990.

WORLD HEALTH ORGANIZATION GUIDELINES

In 1991 a panel of global nutritional experts issued a report, *Diet, Nutrition and the Prevention of Chronic Diseases*, commissioned by the World Health Organization, the

COMPARISON OF CHINESE AND AMERICAN DIETS

Dietary intakes	China	U.S.
Total dietary fibre (g/day)	33.3	11.1
Starch (g/day)	371	120
Plant protein (% of total protein)	89	30
Fat (% of calories)	14.5	38.8
Calcium (mg/day)	544	1143
Retinol (Vit. A retinol equiv/day)	27.8	990
Total carotenoids (retinol equiv/day)	836	429
Vitamic C (mg/day)	140	73
Blood plasma constituents		
Cholesterol (mg/dl)	127	212
Triglycerides (mg/dl)	97	120
Total protein (g/dl)	4.8–6.2	6.4–8.3

Source: China Health Study, 1990

health-care arm of the United Nations. The report called for developing countries around the world to avoid the modern way of eating as the best way to prevent cancer, heart disease, and other degenerative diseases. Highlighted excerpts from the Executive Summary include:

• Anthropoligical studies show that the diet which fueled most of human evolution was low in fat, very low in sugar, and high in fibre and other complex carbohydrates.

• Although a large number of dietary factors have been investigated, those most frequently linked to such diseases [as cancer and heart disease] are embodied in the so called 'affluent' diet, a pattern of eating typified by high consumption of energy-dense foods of animal origin and of foods processed or prepared with added fat, sugar, and salt.

• All of the available evidence suggests that, for cardiovascular disease and for cancer, diet has an influence throughout the life cycle, even though the end-points are manifested in the adult. Thus, policies and programmes directed towards the control of nutritional inadequacies and nutritional excesses in populations need to influence food choices throughout the life cycle.

• As a result, populations in affluent countries now habitually consume a diet unknown to the human species a mere ten generations ago. Compared with the diet that fueled human evolution, today's affluent diet has twice the amount of fat, a much higher ratio of saturated to unsaturated fatty acids, a third of the daily fibre intake, much more sugar and sodium, fewer complex carbohydrates, and a reduced intake of micronutrients. Throughout the world, the adoption of such a diet, foreign to human biology, has been accompanied by a major increase in the incidence of chronic diseases, including coronary heart disease, stroke, various cancers, diabetes mellitus, gallstones, dental caries, gastrointestinal disorders, and various bone and joint diseases.

• Knowledge about the causes of chronic diseases is now sufficiently strong to support the view that changes in dietary practices, rebalanced along the lines recommended in this report, can do much to prevent the premature death and disability caused by these diseases. . . . The population nutrient intakes recommended in this report translate into a diet that is low in fat, and especially low in saturated fat, and high in complex starchy carbohydrates. Such a diet is characterized by frequent consumption of vegetables, fruits, cereals, and legumes, and contrasts sharply with current diets drawing substantial amounts of energy from whole-milk dairy products, fatty meats, and refined sugars.

• Foods of animal origin are no longer viewed as dominant items in an optimum healthy diet.

• Authorities in developing countries are cautioned not to imitate agricultural, farming, food production and promotion policies that were designed to emphasize the production of animal products and are based on nutritional knowledge long since outmoded. The difficulty of altering such policies, now apparent in many wealthy nations, serves as a further warning against their introduction.

• The almost universal increase in chronic diseases, which tend to occur in middle and later adult life, works in developing countries to counteract the gains in life expectancy attributable to an improved food supply and control of infectious diseases. Moreover, evidence suggests that even a modest increase in prosperity can bring on the considerable burden of chronic diseases.

• Though such figures suggest bleak prospects for the health of development, chronic diseases are, to a large extent, manifestations of nutrient excesses and imbalances in the diet and are thus largely preventable. An epidemic of cancers, heart disease and other chronic ills need not be the inevitable price paid for the privilege of socioeconomic progress.

See the accompanying chart for specific dietary recommendations.

Source: "Diet, Nutrition and the Prevention of Chronic Diseases, a Report of the WHO Study Group on Diet, Nutrition and Prevention of Noncommunicable Diseases," *Nutrition Reviews* 49(1991):291–301.

WORLD HEALTH ORGANIZATION
POPULATION NUTRIENT GOALS

	Lower Limit	*Upper Limit*
Total Fat	15% of energy	30% of energy[1]
Saturated fat	0%	10%
Polyunsaturated	3%	7%
Dietary cholesterol	0 mg/day	300 mg/day
Total Carbohydrate	55% of energy	75% of energy
Complex	50%	75%
Dietary fiber		
As nonstarch polysaccharides	16 g/day	24 g/day
As total fiber	27 g/day	40 g/day
Free sugars	0% of energy	10% of energy
Protein	10% of energy	15% of energy
Salt	not defined	6 g/day

[1] An interim goal for nations with high fat intakes; further benefits would be expected by reducing fat intake toward 15 percent.
Source: WHO, 1991

Appendix II
Dietary Guidelines for Tropical and Semitropical Regions and for Polar and Semipolar Regions

TROPICAL AND SEMITROPICAL REGIONS

Traditionally, in South Asia, Southeast Asia, Africa, Central and South America, and other tropical and semitropical regions, people have been eating cooked whole-cereal grains as principal food. The grain, including long-grain rice, basmati rice, sorghum, and others, is complemented with vegetables, as well as soup and broth, beans and sea vegetables, and other categories of food in the standard macrobiotic diet.

Proportions of foods, cooking styles, seasoning, and other factors may differ from standard cooking in temperate regions. For example, the amount of vegetables, fresh raw salad, and fruit may be slightly higher; steaming, stir-frying, braising, and other lighter cooking methods may be used more frequently, including boiling of grain rather than pressure cooking; and less salt, miso, and soy sauce or lighter miso and other seasonings may be used. However, in a hot and humid climate, a salty taste may often be more required than in a temperate climate.

In addition to whole grains, some cultures and island societies such as Hawaii and the Caribbean islands have traditionally consumed cassava, taro, yams, sweet potatoes, and other roots and tubers as staple food. In such cases, these may be included in the grain category as the principal source of complex carbohydrates.

In addition to fish and seafood, a small volume of wild animals, birds, and insects may be eaten if traditionally and commonly consumed. Also a small volume of spices, herbs, and aromatic, fragrant beverages may be taken on occasion to help offset the high heat and humidity. Typical foods in tropical and semitropical regions include:

Whole Grains and Staple Roots and Tubers

Amaranth	Medium-grain brown rice
Barley	Quinoa
Basmati rice	Sorghum
Bulghur	Sweet potato
Cassava (yucca, manioc, tapioca)	Taro (Albi, poi)
Corn	Teff
Couscous	Yam
Long-grain brown rice	

Other grains, grain products, staple roots, and tubers that have traditionally been consumed in tropical and semitropical regions

Vegetables from Land and Sea

Artichoke	Jicama
Asparagus	Okra
Avocado	Plantain
Bamboo shoots	Potato (traditionally processed)
Curly dock	Purslane
Eggplant	Spinach
Fennel	Swiss chard
Green pepper	Zucchini

Other vegetables that have traditionally been consumed in tropical and semitropical
regions

Sea vegetables, water moss, river and lake moss

Fruit, Nuts, and Seeds

All seeds and nuts	Mango
Banana	Orange
Breadfruit	Papaya
Coconut	Pineapple
Grapefruit	Plantain
Guava	Quince
Kiwi	Tangerine

Other fruits that have traditionally been consumed in tropical and semitropical regions

POLAR AND SEMIPOLAR REGIONS

Traditionally, in Alaska, Northern Canada, Greenland, Iceland, Scandinavia, Northern
Russia, Siberia, Mongolia, Tibet, the Andes, and other cold climates and regions, the
standard diet has included proportionately more animal food than in temperate latitudes. Because of the short growing season, grains and vegetables are in shorter supply,
though traditionally hardy strains of buckwheat, mountain barley, and other grains were
harvested, as well as a wide variety of wild plants (including wild burdock, milkweed,
dandelion, mugwort, wild leek, water lily root, wild ginger, and wild beans), sea vegetables and mosses, fruits (including chokeberry, wild cherry, currants, cranberries,
blueberries, wild strawberries, and grapes), seeds and nuts (such as acorns), and roots,
stems, leaves, and flowers of many kinds.

In addition to slightly more fish and seafood (on average from 20 to 30 percent of the
daily diet, especially in colder seasons), people in polar and semipolar regions ate a small
amount of whale, caribou, wild game, and dairy food. Because of the cold weather and
hard physical activity, they were able to digest small amounts of these foods without ill
effects as is the case in other climates and environments and among people observing a
more sedentary lifestyle. Further, pressure cooking, longtime boiling, broiling, baking,
roasting, and other stronger cooking methods may be used more frequently; and more
salt, miso, shoyu, and other seasonings as well as darker miso may be used.

Resources

RECOMMENDED READING

The following books are recommended for further reading and study. Those marked with an asterisk are especially recommended.

AIDS, Macrobiotics, and Natural Immunity by Michio Kushi and Martha Cottrell, M.D., Japan Publications, 1990.

Amber Waves of Grain: American Macrobiotic Cooking by Alex and Gale Jack, Japan Publications, 1992.

The Art of Peace by George Ohsawa, George Ohsawa Macrobiotic Foundation, 1991.

Aveline Kushi's Complete Guide to Macrobiotic Cooking by Aveline Kushi with Alex Jack, Warner Books, 1985.

Aveline: The Life and Dream of the Woman behind Macrobiotics Today by Aveline Kushi and Alex Jack, Japan Publications, 1988.

Barefoot Shiatsu by Shizuko Yamamoto, Japan Publications, 1979.

The Book of Do-in: Exercises for Physical and Spiritual Development, Japan Publications, 1979.

The Book of Macrobiotics by Michio Kushi with Alex Jack, Japan Publications, 1986.

Cancer-free: 30 Who Triumphed over Cancer Naturally by Ann Fawcett and the East West Foundation, Japan Publications, 1992.

Changing Seasons Macrobiotic Cookbook by Aveline Kushi and Wendy Esko, Avery Publishing Group, 1985.

Diet for a Strong Heart by Michio Kushi with Alex Jack, St. Martin's Press, 1985.

Doctors Look at Macrobiotics edited by Edward Esko, Japan Publications, 1989.

Food Governs Your Destiny: The Teachings of Namboku Mizuno by Michio and Aveline Kushi with Alex Jack, Japan Publications, 1991.

Forgotten Worlds by Michio Kushi with Edward Esko, One Peaceful World Press, 1992.

The Good Morning Macrobiotic Breakfast Book by Aveline Kushi and Wendy Esko, Avery Publishing Group, 1991.

The Gospel of Peace: Jesus' Teachings of Eternal Truth by Michio Kushi and Alex Jack, Japan Publications, 1992.

Healing Miracles from Macrobiotics by Jean and Mary Alice Kohler, Parker Publishing, 1979.

Healing Planet Earth by Edward Esko, One Peaceful World Press, 1992.

How to See Your Health: The Book of Oriental Diagnosis by Michio Kushi, Japan Publications, 1980.

Introducing Macrobiotic Cooking by Aveline Kushi and Wendy Esko, Japan Publications, 1987.

Introduction to Macrobiotics by Carolyn Heidenry, Avery Publishing Group, 1984.

Let Food Be Thy Medicine by Alex Jack, One Peaceful World Press, 1991.

Macrobiotic Childcare and Family Health by Michio and Aveline Kushi, with Edward and Wendy Esko, Japan Publications, 1986.

Macrobiotic Cooking for Everyone by Edward and Wendy Esko, Japan Publications, 1980.

Macrobiotic Diet by Michio and Aveline Kushi, with Alex Jack, Japan Publications, revised edition, 1993.

Macrobiotic Family Favorites by Aveline Kushi and Wendy Esko, 1987.

Macrobiotic Home Remedies by Michio Kushi with Marc Van Cauwenberghe, M.D., Japan Publications, 1985.

Macrobiotic Miracle: How a Vermont Family Overcame Cancer, Japan Publications, 1985.

Macrobiotic Palm Healing: Energy at Your Finger-tips by Michio Kushi with Olivia Oredsen, Japan Publications, 1989.

Macrobiotic Pregnancy and Care of the Newborn by Michio and Aveline Kushi, with Edward and Wendy Esko, Japan Publications, 1984.

The Macrobiotic Way of Zen Shiatsu by David Sergel, Japan Publications, 1990.

Macrobiotics and Oriental Medicine by Michio Kushi with Phillip Jannetta, Japan Publications, 1991.

Natural Healing through Macrobiotics by Michio Kushi with Edward Esko, Japan Publications, 1979.

The New Pasta Cuisine by Aveline Kushi and Wendy Esko, Japan Publications, 1992.

Nine Star Ki by Michio Kushi with Edward Esko, One Peaceful World Press, 1991.

One Peaceful World by Michio Kushi with Alex Jack, St. Martin's Press, 1987.

Other Dimensions: Exploring the Unexplained by Michio Kushi with Edward Esko, Avery Publishing Group, 1991.

Out of Thin Air by Alex Jack, One Peaceful World Press, 1993.

Promenade Home: Macrobiotics and Women's Health by Gale and Alex Jack, Japan Publications, 1988.

The Quick and Natural Macrobiotic Cookbook by Aveline Kushi and Wendy Esko, Contemporary Books, 1989.

Physician Heal Thyself by Dr. Hugh Faulkner, One Peaceful World Press, 1992.

Recovery: From Cancer to Health through Macrobiotics by Elaine Nussbaum, Avery Publishing Group, 1992.

Standard Macrobiotic Diet by Michio Kushi, One Peaceful World Press, 1991.

Sugar Blues by William Dufty, Warner Books, 1975.

PERIODICALS

Macro News, Philadelphia, Penn.
Macrobiotics Today, Oroville, Calif.
One Peaceful World, Becket, Mass.

THE KUSHI INSTITUTE

The Kushi Institute is the world's leading macrobiotic educational center, with headquarters on a beautiful 600-acre site in the Berkshires in western Massachusetts and affiliated institutes in other parts of the world. Year-round activities and programs include:

• **Personal Guidance Sessions** with Michio Kushi and other macrobiotic teachers.
• **The Way to Health Seminar,** a seven-day residential program attended by many friends with cancer and their families, featuring daily cooking classes, instruction in theory and practice, and exercise and massage.
• **New Medicine and Human Destiny,** a series of three-and-a-half-day seminars taught by Michio Kushi featuring studies on the origin and development of health, the relation of diet and degenerative disease, and the reorientation of modern society in a healthier, more peaceful direction.
• **Spiritual Development Training Seminars,** a series of three-and-a-half-day seminars taught by Michio Kushi designed to enhance each person's capacity for self-realization and fulfillment, featuring training in meditation, prayer, chanting, and using energy for healing.
• **Leadership Training Program,** a series of three five-week intensives for those wishing to become certified macrobiotic teachers, cooks, or shiatsu practitioners.
• **Kushi Institute Extension,** a series of weekend seminars offered in major North American cities such as Chicago, Cleveland, and Philadelphia, leading to receiving certificates in the Leadership Training Program.
• **Macrobiotic Summer Conference,** a week-long program offering general classes in macrobiotic cooking and health care, diagnosis, ecology, and other topics, presented each summer, usually in early August, featuring the Kushis and faculty of the Kushi Institute.

All seminars and programs feature delicious macrobiotic/vegetarian meals with an emphasis on quiet eating and thorough chewing. For dates and further information, contact:

Kushi Institute
Box 7
Becket, MA 01223
(413) 623-5741
Fax (413) 623-8827

ONE PEACEFUL WORLD SOCIETY

One Peaceful World is an international information network and friendship society founded by Michio and Aveline Kushi. Its members include individuals, families, educational centers, organic farmers, teachers, parents and children, authors and artists, homemakers and businesspeople, and others devoted to the realization of one healthy, peaceful world. Activities include education and spiritual tours, assemblies and forums, international food aid and development, the Children's Shrine in Becket for the spirits of unborn children, One Peaceful World Press, and other activities to help humanity pass safely through this time.

Annual membership is $30 for individuals, $50 for families, and $100 for supporting members. Benefits include the quarterly *One Peaceful World Newsletter,* edited by Alex Jack, with current cancer case history reports and medical-scientific updates, discounts on selected books, cassettes, and videos, and special mailings and communications. For further information, please contact:

One Peaceful World
Box 10
Becket, MA 01223
(413) 623-2322
Fax (413) 623-8827

About the Authors

Michio Kushi, the leader of the international macrobiotic community, was born in Japan and studied international law and political science at Tokyo University. He came to the United States in 1949 and is the founder and chairman of the Kushi Institute, the East West Foundation, and One Peaceful World. He has helped thousands of individuals and families recover their health and happiness and has given seminars on Oriental medicine and philosophy to medical professionals and health-care associates around the world. He has spoken at the United Nations, inspired dietary and nutritional research at Harvard Medical School and other universities and institutions, and served as an adviser to governments in Europe, Asia, Africa, Latin America, and the Middle East. He is the author of several dozen books and the father of five children and lives with his wife, Aveline, in Brookline and Becket, Masachusetts.

Alex Jack is an author, journalist, and teacher. He has worked closely with Michio and Aveline Kushi for nearly twenty years, serving as editor-in-chief of the *East West Journal,* director of the Kushi Institute of the Berkshires, and general coordinator of One Peaceful World. He has taught macrobiotics, holistic health, and planetary medicine around the world, including the New England Acupuncture Center, the Natural Organic Farmers Association, the Buddhist Association in Peking, and the Cardiology Center of Leningrad. His books include *Diet for a Strong Heart, Aveline Kushi's Complete Guide to Macrobiotic Cooking, Let Food Be Thy Medicine,* and *Amber Waves of Grain.* He lives in western Massachusetts with his wife, Gale, and two children, Masha and Jon.

Index